Orthopedic Disorders of the Foal

Editor

ASHLEE E. WATTS

VETERINARY CLINICS OF NORTH AMERICA: EQUINE PRACTICE

www.vetequine.theclinics.com

Consulting Editor
THOMAS J. DIVERS

August 2017 • Volume 33 • Number 2

ELSEVIER

1600 John F. Kennedy Boulevard • Suite 1800 • Philadelphia, Pennsylvania, 19103-2899

http://www.vetequine.theclinics.com

VETERINARY CLINICS OF NORTH AMERICA: EQUINE PRACTICE Volume 33, Number 2
August 2017 ISSN 0749-0739, ISBN-13: 978-0-323-53263-1

Editor: Katie Pfaff
Developmental Editor: Donald Mumford

Veterinary Clinics of North America: Equine Practice (ISSN 0749-0739) is published in April, August, and December by Elsevier Inc., 360 Park Avenue South, New York, NY 10010-1710. Business and Editorial Offices: 1600 John F. Kennedy Blvd., Suite 1800, Philadelphia, PA 19103-2899. Subscription prices are $270.00 per year (domestic individuals), $506.00 per year (domestic institutions), $100.00 per year (domestic students/residents), $315.00 per year (Canadian individuals), $637.00 per year (Canadian institutions), $365.00 per year (international individuals), $637.00 per year (international institutions), and $180.00 per year (international and Canadian students/residents). To receive student/resident rate, orders must be accompanied by name of affiliated institution, date of term, and the signature of program/residency coordinator on institution letterhead. Orders will be billed at individual rate until proof of status is received. Foreign air speed delivery is included in all *Clinics* subscription prices. All prices are subject to change without notice. **POSTMASTER:** Send address changes to *Veterinary Clinics of North America: Equine Practice*, 3251 Riverport Lane, Maryland Heights, MO 63043. Customer Service (orders, claims, online, change of address): Elsevier Health Sciences Division, Subscription **Customer Service, 3251 Riverport Lane, Maryland Heights, MO 63043. Tel: 1-800-654-2452 (U.S. and Canada); 314-447-8871 (outside U.S. and Canada). Fax: 314-447-8029. E-mail: journalscustomerservice-usa@elsevier.com (for print support);** E-mail: **journalsonlinesupport-usa@elsevier. com (for online support)**.

Reprints. For copies of 100 or more of articles in this publication, please contact the Commercial Reprints Department, Elsevier Inc., 360 Park Avenue South, New York, NY 10010-1710. Tel.: 212-633-3874; Fax: 212-633-3820; E-mail: reprints@elsevier.com.

Veterinary Clinics of North America: Equine Practice is covered in *MEDLINE/PubMed (Index Medicus), Excerpta Medica, Current Contents/Agriculture, Biology and Environmental Sciences,* and *ISI*.

Contributors

CONSULTING EDITOR

THOMAS J. DIVERS, DVM
Diplomate, American College of Veterinary Internal Medicine; Diplomate, American College of Veterinary Emergency and Critical Care; Steffen Professor of Veterinary Medicine, Section of Large Animal Medicine, College of Veterinary Medicine, Cornell University, Ithaca, New York

EDITOR

ASHLEE E. WATTS, DVM, PhD
Diplomate, American College of Veterinary Surgeons–Large Animal; Assistant Professor, Equine Orthopedic Surgery, Director of the Comparative Orthopedics and Regenerative Medicine Laboratory, Department of Large Animal Clinical Sciences, College of Veterinary Medicine and Biomedical Sciences, Texas A&M University, College Station, Texas

AUTHORS

MAIA R. AITKEN, DVM
Diplomate, American College of Veterinary Surgeons–Large Animal; Staff Surgeon, University of Pennsylvania, Department of Clinical Studies New Bolton Center, Kennett Square, Pennsylvania

WILLIAM TRUE BAKER, DVM
Diplomate, American College of Veterinary Surgeons; Hagyard Equine Medical Institute, Davidson Surgery Center, Lexington, Kentucky

FRED J. CALDWELL, DVM, MS
Diplomate, American College of Veterinary Surgeons–Large Animal; Diplomate, American College of Sports Medicine and Rehabilitation; Associate Professor of Equine Sports Medicine and Surgery, Department of Clinical Sciences, JT Vaughan Large Animal Teaching Hospital, College of Veterinary Medicine, Auburn University, Auburn, Alabama

MICHELLE C. COLEMAN, DVM
Diplomate, American College of Veterinary Internal Medicine; Department of Large Animal Clinical Sciences, College of Veterinary Medicine and Biomedical Sciences, Texas A&M University, College Station, Texas

JOSÉ M. GARCÍA-LÓPEZ, VMD
Diplomate, American College of Veterinary Surgeons; Diplomate, American College of Sports Medicine and Rehabilitation; Associate Professor, Department of Clinical Sciences, Cummings School of Veterinary Medicine, Tufts University, North Grafton, Massachusetts

EARL M. GAUGHAN, DVM
Diplomate, American College of Veterinary Surgeons; Technical Services Veterinarian, Merck Animal Health, Madison, New Jersey

KATI GLASS, DVM
Diplomate, American College of Veterinary Surgeons–Large Animal; Clinical Assistant Professor, Department of Large Animal Clinical Sciences, College of Veterinary Medicine and Biomedical Sciences, Texas A&M University, College Station, Texas

ROBERT J. HUNT, DVM, MS
Diplomate, American College of Veterinary Surgeons; Hagyard Equine Medical Institute, Davidson Surgery Center, Lexington, Kentucky

DAVID G. LEVINE, DVM
Diplomate, American College of Veterinary Surgeons–Large Animal; Assistant Professor of Clinical Large Animal Surgery, University of Pennsylvania, Department of Clinical Studies New Bolton Center, Kennett Square, Pennsylvania

TARALYN M. McCARREL, DVM
Diplomate, American College of Veterinary Surgeons–Large Animal; Assistant Professor of Large Animal Surgery, Large Animal Clinical Sciences, College of Veterinary Medicine, University of Florida, Gainesville, Florida

STEPHEN E. O'GRADY, DVM, MRCVS
Virginia Therapeutic Farriery, Keswick, Virginia

KYLA F. ORTVED, DVM, PhD
Diplomate, American College of Veterinary Surgeons; Diplomate, American College of Veterinary Sports Medicine and Rehabilitation; Assistant Professor of Large Animal Surgery, Clinical Studies, New Bolton Center, University of Pennsylvania, Kennett Square, Pennsylvania

HEIDI L. REESINK, VMD, PhD
Diplomate, American College of Veterinary Surgeons–Large Animal; Assistant Professor of Large Animal Surgery, Department of Clinical Sciences, College of Veterinary Medicine, Cornell University, Ithaca, New York

STACY A. SEMEVOLOS, DVM, MS
Oregon State University, College of Veterinary Medicine, Corvallis, Oregon

ASHLEE E. WATTS, DVM, PhD
Diplomate, American College of Veterinary Surgeons–Large Animal; Assistant Professor, Equine Orthopedic Surgery, Director of the Comparative Orthopedics and Regenerative Medicine Laboratory, Department of Large Animal Clinical Sciences, College of Veterinary Medicine and Biomedical Sciences, Texas A&M University, College Station, Texas

CANAAN WHITFIELD-CARGILE, DVM
Diplomate, American College of Veterinary Surgery; Diplomate, American College of Veterinary Sports Medicine and Rehabilitation; Department of Large Animal Clinical Sciences, College of Veterinary Medicine and Biomedical Sciences, Texas A&M University, College Station, Texas

Contents

of synovial, bony, and physeal infections with appropriate and aggressive local therapy. Recent literature may indicate that prognosis for survival and potential athleticism in foals that are treated expediently with local therapies and are without comorbidities may be more favorable than has been previously indicated.

 Video content accompanies this article at http://www.vetequine. theclinics.com.

Flexural deformities in young horses are commonly referred to as contracted tendons, which is a term that is not consistent with what is currently understood about their cause. Flexural deformity of the distal interphalangeal joint can be either congenital (present at birth) or acquired (develop at a later stage of growth typically between 1 and 6 months of age). These 2 manifestations are commonly managed differently depending on the cause, age of onset, severity, duration, complicating factors, and owner expectations. Early recognition and appropriate intervention are essential to ensure that it is not performance limiting.

Early recognition and treatment of congenital and acquired flexural deformities of the carpi and fetlocks of foals can lead to conformation correction and an athletic future. Treatment is often based on rigid external coaptation assisted by systemic medical treatment. Foals that readily respond to treatment and correct conformation faults can have normal adult athletic expectations.

Angular limb deformities are seen in young foals and are defined as lateral or medial deviations of the limb in the frontal plane distal to a particular joint. Several factors can contribute to the development of an angular limb deformity. Early assessment of the level of ossification of the cuboidal bones is critical to avoid complications long term. Although most deviations self-correct with minimal intervention other than modifications in exercise and hoof trimming, some require surgical intervention in the form of growth acceleration or retardation. This article focuses on growth augmentation techniques, such as hemicircumferential transection and elevation.

Angular limb deformities are common in foals; however, the importance of the deformity and if treatment is required depend on the degree of deformity relative to normal conformation for stage of growth, the breed and discipline expectations, age, and response to conservative therapies. This article addresses the importance of the foal conformation examination to determine which foals need surgical intervention to correct an angular deformity and when. Techniques for surgical growth retardation include the transphyseal staple, screw and wire transphyseal bridge, and transphyseal screw. Appropriate timing for intervention for each location and complications associated with each procedure are discussed.

This article reviews current knowledge of osteochondritis dissecans (OCD) development in horses, including normal cartilage development, early osteochondrosis pathogenesis, and factors that result in healing or advancement to OCD fragments. Discussion includes current theories, detection, and therapeutic options.

Osteochondrosis is common in young, athletic horses. Some lesions respond to conservative therapy. Surgical management is the mainstay of treatment. Arthroscopic debridement is useful in the femoropatellar joint, tarsocrural joint, fetlock joint, and shoulder joint. Debridement is associated with good outcomes, except in the shoulder joint. Osteochondrosis lesions in the elbow may be difficult to access arthroscopically, thereby transosseous debridement. Surgical management of subchondral cystic lesions of the medial femoral condyle consists of debridement, debridement with grafting, transcondylar screws, and intralesional corticosteroid injection. Surgical management is indicated with lameness and persistent effusion, and in many horses intended for athletic use.

Foals are susceptible to many of the same types of fractures as adult horses, often secondary to external sources of trauma. In addition, some types of fractures are specific to foals and occur routinely in horses under 1 year of age. These foal-specific fractures may be due to the unique musculoskeletal properties of the developing animal and may present with distinct clinical signs. Treatment plans and prognoses are tailored specifically to young animals. Common fractures not affecting the long bones in foals are discussed in this article, including osteochondral fragmentation, proximal sesamoid bone fractures/sesamoiditis, and distal phalanx fractures.

Physeal fractures are common musculoskeletal injuries in foals and should be included as a differential diagnosis for the lame or nonweightbearing foal. Careful evaluation of the patient, including precise radiographic assessment, is paramount in determining the options for treatment. Prognosis mostly depends on the patient's age, weight, and fracture location and configuration.

Kati Glass and Ashlee E. Watts

Many long bone fractures that are not considered repairable in the adult horse are repairable in the foal. This is largely because of reduced patient size and more rapid healing in the foal. When there is no articular communication, the long-term prognosis for athletic function can be very good. Emergency care and transport of the foal with a long bone fracture is different than the adult.

VETERINARY CLINICS OF NORTH AMERICA: EQUINE PRACTICE

FORTHCOMING ISSUES

December 2017
Equine Ophthalmology
Mary Lassaline, *Editor*

April 2018
Advances in the Diagnosis and Management of Equine Gastrointestinal Disease
Henry Stämpfli and Angelika Schoster, *Editors*

RECENT ISSUES

April 2017
Equine Pharmacology
K. Gary Magdesian, *Editor*

December 2016
Advances in Diagnostic and Therapeutic Techniques in Equine Reproduction
Marco A. Coutinho da Silva, *Editor*

August 2016
Geriatric Medicine
Catherine M. McGowan, *Editor*

RELATED ISSUE

Veterinary Clinics of North America: Food Animal Practice
July 2017 (Vol. 33, Issue 2)
Lameness in Cattle
JK Shearer, *Editor*

THE CLINICS ARE NOW AVAILABLE ONLINE!
Access your subscription at:
www.theclinics.com

Preface

Prelude to an Equine Athlete: Foal Orthopedics

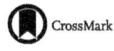

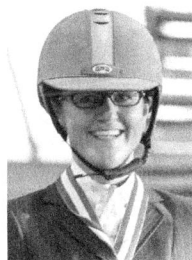

Ashlee E. Watts, DVM, PhD, DACVS
Editor

The goal of any broodmare operation is to raise healthy foals that will grow up to be equine athletes. The future athletic performance of the foal depends largely on the breeding program itself, and the importance of good genetics cannot be overstated. However, without sound limbs, even the best-bred foal will not have a successful athletic career! Thus, care of the musculoskeletal system of foals is of the utmost importance, whether monitoring growth and conformation, managing limb deformities or infections, or fixing fractures and osteochondritis dissecans lesions, veterinarians have an important role in the future athletic success of all foals! My hope for this issue, Orthopedic Disorders of Foals, a first on this topic for *Veterinary Clinics of North America: Equine Practice*, is that the articles will serve as thorough and concise reviews on each topic as well as an update to readers with the latest and greatest ideas, diagnostics, therapies, and understanding of disease mechanisms. My further hope is that the issue will be useful for both the equine veterinarian in a busy broodmare practice and the veterinarian who sees just one to two foals a year, and everyone in between.

I am grateful to Dr Tom Divers, a wonderful equine veterinarian, internist, person, and friend, for the invite to guest edit this issue and to Patrick Manley and Donald Mumford from Elsevier for guidance along the way. It was not difficult to come up with the requested number of articles because foals are not just little horses and they have a number of orthopedic disorders specific to them. Each of the authors is an expert in their

Vet Clin Equine 33 (2017) xi–xii
http://dx.doi.org/10.1016/j.cveq.2017.05.001
0749-0739/17/© 2017 Published by Elsevier Inc.

field, and I am grateful to them for taking the time to put together each article and share their knowledge.

Ashlee E. Watts, DVM, PhD, DACVS
Equine Orthopedic Surgery
Comparative Orthopedics &
Regenerative Medicine Laboratory
Department of Large Animal Clinical Sciences
College of Veterinary Medicine &
Biomedical Sciences
Texas A&M University
4475 TAMU
College Station, TX 77843, USA

E-mail address:
awatts@cvm.tamu.edu

Routine Orthopedic Evaluation in Foals

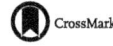 CrossMark

Robert J. Hunt, DVM, MS*, William True Baker, DVM

KEYWORDS

- Foal • Musculoskeletal • Examination

KEY POINTS

- In order to recognize abnormalities on the physical evaluation, it is mandatory to understand normal developmental variations of the musculoskeletal system.
- Many abnormalities are self-limiting and, therefore, it is important to recognize which problems require intervention for a successful outcome and which may be complicated by treatment.
- Physical evaluation of the musculoskeletal system in foals is routinely performed on newborns as a component of an after-foaling examination, or for lameness or conformation evaluation in foals of all ages.

There are a multitude of disorders of the musculoskeletal system of foals that present during the development of the foal from the time of parturition onward. In order to recognize abnormalities on the physical evaluation, it is mandatory to understand normal developmental variations of the musculoskeletal system.[1–5] Many abnormalities are self-limiting[6] and, therefore, it is important to recognize which problems require intervention for a successful outcome and which may be complicated by treatment.[7]

The importance of a complete and thorough physical evaluation cannot be overemphasized and is the most productive diagnostic tool for recognizing most abnormalities of the skeletal system. It should form the basis for a final diagnosis of all orthopedic disorders or guide the clinician toward other diagnostic modalities to arrive at an accurate diagnosis. Physical evaluation of the musculoskeletal system in foals is routinely performed on newborns as a component of an after-foaling examination, or for lameness or conformation evaluation in foals of all ages.[4]

Foals are unique in several regards compared with other age groups of horses. The behavior of foals makes them inherently more challenging to complete a thorough physical and locomotor evaluation. It is important to exercise patience and work slowly when evaluating the foal whether examining the body or the extremities.

Hagyard Equine Medical Institute, Davidson Surgery Center, 4250 Iron works Pike, Lexington, KY 40511, USA
* Corresponding author.
E-mail address: rhunt@hagyard.com

Vet Clin Equine 33 (2017) 253–266
http://dx.doi.org/10.1016/j.cveq.2017.03.011
0749-0739/17/© 2017 Elsevier Inc. All rights reserved.

Becoming familiar with the foal and palpating normal areas to gauge the foal's behavioral response will help differentiate this from a pain response to palpation.

Another unique feature of foals is that they are particularly vulnerable to injury from external sources, such as impact injuries from other horses, running into objects, or sustaining injuries from mal-loading a limb or falling.[8] Foals are also susceptible to septic conditions of the skeletal system, including hematogenous osteomyelitis, septic arthritis, or external wounds resulting in sepsis.[9–17]

Foals are also unique in that they have a relatively rapid progression of pathologic processes in which there may be alarmingly quick deterioration requiring only a few days for permanent degenerative changes to occur in bone and soft tissue. Fortunately, the converse may occur with rapid resolution of a disease process, and it is well recognized that foals appear to be able to restore specific tissues much better than adults.

There are many conditions in foals that are specific to a given age group. There should be a general understanding of which of these are most likely to occur for the individual foal being examined. Disorders resulting in lameness and/or gait deficits in foals are common, and the physical evaluation is the most important means for differentiating the cause. Evaluation for lameness is generally preceded by a history that will often raise suspicion for a given disorder. Factors to consider in the history include awareness of any recent management changes, suspected traumatic events, presence of herd health issues, and a record of the foal's health history.

ORTHOPEDIC EVALUATION

An assessment of the physical health, including temperature, vital parameters, demeanor, overall condition and body score of the foal, stance, any obvious conformational aberrations, swellings, or other physical anomalies, should be noted. It is helpful to observe the foal rising from a recumbent position and unrestrained to determine if there is a gait deficit or reluctance to load a limb or display any positional abnormalities of a limb or body carriage. Initiation of the gait from a standing position is also helpful to detect subtle gait deficits. Observation of the foal at a walk when evaluating for conformation or lameness must be performed with the foal relaxed and not pulling on the handler. It may be necessary to allow the foal to follow the mare as long as the environment is safe.

All evaluations begin with a thorough history and visual inspection at rest and in motion and are followed up with an in-depth and thorough evaluation by palpation when possible. Observation of the gait in a lame foal can be intriguing and very telling in that oftentimes the slower the gait, the easier it is to determine the origin of pain. Even with a moderate lameness, foals often pick the lame limb up and carry it rather that display a limp; therefore, evaluation at the walk may be more productive through observation of limb carriage and flight pattern along with foot placement and lift off. It should be noted if a particular component of the stride is shortened or prolonged. Given that the manifestation of lameness is an avoidance response to pain, it is often relatively simple to determine the component of the gait they are attempting to avoid.

Palpation of foals may be intimidating and seemingly nonproductive if the foal is not acclimated to handling; however, with patience and by gaining trust and confidence from the foal, a thorough palpation may be accomplished. It is important to begin in areas that are normal and gradually ease into suspicious areas. If possible, the contralateral normal structure should be palpated initially to gauge the foal's response before manipulating an area of concern.

For foals reared in production horse operations, it is common to perform an after-foaling physical evaluation on essentially all newborns at approximately 1 to 2 days of age or sooner if a problem is recognized.[4] The orthopedic evaluation is a component of the neonatal physical evaluation and includes observation of the foal at rest, standing, ambulating, and nursing. The lack of the ability to stand and nurse is a routine cause for termination by most contractual arrangements, and the cause should be established on the examination.

Palpation of the extremities is an integral component of the orthopedic evaluation; however, in neonatal foals, a thorough visual inspection is more common because they are not typically used to limb palpation. Physical development, strength, and size of the foal and the demeanor and general activity level are noted. An initial conformation assessment is made taking note of any skeletal anomalies, such as flexural and laxity issues or angular limb deformities, long bone curvature deformities, healed or nonhealed in utero long bone fractures, or spinal deformities. Congenital skeletal deformity, injury, or sepsis while in utero may be detected during the initial evaluation.

Special attention is given to thoracic palpation to detect parturition-associated rib fracture. If detected, ultrasound evaluation should be performed to determine the degree of displacement, proximity to the heart, and damage to lung or the diaphragm.[18,19] Recognition of the position of the fractured ribs and the structures involved is vital for proper management and the ultimate survival of the foal.

As the foal advances in development, so does the likelihood of injury to skeletal structures. Injuries resulting from overexertion in the younger foal are extremely common and include proximal sesamoid bone injuries, coffin bone injuries, cuboidal bone injury, and almost any other imaginable skeletal injury. Changes in management, such as introduction to a larger turnout setting or turnout with new horses, should be noted. Age and temperament of the mare, whether she is multiparous or has had behavioral issues with foals in the past, may raise suspicions for mare-induced injury from external trauma or exertional injury from the mare running.

One of the most common exertional injuries in foals is fracture of the proximal sesamoid bones.[20] There is a broad range of severity in fracture types, clinical presentation, and prognosis. Lameness varies with the severity of the injury and ranges from non-weight-bearing to almost imperceptible only being recognized on sharp turns. The more severe injuries often occur as a younger mare with a foal 1 to 3 weeks of age, which has been introduced to a large field for the first time. One or both forelimbs of the foal may be involved, and there may be total disruption and distraction of the proximal from the distal bone components of the sesamoid. Fractures of the proximal sesamoid bones may involve the base, body, or the apical region (**Fig. 1**), or there may be soft tissue suspensory avulsion, which may result in elongation of the sesamoid or mineralization of soft tissue proximal or distal to the sesamoid.

Clinical detection of proximal sesamoid bone injury may be apparent on initial visual inspection as variable degrees of local swelling over the involved sesamoid; commonly there is an increased digital pulse in addition to warmth, but the area is not as hot as it is with sepsis. Flexion of the fetlock generally yields a pain response, and in the acute injury, digital pressure to the affected sesamoid will yield a pain response (**Fig. 2**). It is possible to differentiate between apical and basilar sesamoid injuries on palpation. If there is suspicion of a fracture of the proximal sesamoids, radiographs are indicated.

The vulnerability of foals to septic conditions is well recognized, and accurate diagnosis is imperative. Septic processes such as septic arthritis or osteomyelitis should be recognized as early as possible in order to provide appropriate treatment and prevent tissue deterioration.[10–17] Differentiation between articular versus nonarticular

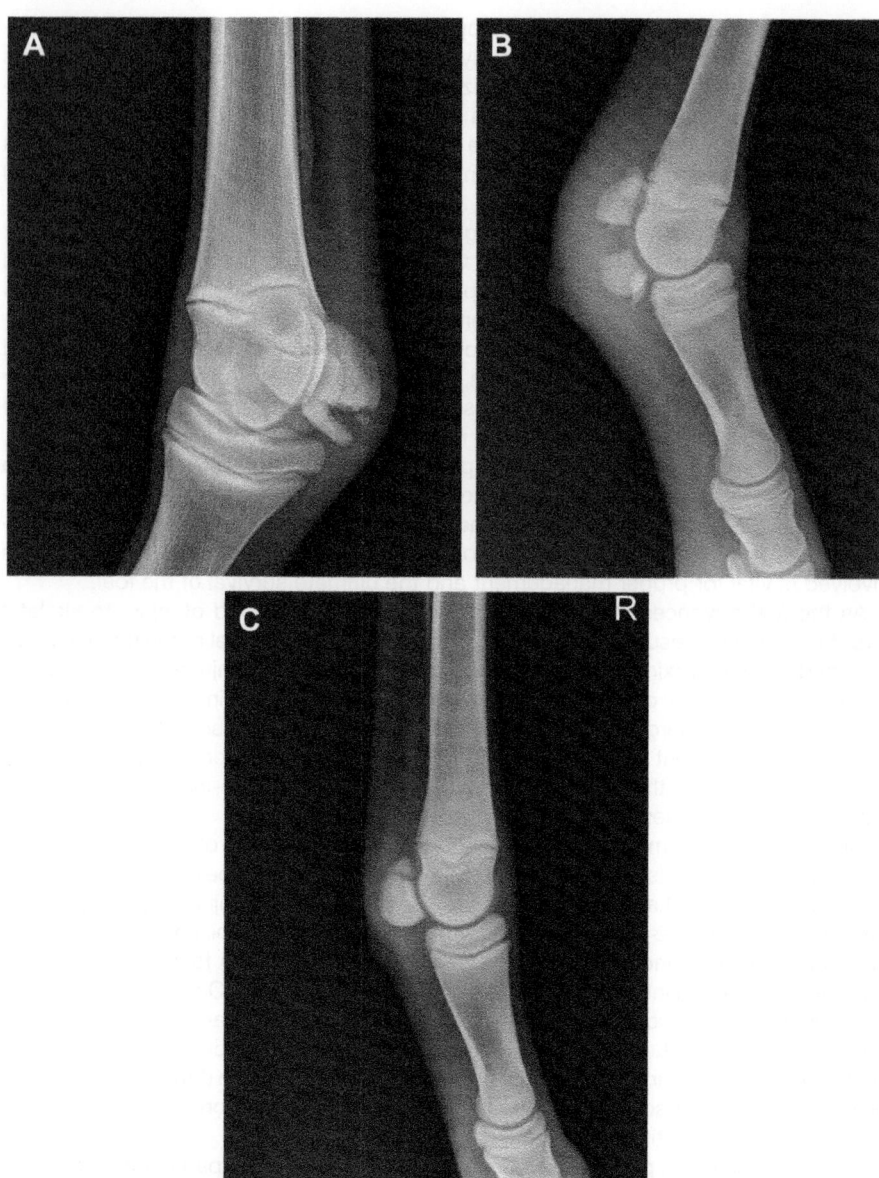

Fig. 1. Examples of various types of proximal sesamoid bone fractures commonly seen in foals. (*A*) Basilar sesamoid fracture. (*B*) Severely displaced midbody biaxial sesamoid fracture. (*C*) Minimally displaced uniaxial apical sesamoid fracture.

sepsis, or involvement of bone or surrounding soft tissue, will dictate specific treatment. The orthopedic evaluation is critical for making this determination through detection of classic signs of inflammation of the involved tissue, including heat, pain, and swelling. Localization to the specific structure may be finalized with radiography, ultrasonography, or other imaging modalities, and possible arthrocentesis or aspiration.[11,15]

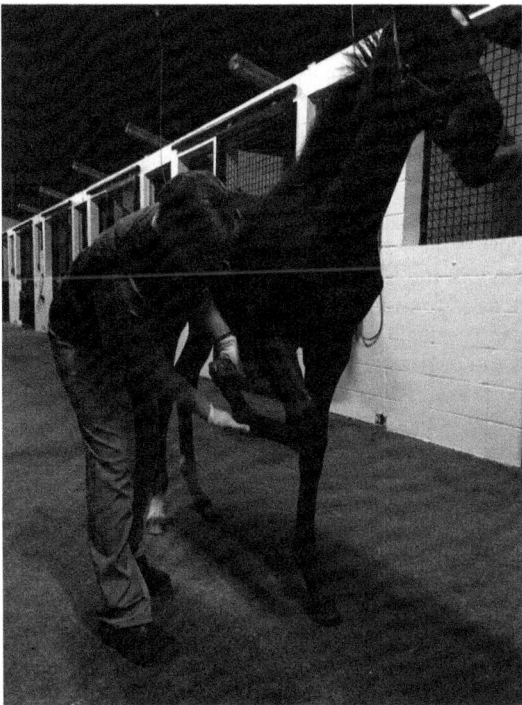

Fig. 2. Palpation of the proximal sesamoids in a foal.

Causes of Lameness

Gait deficits resulting from pain should be differentiated from those resulting from mechanical or structural dysfunction. Functional injuries include peripheral nerve injury,[21,22] scarring of muscle or tendon groups causing limitations on function, rupture of extensor tendon groups such as common and lateral digital extensor tendon rupture, or rupture of a flexor group such as a gastrocnemius muscle group.[23,24] Ruptured common and lateral digital extensor tendon is recognized on the clinical examination by a focal soft tissue swelling over the dorsolateral surface of the carpus in conjunction with knuckling forward of the carpus and fetlock and a lack of ability to advance the limb when attempting to ambulate. In order to differentiate between ruptured common and lateral digital extensor tendons and flexural limb deformities one should apply pressure to the dorsal aspect of the carpus when the foal is standing. With an extensor tendon rupture, the limb is able to be positioned normally, whereas a flexural deformity cannot be positioned into a normal stance and remains flexed at the carpus. Rupture of flexor groups, such as a gastrocnemius rupture, results in a loss of support along a tension surface with a resultant drop of the supported structures. In the event of a ruptured flexor group, a characteristic appearance of a dropped hock and extended stifle along with soft tissue swelling in the musculotendinous region of the gastrocnemius is observed.[23]

Nerve injury may occur during parturition with a difficult delivery and involves the front or hind quarters or may occur from blunt trauma at any time during development.[18,21,22] Nerve injury can be differentiated from lameness by the lack of pain on manipulation of the limb and being able to position the limb in a normal stance folllowing nerve injury. An example is a radial nerve injury, which manifests with a dropped elbow and flexed carpus while keeping a caudally placed limb.[21] The limb may also be placed in a normal stance and maintained in position with pressure applied to the front of the carpus and is nonpainful. In contrast, a structural injury such as fracture of the elbow will also display a dropped elbow and flexed carpus but maintains the limb forwardly placed (**Fig. 3**). Structural injuries are painful on manipulation of the limb, and patients resent forced load bearing when locking the limb in place using pressure on the carpus.[8]

Lameness originating from the foot in foals is common and deserves considerable discussion. Most foot-associated lameness in foals is caused by bruising, abscess/ infection, and fracture. There are several characteristics of these disorders that help differentiate the cause of the lameness. Severe lameness is more commonly associated with infectious causes such as subsolar abscess or abscess of the dorsal lamina that may extend to the coffin joint.[25,26] Bruising or infection is far more common at the toe compared with the palmar region of the foot; as the foal displays a reluctance to load bear on the toe, there is an exaggerated heel-to-toe action, and the foot remains forwardly placed while walking and standing. Accompanying clinical signs include increased digital pulse, heat of the involved area, and sensitivity to compression of the involved region. Exceptions to this include lack of response to hoof testers if there is excessive separation of tissue from purulent material or if there is extensive necrosis that is without innervation. Also, the hoof capsule may be cool to palpate if there is necrosis present. In the presence of dorsal swelling of the coronary band in which there is bulging over the dorsal hoof wall, septic arthritis of the distal interphalangeal joint must be considered and addressed.[10,11,15]

Hind foot bruising and abscess at the toe region are common and result from the young foal traumatizing and bruising the soft noncornified solar horn when introduced to hard ground, which may occur in the front feet as well.[25,26] It is common to have both feet involved, and the foal reluctantly makes contact with the ground, displaying either a drifting or a floating movement of the foot before contact with the ground followed by a jerking action when lifting the foot. Radiographs may disclose a gas pocket or abnormality on the distal tip of the coffin bone, such as fragmentation or demineralization from trauma (**Fig. 4**).

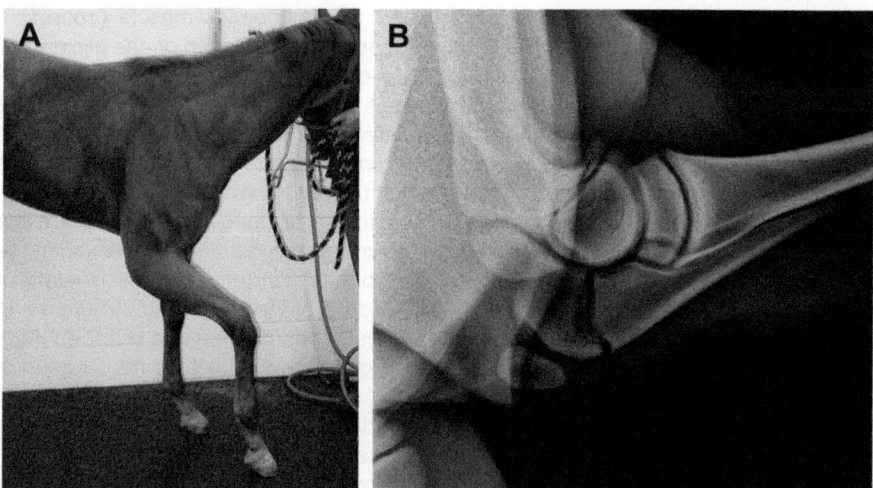

Fig. 3. (*A*) Clinical presentation of a fractured elbow. (*B*) Radiographic presentation of an elbow fracture.

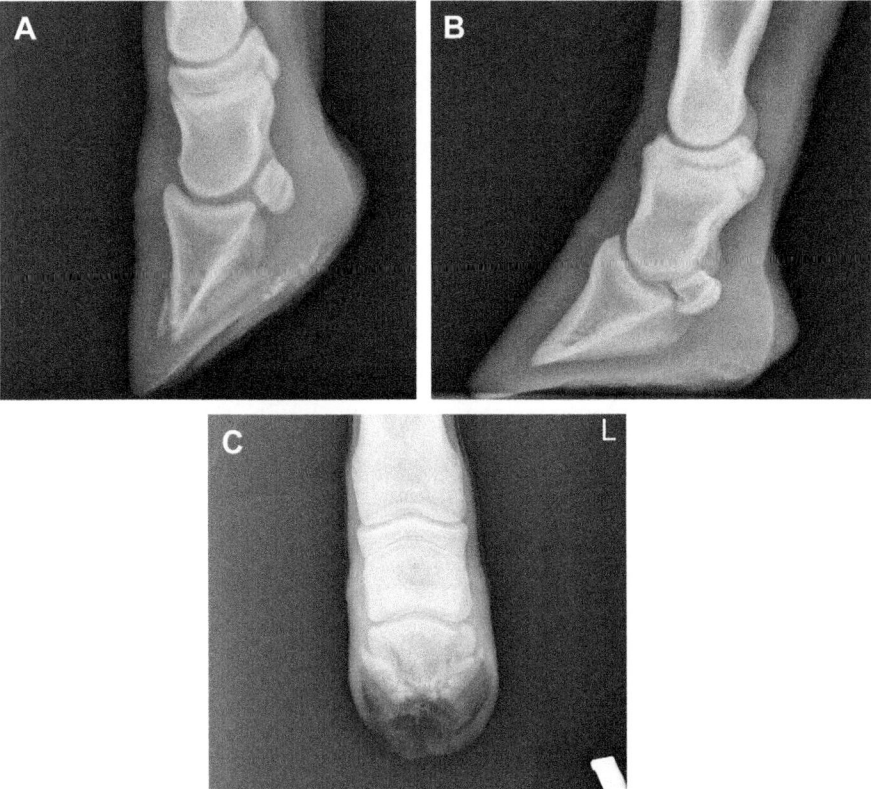

Fig. 4. (*A*) Fracture of the distal tip of the distal phalanx in a 2-week-old foal associated with trauma as a neonate. Note the gas pocket associated with an abscess that was opened and drained. No invasive surgery was performed. (*B*) The same foal at 6 months of age showing healing and normal contour of the distal phalanx after conservative therapy. (*C*) Demineralization and sequestration associated with septic osteitis of the distal phalanx.

Fracture of the lateral palmar process of the distal phalanx (lateral wing fracture) (**Fig. 5**) is extremely common in foals and likely results from malapplied internal or external forces on the foot.[27] Clinical findings of distal phalangeal wing fractures include an increased digital pulse, normal temperature, and a positive pain response with pressure applied across the heels of the foot.[27–29] The most common gait for a foal with a lateral wing fracture is to maintain the contact phase of the stride in an abducted or base-wide stance to avoid loading the involved region of the foot. However, the gait may vary if the medial wing is fractured as well. The diagnosis is generally confirmed radiographically.

Other areas worthy of mention include some of the palpable disorders of the upper hind limb. Injuries to the proximal tibia, such as physeal fractures, or septic conditions are detectable with palpation. Effusion of the femoropatella joint in conjunction with pain and pyrexia is a common sign of septic arthritis. Displaying a straight or upright stance of the stifle with effusion of the medial femorotibial joint is common with medial femoral condyle osteomyelitis or avascular necrosis. Muscle rents of the vastus lateralis or biceps femoris are very common, and the lameness varies based on the severity of the tear. Muscle rents are detectable on palpation and are mostly identified in foals

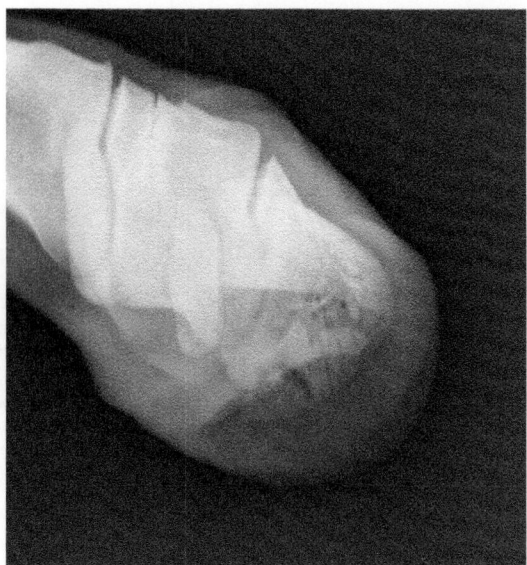

Fig. 5. Type 1 fracture of the lateral palmar process of the distal phalanx.

introduced to new surroundings (**Fig. 6**). Pelvic and hip problems occur frequently and are mostly from traumatic or septic causes. Common areas of injury include the tuber coxae (**Fig. 7**), the coxofemoral region, and the tuber ischia. The location of pain is recognized on palpation and visual observation of contour changes of the region involved and positional alterations of the tail. Palpation of the spinous processes may facilitate detection of early stage osteomyelitis of a vertebral body or traumatic injury. Essentially all parts of the musculoskeletal system of a foal are vulnerable to insult from traumatic, septic, or developmental orthopedic complications. Detection of these abnormalities with a thorough physical evaluation is often the difference in life or death or the future usefulness of the foal.

Conformation Evaluation: Neonate

In addition to evaluation for lameness or pathologic conditions, conformation evaluation is performed on foals at commercial horse operations. The initial conformation examination should be included within the initial after-birth examination to adequately establish a baseline for the foal as well as note any deviations that will need to be followed along. During the first 6 months of their lives, foals display dynamic growth and thus are able to make exceptional changes in their conformation over that time period.[1,2] Many deviations seen within the first days of life have the ability to improve or completely resolve without intervention.[6] Small changes in management combined with a modicum of patience and wealth of communication often result in the desired clinical outcome.

The vast majority of conformational defects seen in the foal are a result of either angular limb deformities or flexural limb deformities, although compound problems with both deformities are seen.[1–5,30,31] Angular limb deformities encompass axial deviations in the longitudinal length of the limb in a medial or lateral direction along the frontal plane. Flexural limb deformities are generally associated with soft tissue laxity or contracture, resulting in deviations centered on joints in a dorsal or palmar/plantar direction in the sagittal plane.

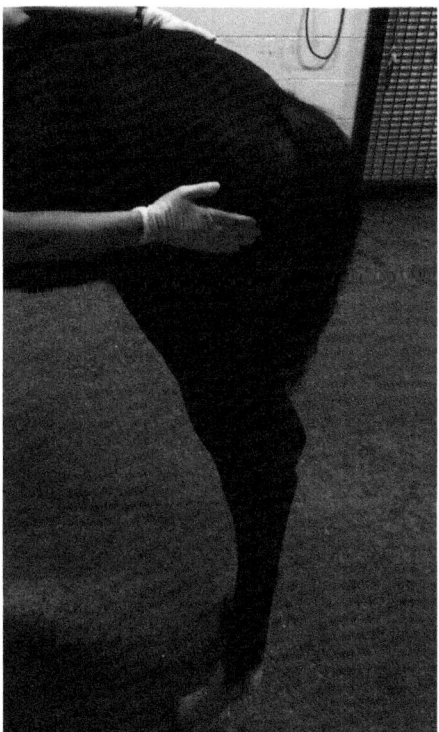

Fig. 6. Palpation of the musculature of the proximal hind limb to detect muscle rents.

It is uncommon for a foal to be born with correct limb conformation because they have been in a flexed intrauterine position and have varying degrees of muscle tone and weakness combined with postnatal laxity in their periarticular structures. A small amount of carpal valgus should be considered normal as correct carpal conformation is identified in only 3% of Thoroughbred foals evaluated in their first week of life.[31]

With the foal in lateral recumbency, all long bones and joints should be palpated for heat, pain, or swelling and manipulated not only in their normal anatomic direction of movement but also in a medial to lateral direction to judge laxity of the periarticular supporting structures. Restriction of the joint from a full range of motion should be noted. The cause of that restriction is best found by firm extension of the joint in question and concurrent palpation of the tendons for tension. The foal should then be made to rise, watching for any specific weakness in the attempt. Once up, the foal should be evaluated on flat ground without bedding to allow for full visualization of the foot. The foal should be evaluated for any subtle sign of joint contracture or weight-bearing laxity. With the foal standing square, it should be evaluated from the front for any angular deviations of the extremity. Carpal valgus of 4° is considered within normal limits for neonatal foals.[1,2,30,31] The front limbs should be rotated out from the chest so that the face of the knees and the fetlocks are facing slightly lateral to the sagittal plane. Evaluation from behind should assess pelvic symmetry as well as tarsal and fetlock angular deviations. The hind limbs should also be facing slightly lateral from the sagittal plane, and mild tarsal valgus deviation is normal. The foal should then be observed from each side examining each limb for contracture or laxity and noting what joint it is centered around. The foal should be walked, or allowed to walk beside

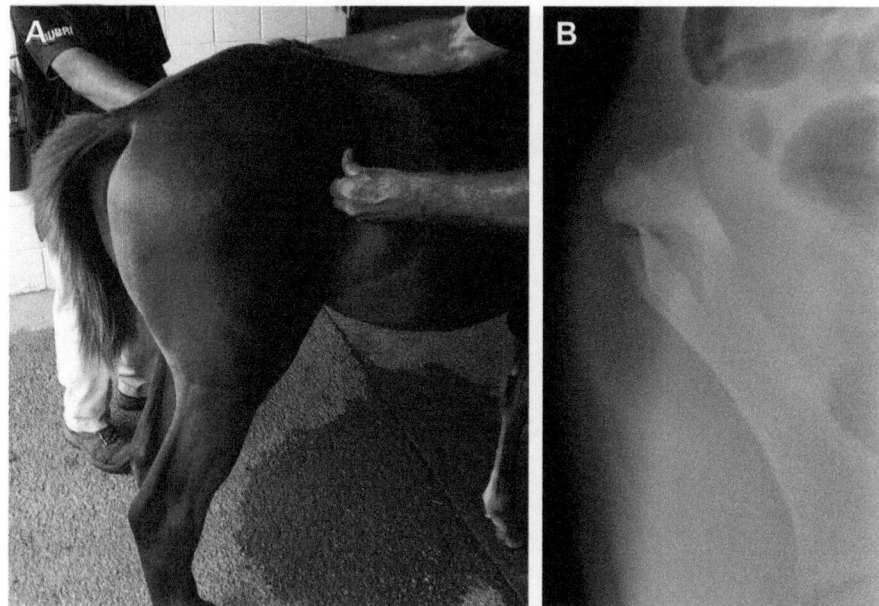

Fig. 7. (*A*) Elicitable pain response on palpation of the tuber coxae. Note the displacement of the tail head. (*B*) Fracture of the tuber coxae in the same foal.

the mare, toward and away from the practitioner evaluating the foal to gauge the flight of the limbs.

There is a wide range of limb contracture, or flexural deformity, seen in the neonate that ranges from innocuous to life threatening. The carpus is most often affected with some degree of fetlock involvement as well. Significant carpal contracture can first be noted at the time of parturition and can severely compromise the delivery resulting in dystocia (**Fig. 8**).[32] Carpal contracture is usually bilateral, although often of slightly different degrees.[2–6,30,31] Carpal contracture to an angle of less than 100° that is not able to be manually straightened to 180° carries a poor prognosis and may warrant

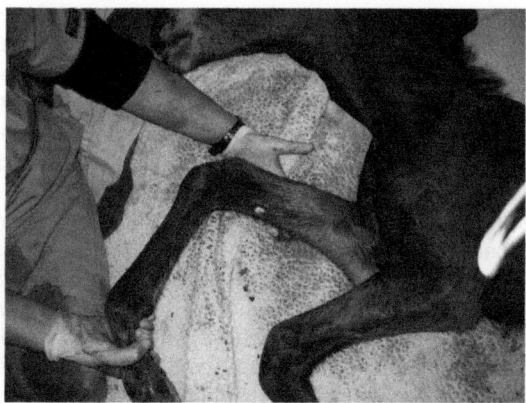

Fig. 8. Severe carpal and fetlock contraction contributing to dystocia.

euthanasia.[7] Minor contracture will generally respond to conservative therapy and restricted exercise in less than 1 week.[5,7,30] For foals unable to stand, intensive nursing care is indicated, and the reader should refer to Earl M. Gaughan's article, "Flexural Limb Deformities of the Carpus and Fetlock in Foals," in this issue for management alternatives.

Musculotendinous laxity is common in the neonatal foal, and visual recognition of joint hyperextension is sufficient for an initial diagnosis.[2,3,31] A full examination of the limb should be performed to rule out extensor tendon contracture or anatomic malformations of the joint in question. For mild to moderate laxity, a conservative approach of stall rest with limited turnout should be instituted. The foal should be monitored closely for abrasions of the heal bulbs, and protective dressing should be used if necessary.[30] For severe laxity or moderate laxity that fails to respond to conservative management, glue-on heel-extension shoes may be applied to the foal's foot. Caution should be exercised so that the extensions are long enough to prevent distal interphalangeal joint luxation. The feet should be closely monitored for wall distortion from heel overload and addressed accordingly. Excessive bandaging of the limb should be avoided if possible because it can exacerbate laxity.

Many angular limb deviations in newborn foals are the result of periarticular laxity.[1–4] The resultant uneven stress across a joint and uneven loading of the articular surface within the joint may, when combined with excess exercise, cause irreversible changes to the cuboidal bones of the carpus and tarsus.[2,5,7,33] Angular limb deviations of the tarsus are commonly seen in the neonate and may be associated with intrauterine fetal positioning and joint laxity.[5] Most will respond to controlled exercise and strengthening of the foal's hind end.[34] Deviations of the tarsus in the sagittal plane are often seen in the premature/dysmature foal with incomplete ossification of the tarsal bones.[33] Stall rest is indicated until adequate ossification is seen radiographically.

Windswept conformation is common, and the foal may present with one hind limb with valgus deviation at the tarsus and fetlock while the other limb has varus deviations at the tarsus and fetlock. This results in both feet pointing in the same direction. The conformation is usually transient and will improve with strengthening of the musculoskeletal system during the first 4 to 6 weeks of life. Caution should be exercised in the degree of activity allowed typically beginning with stall-sized restriction for the first 2 to 3 weeks before advancing to a paddock for another 2 to 3 weeks. It is not common to require surgery for limb correction, with the exception of varus deviation of the fetlock, which is still evident and not improving by 8 weeks of age.

Conformation Evaluation: One Month and Older

Evaluation of the 1-month and older foal should proceed as previously described because the basics for evaluation of conformation remain the same, although some developmental transitions may be expected. The foal should have aged enough at this point to begin to show its true skeletal conformation unclouded by soft tissue laxity. Initial examination at rest should take into account any residual flexural deformities or laxity disorders. Some foals will maintain some mild carpal contracture through this period or may develop flexural disorders that worsen with rapid weight gains and increased exercise.

Special attention should be made to evaluate the foal both in line with its axial spine and also at a slightly oblique angle that is in line with the face of the carpus or the line of the hocks behind. From this oblique angle, the practitioner can better judge any deviations of the limb centered on the joints. Mild carpal valgus conformation with slight outward rotation of the forelimbs is normal.[1,30,31] Correct conformation but offset carpus should be monitored for development of fetlock and carpal varus. Standing in front of the face of the carpus, a line bisecting the cannon bone should ideally also bisect the fetlock joint and all the phalanges into the foot. Any inward deviations of the phalanges from the cannon that are centered on the fetlock are considered fetlock varus. The foal is evaluated in motion taking special note of the flight pattern of the limb, and contact and lift-off of the foot, and if there is base narrow, normal, or base wide stance during locomotion. A flight pattern toward midline or base narrow distal to the fetlock often accompanies fetlock varus and pigeon-toed conformation of the foot. With this conformation, the foal contacts the lateral aspect of the heel and lifts off the lateral wall of the toe at the end of the stance phase. Offset carpi with correct alignment can exacerbate this finding. Fetlock varus and pigeon toe is exaggerated if the foal is upright in the fetlocks; as often occurs, with relaxation of the angle of the fetlock, the varus deviation and pigeon toe conformation frequently improve. A 1- to 2-month-old foal with offset knees that initially was correct in the axial plane and begins tracking base narrow is at high risk for developing fetlock varus. As there is greater wear on the lateral wall of the heel, quarter, and toe, the result is an imbalanced foot that toes in (pigeon-toe). The imbalance that develops from uneven wear on the foot forms the basis for corrective trimming of the varus deviation foal. The goal is to provide balance to the foot and lateral support to the heel and quarter in order to encourage a correct or base wide stance.[25] Mild correction may be applied to the foal's hoof by slightly lowering the medial heel and hoof wall so that the lateral aspect of the hoof capsule is effectively longer to induce lateral rotation on the distal limb during weight bearing. A variety of composite materials and hoof appliances are available for use as wall extensions in the event there is not adequate hoof mass to accomplish correction. Hoof wall manipulation should be performed judiciously, taking care not to induce permanent hoof wall distortion.

Foals that develop rapid onset varus deviation between 90 and 120 days of age are problematic in that there may be limitations on the amount of correction that may be achieved by either conservative or surgical measures. The deviation occurs in a matter of days concomitant with the onset of severe physeal dysplasia of the distal metacarpus. Even with immediate surgical intervention, there are limitations on the amount of correction with undesirable results. The most favorable outcome is achieved through close monitoring and detection of high-risk individuals, early intervention with conservative measures to address physeal dysplasia along with rapid surgical intervention.

Valgus deviations and rotational deviations are common, and based on their clinical progression, accompanying flight pattern of the lower limb, and other conformational issues or maturity of the foal, may require management changes or intervention. Most foals with carpal valgus that track with an inward sweeping pattern have a tendency to land and lift off the medial wall of the foot and require subsequent balance. Outward rotational deviations may appear as carpal valgus when standing but when in flight tend to displace the carpus laterally, thus appearing as a midflight varus deviation. The foot also wears mostly on the lateral wall and therefore should be maintained in balance. Surgical intervention is contraindicated for rotational deviations, whereas carpal valgus deviations with the described alteration in the limb flight pattern respond favorably to surgical manipulation.[7]

SUMMARY

Orthopedic evaluation in foals can be performed at multiple times and for multiple reasons. It is important to physically evaluate the foal from birth through the first months of life to screen for any musculoskeletal injuries or pathologic conditions, and it is also a critical time to address any conformational issues that may be present. The same principles of thoroughness and attention to detail should be adhered to irrespective of the reason for evaluation or the age of the foal. The orthopedic evaluation should be the primary tool used to help guide the practitioner toward further diagnostics or therapeutic intervention.

REFERENCES

1. Robert C, Valette JP, Denoix JM. Longitudinal development of equine forelimb conformation from birth to weaning in three different horse breeds. Vet J 2013; 198:e75–80.
2. Levine DG. The normal and abnormal equine neonatal musculoskeletal system. Vet Clin Equine 2015;31:601–13.
3. Bohanon TC. Developmental musculoskeletal disease. In: Kobluk CN, Ames TR, Geor RJ, editors. The horse: diseases & clinical management, vol. 2. Philadelphia: WB Saunders; 1995. p. 815–58.
4. McIlwraith CW, Anderson TM, Sanschi EM. Conformation and musculoskeletal problems in the racehorse. Clin Tech Equine Pract 2003;2(4):339–47.
5. Witte S, Hunt R. A review of angular limb deformities. EVE 2009;21(7):378–87.
6. Baker WT, Slone DE, Ramos JA, et al. Improvement in bilateral carpal valgus deviation in 9 foals after unilateral distolateral radial periosteal transection and elevation. Vet Surg 2014;44:547–50.
7. Getman LM. Surgical treatment of severe, complex limb deformities in horses. EVE 2011;23(8):386–90.
8. Watkins JP. Etiology, diagnosis, and treatment of longbone fractures in foals. Clin Tech Equine Pract 2006;5:296–308.
9. Hance SR. Hematogenous infections of the musculoskeletal system in foals. Proc Am Assoc Equine Pract 1998;44:159–66.
10. Hanson R. Septic joints in foals. Proc North Am Vet Conf 2006;110–2.
11. Morton AJ. Diagnosis and treatment of septic arthritis. Vet Clin North Am Equine Pract 2005;21(3):627–49.
12. Neil KM, Axon JE, Begg AP, et al. A retrospective study of 108 foals with septic osteomyelitis: 1995-2001. Proc Am Assoc Equine Pract 2006;52:567–9.
13. Vatistas NJ, Wilson WD, Pascoe JR, et al. Septic arthritis in foals: bacterial isolates, antimicrobial susceptibility, and factors influencing survival. Proc Am Assoc Equine Pract 1993;39:259.
14. Wagner PC, Watrous BJ, Darien BJ. Septic arthritis and osteomyelitis. In: Robinson NE, editor. Current therapy in equine medicine. 3rd edition. Philadelphia: WB Saunders; 1992. p. 455–62.
15. McIlwraith CW. Treatment of septic arthritis. Vet Clin North Am Large Anim Pract 1983;5:363–421.
16. Steele CM, Hunt AR, Adams PL, et al. Factors associated with prognosis for survival and athletic use in foals with septic arthritis (1987-1994). J Am Vet Med Assoc 1999;215(7):97.
17. Schneider RK, Bramlage LR, Moore RM, et al. A retrospective study of 192 horses affected with septic arthritis/tenosynovitis. Equine Vet J 1992;24:436.
18. Jean D, Laverty S, Halley J, et al. Thoracic trauma in newborn foals. Equine Vet J 1999;31(2):149–52.
19. Bellezzo F, Hunt RJ, Provost P, et al. Surgical repair of rib fractures in 14 neonatal foals case selection, surgical technique, and results. Equine Vet J 2004;36(7): 557–62.

20. Ellis DR. Fractures of the proximal sesamoid bones in thoroughbred foals. Equine Vet J 1979;11(1):48–52.
21. Tyler CM, Davis RE, Begg AP, et al. A survey of neurologic diseases in horses. Aust Vet J 1993;70(12):445–9.
22. Adams R, Mayhew IG. Neurological examination of newborn foals. Equine Vet J 1984;16(4):306–12.
23. Jesty SA, Palmer JE, Parente EJ, et al. Rupture of the gastrocnemius muscle in six foals. J Am Vet Med Assoc 2005;227(12):1965–8, 1929.
24. Aleman M. A review of equine muscle disorders. Neuromuscul Disord 2008;18: 277–87.
25. Greet TR, Curtis SJ. Foot management in the foal and weanling. Vet Clin Equine 2003;19:501–17.
26. Agne B. Diagnosis and treatment of foot infections. J Equine Vet Sci 2010;30(9): 510–2.
27. Faramarzi B, Dobson H. Palmar process fractures of the distal phalanx in foals: a review. EVE 2015. http://dx.doi.org/10.1111/eve.12509.
28. Faramarzi B, McMicking H, Halland S, et al. Incidence of palmar process fractures of the distal phalanx and association with front hoof conformation in foals. Equine Vet J 2014;47(6):675–9.
29. Yovich JV, Stashak TS, DeBowes RM, et al. Fractures of the distal phalanx of the forelimb in eight foals. J Am Vet Med Assoc 1986;189(5):550–4.
30. Adams SB, Santschi EM. Management of congenital and acquired flexural limb deformities. AAEP Proc 2000;46:117–25.
31. Santschi EM, Leibsle SR, Morehead JP, et al. Carpal and fetlock conformation of the juvenile thoroughbred from birth to yearling auction age. Equine Vet J 2006; 38(7):604–9.
32. McCue PM, Ferris RA. Parturition, dystocia and foal survival: a retrospective study of 1047 births. Equine Vet J 2012;44(41):22–5.
33. Dutton DM, Watkins JP, Walker MA, et al. Incomplete ossification of the tarsal bones in foals: 22 cases (1988-1996). J Am Vet Med Assoc 1998;213:1590.
34. Dutton DM, Watkins JP, Honnas CM, et al. Treatment response and athletic outcome of foals with tarsal valgus deformities: 39 cases (1988-1997). J Am Vet Med Assoc 1999;215:1481.

Routine Trimming and Therapeutic Farriery in Foals

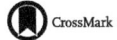 CrossMark

Stephen E. O'Grady, DVM, MRCVS

KEYWORDS

- Foals • Farriery • Hoof trimming • Tendon laxity • Flexural deformity
- Angular limb deformity

KEY POINTS

- Hoof care in the first few months of the foal's life is serious business and should never be taken lightly.
- Overall hoof care is a joint venture between the veterinarian and the farrier.
- Farriery plays a vital role in both the development of the hoof and the conformation of the limb.
- Management of the feet and limbs during this period will often dictate future hoof and limb conformation, which in turn will play a role in the success of the foal as a sales yearling or mature sound athlete.
- A sound foot care program is time-consuming, whereas assembly-line trimming is quick and easy, but the former is much more beneficial.

INTRODUCTION

Among the many factors that dictate the success of the foal as a sales yearling or a mature sound athlete are decisions and management concerning feet and limbs during the first few months of life. This is the period when hoof care helps to produce a strong foundation (hoof) for the animal's future athletic career while influencing the growth and angulation of the limb above the hoof to some degree. Realizing that there are potential complications associated with interventional measures, it is important to understand their principles, as well as the indications, contraindications, and appropriate treatment measures. It is important to remember to avoid causing damage to the foot or other skeletal structures with the various farriery methods used and not allow the foot to become a "victim" of treatment.

Many breeding farms have developed foot care programs that use the skills of a veterinarian with an interest in podiatry and a farrier working together as a team.

Virginia Therapeutic Farriery, 833 Zion Hill Road, Keswick, VA 22947, USA
E-mail address: sogrady@look.net

The veterinarian uses medical and anatomic knowledge, whereas the farrier uses technical and mechanical skills. This joint venture allows a faster and more accurate diagnosis, treatment, possible resolution, and prognosis for foot problems. Unless an orthopedic problem is noted at birth or shortly thereafter, all foals are examined by the veterinarian, farrier, and the manager/owner at the time of the first trim, which is generally performed at a month of age. Problem or suspect foals are identified and are then examined on a monthly or bimonthly basis and followed through weaning. Many subtle problems or indications of potential problems can be detected early, leading to immediate treatment. If this program corrects the limb alignment or increases the athletic potential of one animal on the farm, then the program becomes cost-effective. This article focuses on routine farriery in young horses and those limb deformities that can be addressed through therapeutic farriery or farriery combined with surgery. Surgery associated with limb deformities in the young horse is discussed elsewhere in this issue.

EVALUATING THE FOAL

Good record keeping is vitally important. Records are designed for the individual needs of a given farm/owner and should reflect the physical appearance of a foal's feet and limbs at birth and any subtle changes that occur during development on at least a monthly basis. Digital images (pictures and radiographs) can be taken and added to the foal's record.

Digital pictures are very helpful in determining progress or regression in the foal's feet/limbs. Foals should always be observed walking each time they are evaluated and trimmed. The author prefers to observe the foal walking before the feet and limbs are examined. Watching the young foal walk can be challenging, as they seldom walk in a straight line. This can be remedied by walking the mare along a fence or wall and letting the foal walk on the opposite side of the mare or follow the mare. The foal is observed as it walks toward and away from the examiner. Here the foal is evaluated for any lameness that may be present, the pattern of the foot flight, how the foot breaks over at the toe, and how the foot contacts the ground. When examining the feet and limbs from the front, using an imaginary dot system may be helpful. Starting at the ground surface of the foot, an imaginary dot is placed at the middle of the toe of the foot, the coronary band, the fetlock, proximal third metacarpal bone (MC3), carpus, and distal radius. When these dots are connected with an imaginary line, it is easy to see if and/or where an angular limb deformity exists. In the ideal situation, when viewed from the front, the dots should form a straight line. However, one must be careful to rule out the presence of a rotational deformity. In this case, both carpi are rotated outward (laterally) leading to a toe-out or splay-footed conformation, yet when the dots are connected, the axial alignment of the limb forms a straight line. When viewed from the side, the dots should again form a straight line from the distal radius to the fetlock and from the fetlock through the digit to the ground. The coronary band is observed from the front to see if it is level or parallel with the ground. Examining the feet and limbs from the side should note whether the carpus is flexed or hyperextended. The hoof-pastern axis is evaluated to determine if the bones of the digit are aligned and not broken forward (flexure deformity) or broken backward (flexor flaccidity). Any swellings along the limb or involving the physis are noted and recorded. Each deformity is noted and scored on a scale of 1 to 5; grade 1 being mild whereas grade 5 is severe. Finally, the foot is evaluated off the ground, observing the position of the hoof relative to the bones of the digit (offset foot), symmetry of the foot, and the integrity of the horny structures of the hoof capsule. When viewing the solar surface of the foot, it is important to place the dorsal surface of MC3 in the palm of the examiner's hand and allow the limb to hang loose; this places the limb in relaxation and allows the examiner to view the solar surface of the foot in relation to the ground. The author pays strict attention to the length of both heels as measured from the end of the hoof wall at the heel to the hair line at the bulbs. A disparity in this distance is an indication of disproportionate weight distribution being placed on the foot as it lands. This evaluation enables the examiner to evaluate the feet, limbs, and movement in a systematic manner.

TRIMMING THE FOAL
Birth to 1 Month

At birth, the foal's hooves are enveloped in a gelatinous perioplic membrane (eponychium), which reduces the risk of trauma to the mare's reproductive tract during birth (**Fig. 1**).

Shortly after birth, with the first steps of life, the perioplic membrane on the solar surface of the foot wears and retracts proximally on the hoof wall, dries out, and tends to create a sulcus of varying depths just below the coronary band. This depression, termed the subcoronary groove, is considered normal, grows distally over the next 3 to 4 months, and will often cause a defect when it reaches the ground surface of the foot if the toe length grows excessively long (**Fig. 2**). The foal's foot will be tapered, being wider at the coronet and becoming narrower distally at the ground surface (**Fig. 3**). A foal's foot does not only grow in a distal direction, but it also expands as it develops. As the foal's feet are tapered, expansion occurs proximally and as the ground surface of the distal hoof is relatively small, the weight-bearing area is positioned dorsally. Exercise and trimming will enlarge the area on the ground surface of the foot and move it in a palmar/plantar direction. The pointed or tapered appearance will gradually disappear in the first few months of life. In foals with acceptable limb conformation, there is little need for trimming during the first month of life.

One Month

Foals should be presented to the farrier at 1 month of age for routine trimming. All that will generally be necessary at this time is to square the toe of the hoof with a rasp to encourage the foal to break over in the center of the foot. At this age, due to the

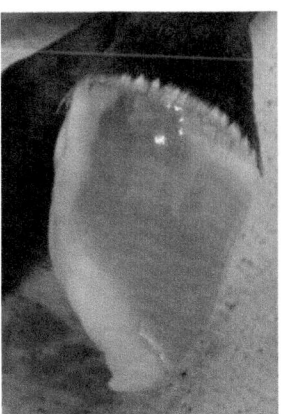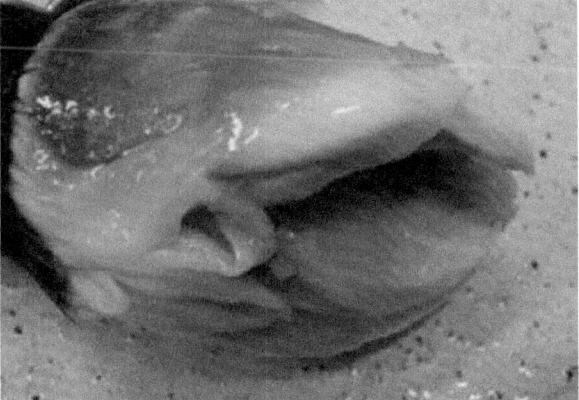

Fig. 1. Perioplic membrane. Note the attachment just below the hairline that forms the sub coronary groove.

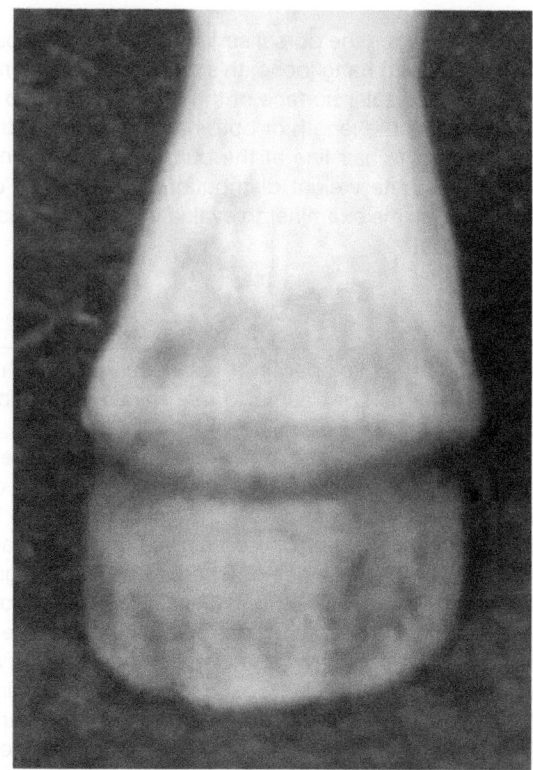

Fig. 2. Sub coronary sulcus in a 10-day-old foal.

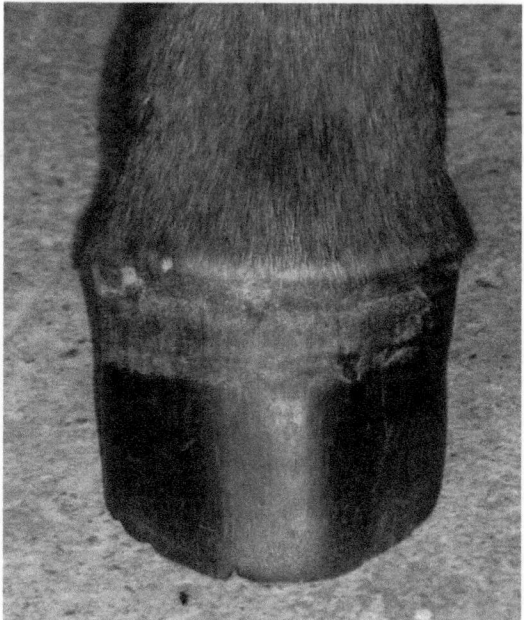

Fig. 3. The width is wider at the coronet than at the ground surface of the foot in this 1-month-old foal. Also note the pointed toe.

pointed toe, the foal may break over to either the outside or inside of the toe (see **Fig. 3**). If the frog has receded below the level of the hoof wall, the heels should be rasped lightly by using the smooth side of the rasp until the hoof wall and the frog are on the same plane. As discussed later in this article, the use of a hoof knife or hoof nippers is discouraged when trimming foals. This first farrier examination also will allow the foal to get used to having its feet handled. The farrier should be patient and the trimming procedure should be performed as gently and efficiently as possible. To expedite trimming, the mare should be backed into a corner of the stall and the foal is positioned against the side of the mare. An experienced handler who is gentile but firm is indispensable during the trimming process and removes any reliance on chemical restraint. The use of sedation when trimming foals should be discouraged. This technique also acts as a form of imprinting for future farrier sessions.

Two Months and Onward

In the first few months of life, attention should be directed toward the structural integrity of the hoof (foot mass/density) rather than to cosmetics. The important issues here are to promote the growth of thick, durable hoof wall, to ensure maximum sole depth to protect the vulnerable sole-wall junction and the developing distal phalanx and to develop the structures in the palmar/plantar section of the foot. The structural mass of the foot, defined as a strong hoof wall, adequate sole depth, and a solid heel base, is vital for future soundness. It is the author's opinion that a *hoof pick, wire brush, and a rasp* are the only tools necessary to trim foals that are kept on a monthly schedule. Furthermore, if the foal has proper exercise, there is generally minimal hoof growth, which makes the use of a hoof knife and hoof nippers unnecessary. The goal is to not have the foal walk entirely on the hoof wall, but to load all the structures on the solar surface of the foot, which makes the foot load sharing. Foals that are trimmed frequently and have a lot of horn removed tend to develop weak and fragile hoof capsules.

The method of trimming foals used by the author may differ from traditional farriery. Dirt and debris is removed from the sole and sulci of the frog using a hoof pick. The bottom of the foot is then cleaned vigorously by using a wire brush to remove any loose exfoliating horn. Otherwise, the ground surface of the foot and the frog are left untouched, which affords the foal ample protection on the ground surface of the foot. Exfoliating horn from the sole will be continuously shed through the abrasive friction with the ground as the foal exercises. The sole of a foal is relatively thin and needs as much thickness as possible to protect the immature developing structures above. Removing excess sole with a hoof knife is a primary cause of sole bruising in foals and may potentially lead to flexural deformities as a result of the pain response. The health of the foot throughout the animal's life is based on good solid heel structures. The heel base includes the hoof wall at the heel, the bars, the angle of the sole, a thick digital cushion, and a wide frog. The bars should not be removed, as they are needed for strength and to stabilize the palmar section of the hoof capsule. The heels are rasped gently from side to side until the rasp just comes in contact with the frog. The hoof wall at the heels will now be on the same plane with the frog. The excess hoof wall at the toe and quarters is then reduced as necessary by using a rasp placed at a 90° angle just dorsal to the sole-wall junction (white line) (**Fig. 4**A). When the desired amount of hoof wall is removed, the outer sharp edge of the angle formed by the angulation of the rasp is removed by running the rasp around the perimeter of the hoof, thus creating a rounded edge (**Fig. 4**B). This round edge will help to prevent cracks and chips in the hoof wall. The method of using the rasp on an angle leaves the hoof wall and the adjacent sole on the same plane, allowing both structures to share the bulk of the weight when the animal moves. This appears to stimulate the horn to grow thicker and

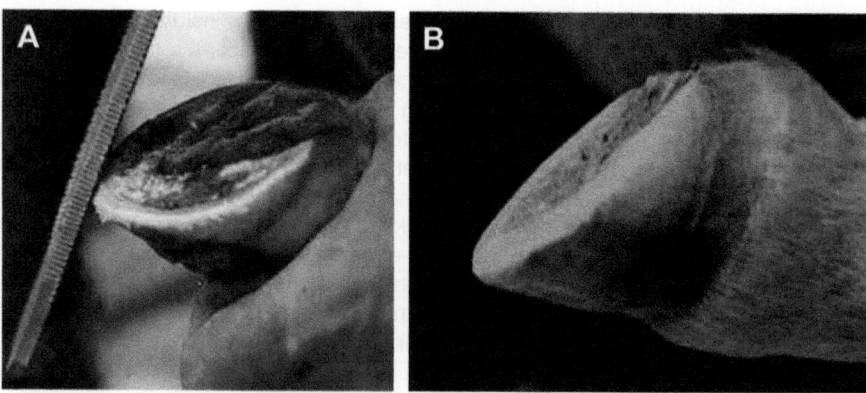

Fig. 4. (*A*) Rasp being used at 90° angle to trim the hoof wall. (*B*) Rasp used in a horizontal direction to create a rounded perimeter.

stronger. *Foals do not grow an excessive amount of hoof wall in the first few months of life, and our ability to influence the foot/limb by excessive trimming on one side of the foot in the horizontal plane is limited.* If it becomes necessary to lower one side of the foot past the point of being level due to a developing hoof capsule distortion or to affect landing, it should not be lowered any more than 2 to 3 mm at one time. Trimming at 2-week intervals may be useful in this situation.

The traditional theory of lowering the lateral side of the foot on a foal that stands toed-out or lowering the medial side of the foot on a toed-in foal is unrealistic. In fact, it may be detrimental. The cause of the foal having a toe-in or toe-out stance generally reflects the conformation of the limb and is rarely limited to the foot. The problem is generally found in the axial alignment of the limb above the foot, such as a rotational deformity of the limb below the carpus or the fetlock; therefore, when one side of the foot is lowered excessively, the cosmetic appearance may be improved but over time will lead to a distortion of the hoof capsule resulting from an unequal load on the foot. This practice also will place excessive and unequal forces on the physes and the joints on the side that is being lowered. The effects of excessive trimming can be seen radiographically a few days after the trim.

Rotational deformities are very common in foals and should not be considered abnormal. For example, a narrow chest coupled with relatively long limbs will cause many foals to adopt a base-wide stance in front, which is often accompanied by outward rotation of the entire limb. When viewed from the frontal plane, the entire limb will be rotated outward, but the axial alignment of the limb will be relatively straight (**Fig. 5**). This stance, which can be considered normal in foals, confers a higher degree of stability and is gradually modified as the transverse diameters of the upper body increase with growth. As the foal moves, it is quite noticeable that the lateral side of the hoof wall contacts the ground initially as a result of the flight pattern caused by the rotated position of the limb. These foals should be trimmed flat or level and not have their feet lowered on the outside wall, which is the traditional practice. A base-wide stance in a 3-month-old to 4-month-old foal results naturally in asymmetric hoof capsules in the frontal plane with the medial side of the hoof capsule slightly lower than the lateral aspect. If this stance is not recognized as physiologic for the age and an attempt is made to "correct" it by lowering the lateral wall, there may be a risk of creating an angular limb deformity where none

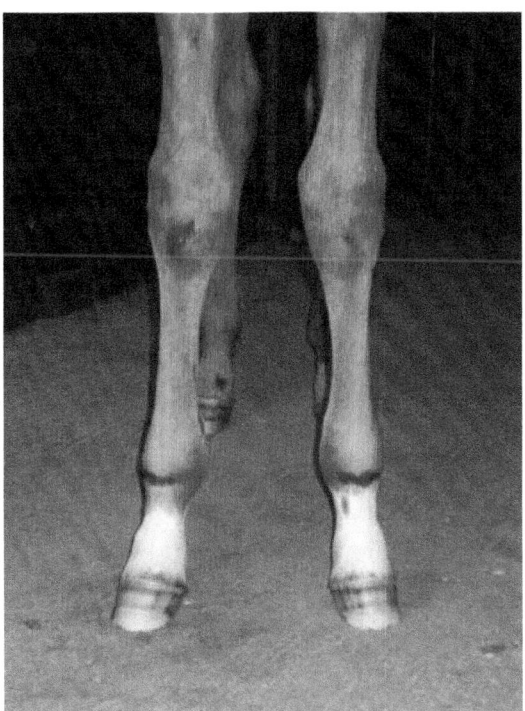

Fig. 5. Rotational deformity, Note the narrow chest, carpi rotated laterally and medial hoof wall beginning to roll axially.

existed previously. In cases in which the medial heel bulb has been displaced proximally as a result of the asymmetrical landing pattern, the medial hoof wall is trimmed slightly lower to create additional ground surface, and if the medial hoof wall begins to roll axially, a small composite extension to increase the ground surface can be used to address this hoof capsule distortion. Therapeutic trimming does not offer favorable results in the malpositioned limb, as this deformity is corrected through growth. As the musculature of the chest increases, the chest widens and the elbows are pushed outward, rotating the limbs inward.

FLEXOR TENDON FLACCIDITY, FLEXURAL DEFORMITIES, AND ANGULAR LIMB DEFORMITIES IN FOALS
Flexor Tendon Flaccidity

Excessive (flexor tendon) laxity most commonly affects the fetlocks of the hind limbs, whereas in the forelimbs, it generally involves the fetlocks and carpi; the vast majority will improve spontaneously with no treatment and will have a good prognosis. This condition is often seen in premature, dysmature, or septic foals. When encountered in the forelimbs, there is a "bowed" appearance to the limb resulting from a laxity of the flexor apparatus. The carpus is in hyperextension and the fetlock is in dorsiflexion, with the palmar surface of the pastern and fetlock on or close to the ground. There may be subluxation of the distal interphalangeal joint (DIPJ) associated with deep digital flexor tendon laxity allowing the toe of the foot to elevate off the ground. In hind limb laxity, the DIPJ is almost always involved, along with laxity noted in the pastern and fetlock (**Fig. 6**). Initial treatment is aimed at

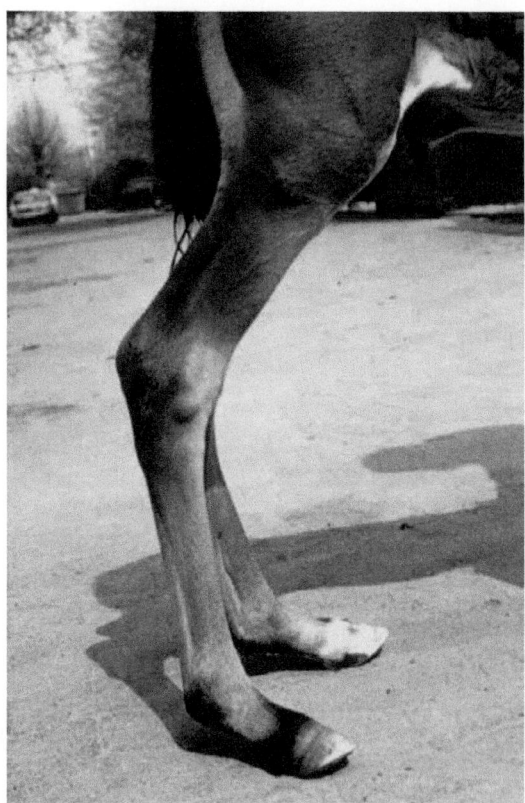

Fig. 6. Flexor laxity of hind limbs in a 1-week-old foal.

protecting the soft tissues of the heels without oversupporting the fetlock, which will further promote the laxity. This can be accomplished by applying an adhesive pad cut in the shape of the heel bulbs (Moleskin; Bayer HealthCare LLC, Whippany, NJ). The condition tends to be self-limiting within days after birth as the foal gains strength and is allowed moderate exercise. However, the tendon laxity often persists, and it is not uncommon to see a foal that still has digital hyperextension at 3 to 4 weeks of age. Treatment is sequential depending on the severity of the tendon laxity and the initial response of the foal to treatment. Therapy begins with controlled exercise allowing the foal access to a small area with firm footing for 1 hour, 2 to 3 times daily. If there is no response by the third day postpartum, the author will place the foot on a piece of one-quarter-inch plywood and trace the foot, leaving 2 to 3 cm of extension beyond the heels. The plywood is attached to the foot by using a soft Kling gauze (Johnson & Johnson, Skillman, NJ) and 2-inch elastic tape (Elasticon; Johnson & Johnson) (**Fig. 7**). The laxity will generally resolve in 7 to 10 days. When presented as an older foal, the toe of the hoof capsule should be reduced from the outer hoof wall; the heels can be rasped gently from the middle of the foot palmarly/plantarly to create additional ground surface in that section of the foot. Some form of a palmar/plantar extension should now be applied that extends approximately 3 to 4 cm beyond the bulbs of the heels to relieve the biomechanical instability of the digit (**Fig. 8**). A cuff-type extension shoe (Dalric heel extension;

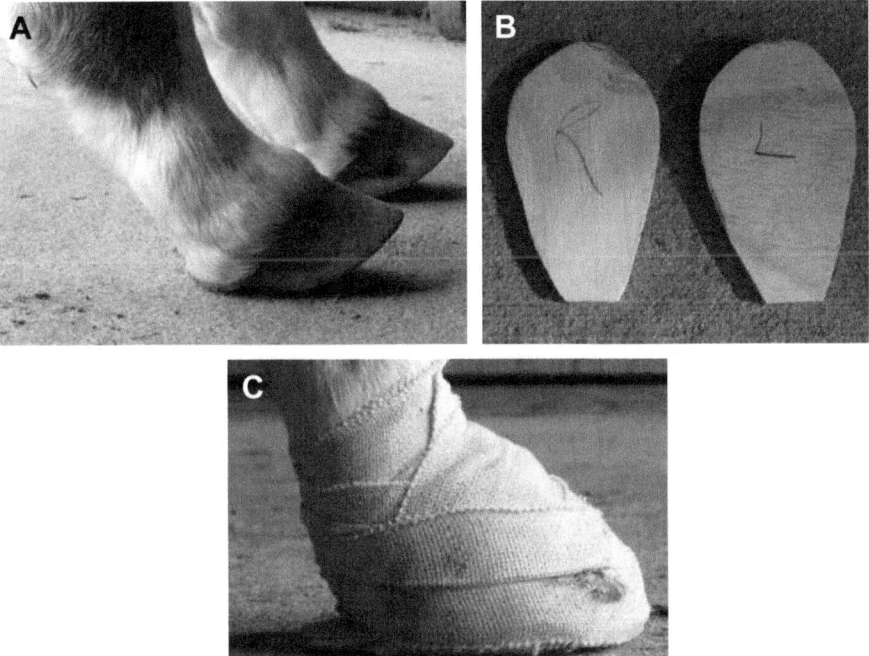

Fig. 7. (*A*) Flexural laxity in a 3-day-old foal. (*B*) Foot is traced on plywood used to create heel extensions. (*C*) Extension is taped on foot.

Nanric, Lawrenceburg, KY) is commercially available, or a thin aluminum plate can be fabricated as a heel extension with the toe bent to align with the dorsal hoof wall to hold it in place. The author believes that with either type of extension used, it should be attached with gauze and elastic tape rather than a composite if the foal is younger than 3 weeks of age. This manner of attachment avoids excessive heat being applied to the fragile hoof capsule when the composite cures and it also prevents contracture of the hoof capsule, which occurs at the heels. Heel

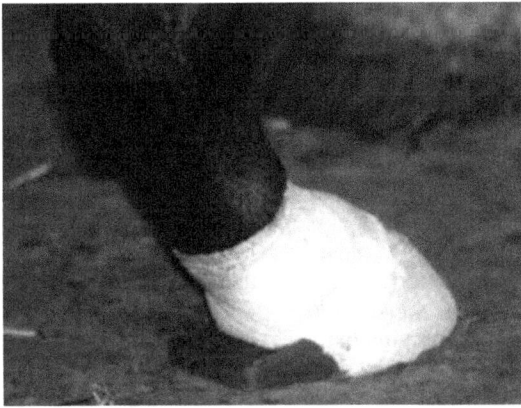

Fig. 8. Commercial heel extension taped on the foot.

extensions should extend beyond the heel bulbs or farther; if not of sufficient length, the extension will serve as a fulcrum and worsen the subluxation of the DIPJ and damage the heels of the hoof capsule.

Regardless of the method of application, the extensions should be changed at 7-day to 10-day intervals.

Bandaging the limb is contraindicated, as this will further weaken the flexor tendons and promote laxity.

Care should be taken to maintain the condition of the feet with trimming while the tendon laxity is being addressed, and long-term rehabilitation of the feet may be necessary. During treatment, the heels become distorted and the hoof wall growth is oriented dorsally, which requires gradual reshaping once the limb laxity is resolved. The heels should be trimmed to the level of normal tubular alignment, if possible, and the heels of the hoof capsule should be on the same plane as the frog; the toe should be trimmed or reduced from the dorsal hoof wall surface in a plantar direction. This process may require 3 to 4 months to accomplish, but over time, a normal foot should be the end result.

Flexural Deformities

Flexural deformities have been traditionally referred to as "contracted tendons." The primary defect is a shortening of the deep digital flexor musculotendinous unit rather than a shortening of just the tendon portion, making "flexural deformity" the preferred term.[1–3] This shortening produces a unit of functional length that is less than necessary for normal limb alignment of the digit; this results in fixed flexion of the various joints of the distal limb, especially the DIPJ.

Flexural deformities may be congenital or acquired. Outcome and prognosis will vary with the severity of the flexural deformity.

Congenital flexural deformities

Congenital flexural deformities are present at birth, may involve a combination of joints (eg, carpal, metacarpophalangeal, and DIPJs) and are characterized by abnormal flexion of these joints and their inability to extend. Proposed etiologies of congenital flexural deformities include malpositioning of the fetus in utero, nutritional mismanagement of the mare during gestation, teratogens in various forages ingested by the mare, and maternal exposure to influenza virus or the deformities could be genetic in origin.[2] The affected foal tends to stand and walk on the toe of the hoof capsule, is unable to place the heel on the ground and assumes a so-called "ballerina" stance. Treatment of foals with a congenital flexural deformity varies with the severity of the deformity. A mild to moderate flexural deformity in which the foal can readily stand, nurse, and ambulate is generally self-limiting and resolves without treatment. Brief intervals of exercise for 1 hour once or twice daily in a small paddock on firm footing for the first few days of life may be all that is necessary for the deformity to resolve. If the condition is severe or has not improved by the third day post foaling, intravenous (IV) administration of oxytetracycline (2–3 g) repeated every other day if necessary is frequently beneficial.[4] A variety of bandaging techniques and splints are often used, along with physical therapy to "stretch" the involved soft tissue structures; this may hasten recovery. Foals with severe congenital flexural deformities usually will have more than just 1 isolated structure or joint that is responsible for the deformity; therefore, in the author's opinion, the use of a toe extension is not indicated. Applying a toe extension will generally result in the neonate stumbling and being unable to ambulate. The "lever arm" principle of the toe extension in an attempt to stretch the tendon is unrealistic and does not come without a price, which is the likelihood of damage to the hoof capsule.

Acquired flexural deformities

Acquired flexural deformities develop when the foal is between 2 and 6 months old and generally involves the DIPJ initially. It is commonly a unilateral condition but occasionally affects both limbs. The etiology of this deformity is unknown, but speculated causes include genetic predisposition, improper nutrition (ie, over-feeding, excessive carbohydrate [energy] intake, unbalanced minerals in the diet), and excessive exercise.[1–3] A recent study looking at grazing patterns in a small number of foals showed that foals with long legs and short necks had a tendency to graze with the same limb protracted.[4] Fifty percent of the foals in this study developed uneven feet with a higher heel on the protracted limb, leading researchers to believe there may be a possible correlation between conformational traits and an acquired flexural deformity. It is the author's opinion that a large contributing factor to this syndrome is contraction of the muscular portion of the musculotendinous unit caused by a pain response; the source of which could be discomfort anywhere along the limb, physeal dysplasia, or trauma from foals exercising on hard ground. Discomfort may follow aggressive hoof trimming in which excessive sole is removed, thus rendering the immature structures within the hoof capsule void of protection. The foal then becomes unwilling to bear full weight and is susceptible to trauma and bruising. Any discomfort or pain in the foot or lower portion of the limb coupled with reduced weight-bearing on the affected limb appears to initiate a flexor withdrawal reflex; this causes the flexor muscles proximal to the tendon to contract, leading to a shortened musculotendinous unit and an altered position of the DIPJ. This shortening of the musculotendinous unit shifts weight-bearing to the dorsal section of the foot causing increased load on the dorsal sole, bruising of the sole, reduced growth of the dorsal aspect of the hoof wall, and excessive hoof wall growth at the heel to compensate for the shortening. As the flexural deformity may be secondary to pain in these cases, it is essential that a possible source of pain should be carefully evaluated and localized by physical examination and, if necessary, by regional analgesia and diagnostic imaging. A genetic component also should be considered for acquired flexural deformities, as some mares consistently produce foals that develop a flexural deformity in the same limb of the dam or grand dam in which a similar deformity is present.[2] However, at present, there is no conclusive scientific evidence to substantiate a genetic basis.

Mild acquired flexural deformities

The initial clinical sign of a flexural deformity may only be abnormal wear of the hoof at the toe, which is often discovered by the farrier during routine hoof care. Closer or subsequent investigation may reveal that the dorsal hoof wall angle is increased and that after the heels of the hoof capsule have been trimmed to a normal length, the heels may no longer contact the ground. A prominent coronary band may become apparent at this stage. Most foals affected to this degree may already have a mildly broken forward hoof-pastern axis. Increased palpable digital pulse, heat in the affected foot, and signs of pain when a small hoof tester is applied to the solar aspect of the toe dorsal to the frog are not uncommon clinical findings. Hoof tester pain is generally the result of trauma or excessive weight-bearing on the toe.

Conservative treatment, such as restricting exercise to reduce further trauma is paramount. Correcting the nutritional status of the foal (ie, weaning the foal to avoid possible excessive nutrition from the mare and/or decreasing carbohydrate intake), administering an anti-inflammatory agent (nonsteroidal anti-inflammatory drug [NSAID]) to relieve pain, administering oxytetracycline to facilitate muscle relaxation, and carefully trimming the hoof are, in the author's opinion, a good starting point. The NSAIDs should be administered short-term and judiciously in foals due to the potential side effects, such as gastroduodenal irritation and nephrotoxicity. For analgesia, the author will administer firocoxib (0.1 mg/kg body weight every 24 hours) or flunixin meglumine (1.1 mg/kg body weight every 24 hours) orally combined with a gastric protectant. Hoof trimming is directed toward improving the hoof angle by lightly trimming the heels from the middle of the foot palmarly until the hoof wall at the heels and the frog are on the same plane. The bars can be thinned in this instance in an attempt to spread and possibly improve heel expansion. The heels adjacent to the sulci should also be rasped to a 45° angle to promote spreading. Breakover is moved palmarly by creating a mild bevel with a rasp, which begins just dorsal to the apex of the frog and extends to the perimeter of the dorsal aspect of the hoof wall (**Fig. 9**). If improvement is noted, this trimming regimen is optimally performed at 2-week intervals. If the toe is constantly being bruised or undergoing abscessation, a hoof composite (Equilox, Equilox Int. Pine Island, MN) can be applied to the dorsal aspect of the sole and the distal dorsal aspect of the hoof wall to form a protective toe "cap." The acrylic composite-impregnated fiberglass or urethane composite used to form the toe cap covers the solar surface to the apex of the frog, protecting that area from further damage. A bevel toward the toe can be created in the composite with a rasp or Dremel tool to facilitate breakover. If there is adequate integrity of the dorsal section of the hoof wall, the author believes that application of a toe extension to be unwarranted and actually contraindicated. Farriers have traditionally applied toe extensions to create a lever arm using a shoe or a composite, but they only exacerbate hoof wall separation and delay breakover. Furthermore, extensions may contribute to lameness due to excessive stresses on the deep digital flexor tendon (DDFT) when the foal puts full weight on its foot and at the initiation of breakover. This treatment is often temporary, and appears to work best when initiated at the first sign of a foot deformity before a marked flexural deformity is noted. Whenever possible, the elimination of any inciting causes should be pursued. The farriery should always be combined with restricted exercise. If the affected foot continues to improve or does not digress, conservative treatment is continued. However, if a mild flexural deformity progresses in severity to the stage in which a marked radiographic flexural deformity is noted, the foal becomes a surgical candidate.

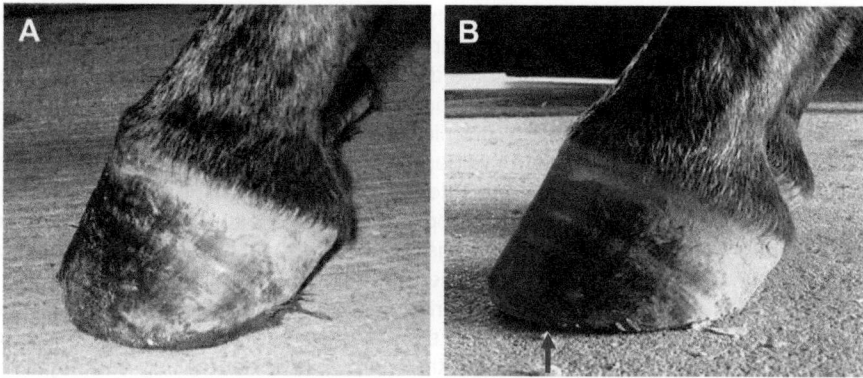

Fig. 9. (*A*) Grade 1 flexural deformity. (*B*) After the foot is trimmed. Note the bevel created under the toe (*Red arrow* denotes the point of breakover).

Severe acquired flexural deformities

A mild acquired flexural deformity may progress in severity despite conservative treatment or a severe acquired flexural deformity may be acute in onset. A severe acquired flexural deformity is characterized by a foot with a hoof angle greater than 80°, a prominent fullness at the coronary band, a broken forward pastern-axis, and disparity in hoof wall growth distal to the coronet at the heel relative to growth at the toe and heels that fail to contact the ground (**Fig. 10**). If the flexural deformity is allowed to persist, the foot eventually assumes a boxy, tubular shape due to the overgrowth of the heels to accommodate the lack of ground contact; heel length will approach the length of the toe (**Fig. 11**). Increased stress on the toe will eventually cause a concavity along the dorsal surface of the hoof wall. Stress exerted on the sole-wall junction in the toe area will cause it to widen, allowing separations to occur.

The diagnosis is straightforward and based on the characteristic foot and limb conformation described previously. Radiographs should be used to confirm the diagnosis and assess changes in the joint. The author will administer mild sedation (half the recommended dose of xylazine [0.33–1.44 mg/kg, IV] combined with butorphanol [0.022–0.066 mg/kg, IV]) and place each of the foal's feet on separate wooden blocks of equal height, which allows normal or equal loading of both forefeet. Lateral-to-medial weight-bearing images of both forefeet should be obtained. The degree of flexion of the DIPJ, the angle of the dorsal hoof wall, and abnormalities at the margin of the distal phalanx should be assessed (**Fig. 12**).

When a marked flexural deformity is present and confirmed by radiographic examination of the feet, conservative treatment and hoof trimming alone are generally unsuccessful in resolving the problem. Elevating the heels has been advocated to reduce tension in the DDFT and to promote weight-bearing on the palmar section of the hoof. However, although elevating the heels improves the hoof-pastern axis and makes the foal more comfortable initially, the author has not been able to subsequently lower the heel or remove the wedge and establish a normal hoof angle with the heel on the ground. Once a marked flexural deformity of the DIPJ and distortion

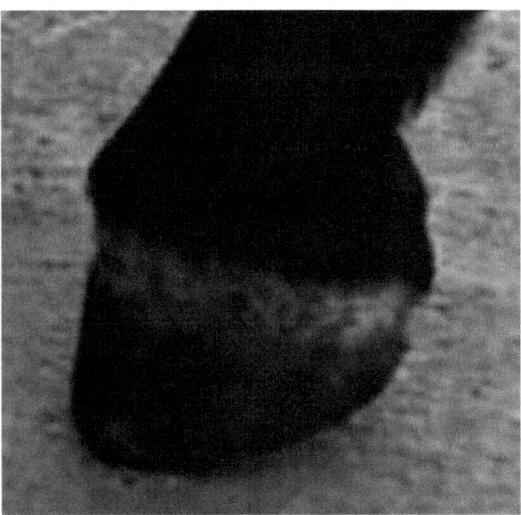

Fig. 10. Grade 3 flexural deformity.

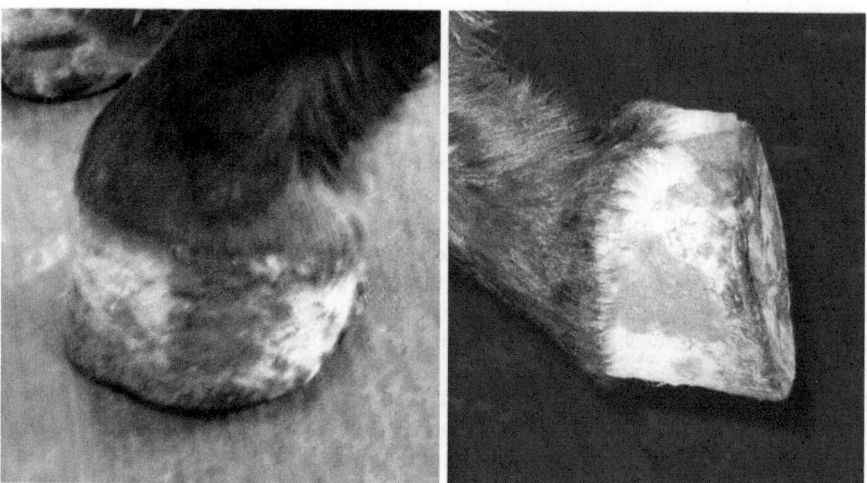

Fig. 11. Chronic flexural deformity in a 3-month-old foal that has acquired a tubular shape with the coronet becoming horizontal.

of the hoof capsule is apparent or progressing, the author recommends transection of the accessory ligament of the DDFT combined with the appropriate farriery.

The author does not recommend a toe extension; rather, an acrylic composite is applied to the solar region of the toe to create a reverse wedge.[5] The wedge affords protection for the toe region and appears to redistribute the load to the palmar aspect of the foot, thus mildly increasing the stresses on the DDFT, and appears to restore the concavity to the sole. The farriery is generally performed before the surgery either before or while the foal is anesthetized to prevent manipulating the limb and handling the surgical site following the procedure. The heels are lowered with a rasp from the point of the frog palmarly, until the sole adjoining the hoof wall (sole plane) at the heels becomes solid. Any concavity in the dorsal aspect of the hoof wall is removed with a rasp. The ground surface of the foot dorsal to the frog and the perimeter of the dorsal hoof wall are prepared for a composite by using a rasp or Dremel tool. Deep

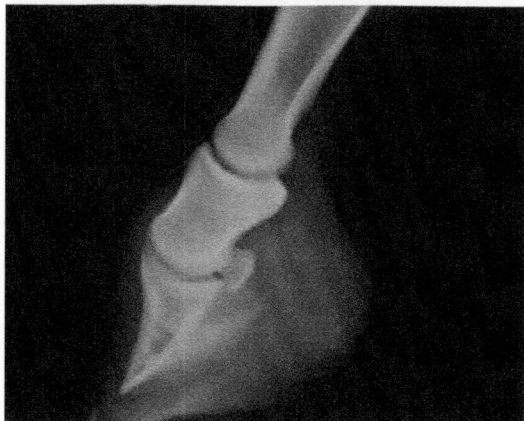

Fig. 12. Radiograph shows a the marked flexural deformity involving the DIPJ.

separations in the sole-wall junction at the toe are explored and filled with clay, if necessary, to prevent infection beneath the composite. Foals undergoing this procedure are usually between 3 and 5 months old; because of their size and weight, reinforcing the composite with fiberglass is necessary to prevent excessive wear. A small section of fiberglass is separated into strands and mixed with the composite. An acrylic composite is applied to the solar surface of the foot beginning at the apex of the frog and extending to the perimeter of the hoof wall where a thin lip is formed. The composite is molded into a wedge starting at 0° at the apex of the frog and extending to 2° to 3° at the toe[2] (**Fig. 13**). If desired, a piece of one-eighth-inch aluminum plate can be cut out in the shape of the dorsal aspect of the sole. Multiple holes are drilled in the plate, and it is gently placed into the composite. The aluminum is pushed down so that the composite material extrudes through the holes, and the aluminum plate is then covered with additional composite. This additional reinforcement allows the older foals to be walked daily or turned out in a small paddock without the composite wearing out. The foal is placed under general anesthesia, and the surgery is performed in a routine manner, as described elsewhere in this issue.

The surgical aftercare is at the discretion of the attending clinician. Controlled exercise in the form of daily walking or turnout in a small paddock with firm footing, such as a round pen, is essential. There is the potential for pain with the initiation of exercise, requiring close monitoring of the foal, and exercise should be increased sequentially. The foal is trimmed at roughly 2-week intervals, based on the amount of hoof growth at the heels with the objective of establishing normal hoof capsule conformation. The composite wedge is removed 1 month after the surgery. At each subsequent trimming, the heels are lowered as necessary from the middle of the foot palmarly, and the hoof wall at the toe is trimmed from the dorsal aspect of the hoof wall until the desired conformation is attained. No sole dorsal to the frog is removed. When the desired conformation is reached, the foot is trimmed in a routine manner on a monthly basis. It is important to emphasize that when the hoof capsule returns to an

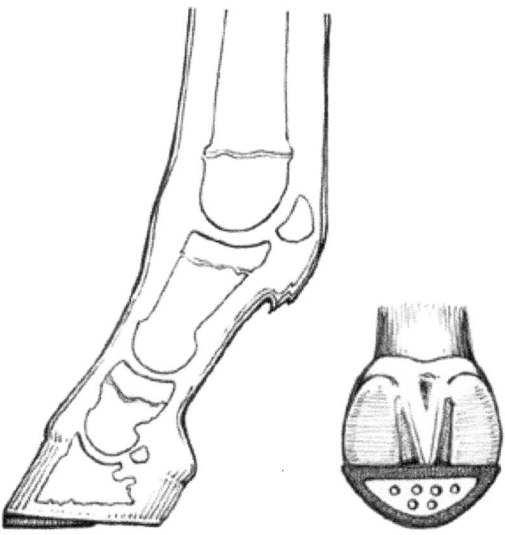

Fig. 13. Reverse wedge created from a composite. An aluminum plate can be imbedded in the composite to prevent wear.

acceptable conformation, only that portion of the sole that is shedding should be removed. This avoids causing discomfort in the dorsal solar area that can result in the horse redeveloping, to some degree, the original deformity.

Angular Limb Deformities

Angular limb deformities are common in foals and require early recognition and treatment.[6–8] This subject receives tremendous attention in any discussion of foal conformation and it refers to a deviation in axial alignment of the limbs when the animal is viewed from the frontal plane. It is understood that a certain amount of deviation is normal in young foals and does not require any special farriery or surgical intervention. Objective data is lacking regarding the dynamics involved in the development of acquired angular limb deformities; however, it is recognized that many foals change axial alignment during various stages of their development. Serial evaluation and treatment of limb deviations is an integral component of management on most breeding operations. Angular limb deformities can be classified as either congenital or acquired during the first few weeks of life. The primary lesion is an imbalance of physeal growth; for various reasons, growth proceeds faster on one side of the physis versus the other. Angular limb deformities can be further classified into 2 categories: valgus deformities occur when the deviation occurs lateral to the axis of the limb (away from the midline) and varus deformities occur when the deviation is medial to the axis of the limb (toward the midline) (**Fig. 14**). The most common location of valgus angular limb deformities is the carpus/tarsus, whereas varus deformities are most often seen at the fetlock.

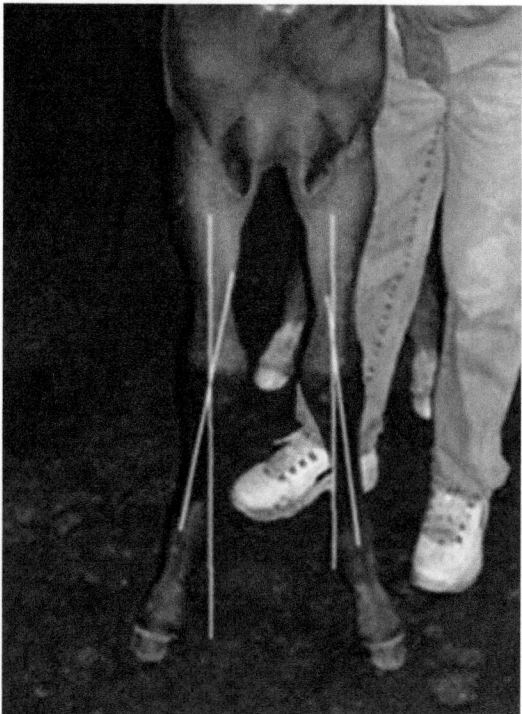

Fig. 14. Carpal valgus. Note the limb below the carpus deviates away from the midline.

Limb alignment of young foals should be observed standing and walking without restriction on the head and neck (not leaning) toward and away from the examiner. Overall body development and maturity should be noted. It is important to take note of foot placement especially when working with distal limb deviations. This will determine the necessity for corrective measures on the feet, such as trimming or placement of a composite extension on the hoof capsule to alter the load on the physis and change the rotation of the limb on contact with the ground. This practice is especially beneficial with a fetlock varus deviation with inward rotational deformities in foals 2 to 4 weeks of age in which there is a limited time frame.

Carpal/tarsal valgus

It is apparent that a mild carpal valgus of 2° to 5° offers the newborn foal a comfortable stance while nursing and eating off the ground and is considered acceptable. If the deviation exceeds 5° to 8°, then it becomes a concern and should be monitored. A few days of stall confinement on firm bedding or limited exercise in a small paddock (2–3 times a day) is a rewarding, cost-effective treatment for early carpal or tarsal valgus.

It may be helpful to digress and briefly mention routine hoof care before discussing angular limb deformities. The technique for using the tools when trimming foals was discussed earlier under the trim. The veterinary and farriery literature abounds with various trimming methods that are thought to affect the various limb conformations; however, none of these methods have been substantiated. The author trims the heels such that the heels of the hoof wall and the frog are on the same plane, visualizes a line across the middle of the foot, and then reduces the toe to make the foot proportional on either side of the line. When the trim is complete, the solar surface of the foot will be level rather than having the lateral-to-medial orientation of foot changed by lowering one side of the foot (**Fig. 15**). Farriery texts describe trimming a foal lower on the outside of the foot when the foot turns out and trimming the foal lower on the inside of the foot when the foot turns in; however, remembering that a toe-out or toe-in

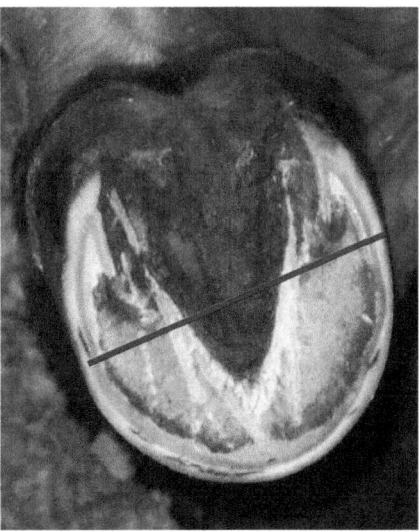

Fig. 15. A 2-month-old foal trimmed to show the proportionality of the foot on either side of a line drawn across the widest part of the foot. Note the hoof wall at the heels and the frog trimmed to the same plane.

stance originates from the limb, therefore, this practice will do nothing more than place excessive stress on one side of the hoof capsule.

If the angular limb deformity is greater than 5° to 8° or shows no improvement in the first few days of life, radiographs should be part of the physical examination.

Occasionally, osseous abnormalities, such as hypoplastic carpal/tarsal bones will preclude correction of the problem without splints or a cast. Radiographs also will reveal the site and degree of deviation, and allow comparison at a later date. Carpal valgus deformities of less than 10° are generally handled successively with conservative treatment.

Conservative therapy for the management of many mild to moderate congenital angular limb deformities may be successful in the newborn foal. Restricted exercise would be either strict stall confinement or brief periods of turnout (1 hour, 2 times daily) in a small area with firm footing. This allows the physis to be stimulated but prevents stress and compression on the overloaded side of the growth plate from excessive exercise. If the knee can be corrected by applying pressure with one hand on the inside of the carpus and counter pressure with the other hand applied to the outside of the fetlock, then a splint made from polyvinylchloride (PVC) pipe fitted from the elbow to below the fetlock applied for a few hours 1 to 2 times daily may be useful. It is labor intensive, but the splints must be removed and replaced periodically to prevent laxity. A full-length thick cotton bandage is applied to the limb first, and then the PVC pipe is placed on the outside of the limb and secured with elastic tape. This will distract the carpus laterally and load the limb more appropriately. The splint is often the most cost-effective treatment available but must be applied with caution, paying strict attention to the details of application. Meticulous attention to applying the splint is essential to prevent focal pressure and the propensity of the foal to develop decubital ulcers from excessive pressure.

Acquired carpal/tarsal valgus deformities can be graded from 1 to 4 according to severity (**Fig. 16**). Angular limb deformities can be present at birth or occur

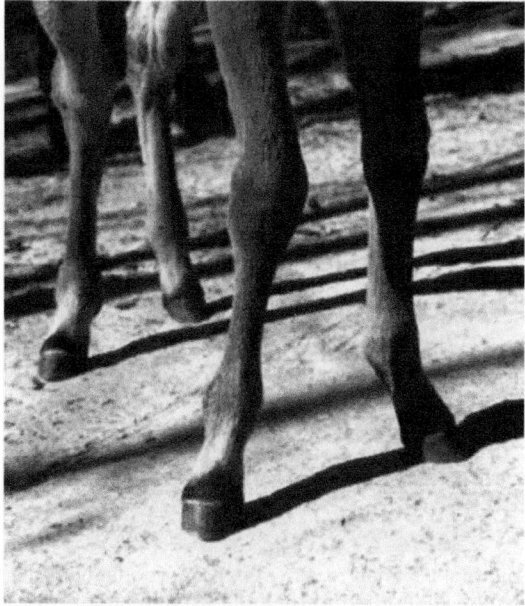

Fig. 16. Grade 3 carpal valgus in a 2-month-old foal.

anywhere from a few days onward. Mild to moderate valgus will generally respond to restricted exercise and the use of a composite extension applied to the medial side of the foot, whereas the more severe cases require surgical intervention combined with farriery.[8,9] Various clinicians have described trimming the lateral side of the foot aggressively when there is a valgus deformity in an attempt to increase the ground surface on this side of the foot. However, it is this author's opinion that the foal does not grow enough horn at this stage to make an appreciable difference, and changing the medial to lateral orientation of the foot may have detrimental effects on the immature hoof capsule. Using some form of extension to increase the ground surface of the foot seems to be more beneficial.[10,11] The author prefers some type of composite applied to the hoof wall rather than a cuffed shoe, which restricts movement of the hoof capsule and contracts the foot, especially the heels. As noted previously, the author will not apply a composite to a foal's foot before 3 weeks of age. The composite extension is placed on the medial side of the hoof and toward the heels, which appears to redirect the forces on the physis on the overloaded side of the limb by moving the axis of weight-bearing toward the center of the limb (**Fig. 17**). The extension also appears to promote centerline breakover. The extension is made from an acrylic composite (Equilox; Equilox Int) mixed with fiberglass strands or a urethane composite (Vettec Super Fast; Vettec) applied directly to the foot and shaped to the desired width. Properly applied for maximum results, the extension should begin at the contact point of the heel and feather up most of the length of the wall. It should not extend dorsally beyond the junction of the quarter and toe to be of any benefit and it should not be built up on the sole but only tapered along the sole toward the frog. The extension should be no wider than a vertical line drawn from the coronet to the ground. If the extension is too wide, it applies leverage that will invariably distort the hoof capsule. The extension should be removed every 2 to 3 weeks to allow the hoof wall to dry out and not break up. Also with chronic use, there may be a restriction of hoof wall growth that may contribute to long-term distortion of the wall.

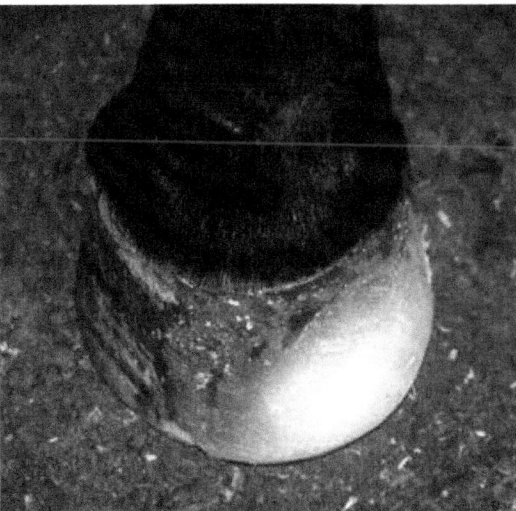

Fig. 17. Extension placed on medial side of hoof on foal in **Fig. 16**.

Strict controlled exercise is essential for this conservative approach to be successful. In severe cases of carpal/tarsal valgus in which surgery is necessary, a medial extension is combined with the surgery.

In many cases, a surgical procedure may be performed too early before conservative therapy is allowed to correct the problem. It appears that valgus angular limb deformities involving the carpus/tarsus will respond to surgery up to 4 months of age or may even be much later for the carpus with full correction. Obviously, if the valgus deformity renders the carpus unstable, then surgery will be required sooner.

Fetlock varus

Varus deformities involving the fetlock are common in either the front or hind limb of newborn foals (**Fig. 18**). This deformity can be congenital or acquired within the first week of life. Fetlock varus is often confused with a foal that has a toe-in conformation. The digit will deviate axially (toward the midline) relative to the fetlock with fetlock varus; a foal with a toe-in conformation will have a rotational deformity at or above the fetlock but the digit will follow the alignment of the limb. However, both conditions may occur concomitantly. A fetlock varus deformity requires early detection and treatment because functional closure of the distal physis of the third metacarpal/metatarsal bone is at approximately 12 weeks of age. Foals with fetlock varus should have their exercise restricted and will generally respond to an extension applied to the lateral side of the foot. The window of opportunity for treatment

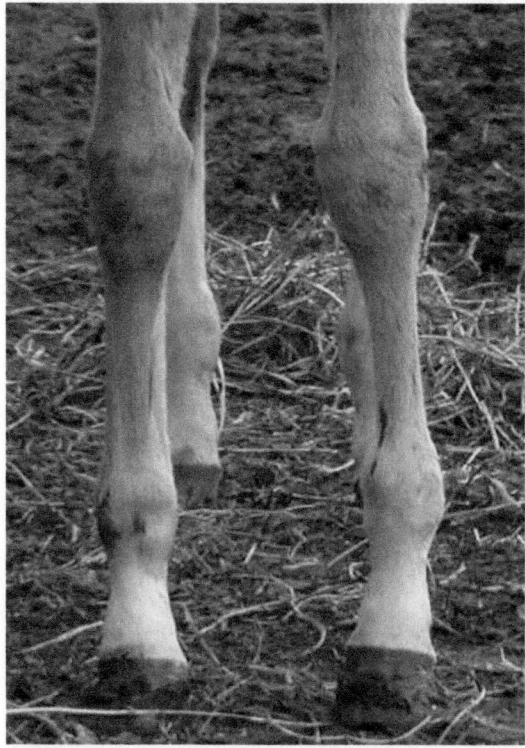

Fig. 18. Left forelimb fetlock varus in a 2-week-old foal. Note the varus deformity and the toe-in stance.

is small and the extension should be applied at 1 to 3 weeks of age. Again, the author is reluctant to apply a composite to a foal's foot before 3 weeks of age. In this case, the author uses a firm impression material (Equilox Pink impression material; Equilox International, Inc, Pine Island, MN), and molds it to the solar surface of the foal's foot, forming an extension on the lateral side (**Fig. 19**). The impression material is molded into the concavity of the sole and the sulci of the frog, which holds it in place, and is then taped on the foot with Kling gauze and 2-inch elastic tape. In severe cases, surgical intervention will be necessary combined with an extension. If the foal is presented for treatment after 30 days of age, treatment becomes difficult, as surgery will be necessary and the overall treatment is less effective and not as cosmetic.

Varus deviations involving the carpus are also recognized in young foals and weanlings. Foals that develop carpal varus from birth to 1 to 2 months of age often have an "over at the knee" appearance and buckle forward when standing. These typically worsen with exercise and improve with rest. Dietary control is important, as is the judicious use of analgesics and controlled exercise. Lateral extensions may be useful, but surgical intervention may be necessary if the varus condition is severe. Weanlings that develop carpal varus are typically offset at the carpus, sometimes pigeon-toed, and often have accompanying physeal dysplasia, which, if kept under control, may resolve the deviation. If the condition fails to respond, surgery, such as transphyseal bridging or placement of a transphyseal screw in the physis of the distal lateral radius, may be necessary. In general, valgus deviations are far easier to manage and are more prone to spontaneously correct and appear much more forgiving from a soundness standpoint than varus deviations.

In summary, management of angular limb deformities, irrespective of the type, severity, or origin, are best managed through a coordinated effort among the owner, farm manager, farrier, and veterinarian. When treating valgus and varus limb deformities, early treatment is best for correction. Flexural and angular limb deformities are often controversial and have a multitude of purported treatments; it is therefore essential that appropriate communication be conveyed among the responsible parties to avoid any misunderstanding and unnecessary or job-threatening miscommunications. Most veterinarians are not able perform the farriery required to address foot and limb issues in foals, so their reliance on a farrier becomes obvious. An avenue of communication between the professions is not only necessary, but mandatory.

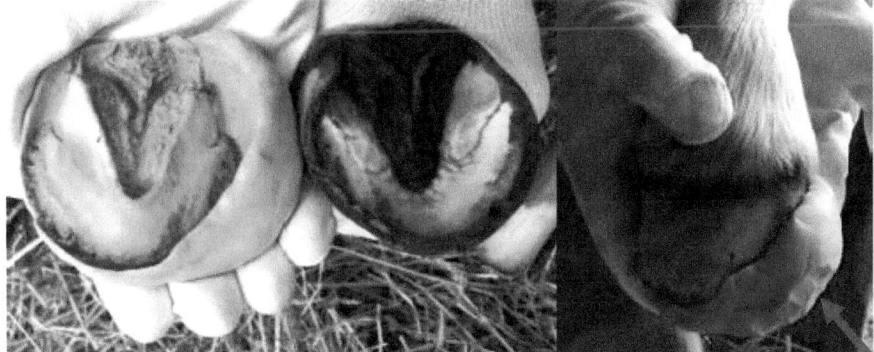

Fig. 19. Impression material is formed to match the concavity of the sole. Impression material can be trimmed to the desired width of the lateral extension (*arrow*).

SUMMARY

Hoof care in the first few months of life is serious business and should never be taken lightly. Farriery plays a vital role in both the development of the hoof and the conformation of the limb. Management of the feet and limbs during this period will often dictate the success of the foal as a sales yearling or mature sound athlete. A planned foot care program is time-consuming, whereas assembly-line trimming is quick and easy, but the thoughtful approach is much more rewarding.

REFERENCES

1. Adkins A. Flexural limb deformity. Proc Br Equine Vet Assoc Congress 2008;47: 41–2.
2. O'Grady SE. Flexural deformities of the distal interphalangeal joint (clubfeet): a review. Equine Vet Educ 2012;24(5):260–8.
3. Hunt RJ. Flexural limb deformities in foals. In: Ross MW, Dyson SJ, editors. Diagnosis and management of lameness in the horse. 2nd edition. Philadelphia: W.B. Saunders; 2011. p. 645–9.
4. van Heel MC, Kroekenstoel AM, van Dierendonck MC, et al. Uneven feet in a foal may develop as a consequence of lateral grazing behavior induced by conformational traits. Equine Vet J 2006;38:646–51.
5. O'Grady SE. How to manage the club foot—birth to maturity. Proc Amer Assoc Equine Pract 2014;60:60–72.
6. Greet TRC. Managing flexural and angular limb deformities: the Newmarket perspective. Proc Amer Assoc Equine Pract 2000;46:130–6.
7. Madison JB, Garber JL, Rice B, et al. Effects of oxytetracycline on metacarpophalangeal and distal interphalangeal joint angles in newborn foals. J Am Vet Med Assoc 1994;204:240–9.
8. Auer JA. Angular limb deformities. In: Auer JA, Stick JA, editors. Equine surgery. 3rd edition. St Louis (MO): Sanders; 2006. p. 1130–49.
9. Greet TRC, Curtis SJ. Foot management in the foal and weanling. In: O'Grady SE, editor. The veterinary clinics of North America, vol. 19. Philadelphia: W.B. Saunders; 2003. p. 501–17, 2.
10. Hunt RJ. Management of angular limb deformities. Proc Amer Assoc Equine Pract 2000;46:128–9.
11. Cheramie HS, O'Grady SE. Hoof repair and glue-on shoe technology. In: O'Grady SE, editor. The veterinary clinics of North America, vol. 19. Philadelphia: W.B. Saunders; 2003. p. 519–30, 2.

Orthopedic Conditions of the Premature and Dysmature Foal

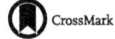 CrossMark

Michelle C. Coleman, DVM*, Canaan Whitfield-Cargile, DVM

KEYWORDS

- Incomplete ossification • Premature • Dysmature • Hypothyroid • Cuboidal bones

KEY POINTS

- Incomplete ossification of the cuboidal bones is a common finding in premature and dysmature foals, and possibly in foals with hypothyroidism.
- Radiographs of the carpus and tarsus should be performed in any high-risk foal to obtain a diagnosis.
- Goals of treatment include limiting weight bearing and exercise.
- Complications including angular limb deformities, degenerative joint disease, and osteochondrosis dissecans may occur.
- Prognosis is guarded depending on the degree of incomplete ossification.

PREMATURITY AND DYSMATURITY OF THE FOAL

Gestational length of the horse is variable, ranging from 310 days to 370 days. Traditionally, the term *premature* is defined as a preterm birth of less than 320 days' gestation; however, given the inherent variability of gestational length, foals with signs of prematurity may be born following a gestational length of more than 320 days. Foals born postterm are considered *dysmature*. These foals have clinical characteristics of a premature foal despite a normal gestational length.[1]

The cause of prematurity and dysmaturity is typically unknown, although they may occur as a result of a high-risk pregnancy. Causes of high-risk pregnancy are included in **Box 1**. Multisystemic failure of the foal is possible, and thus a full physical examination of the foal is warranted. Common clinical signs of prematurity/dysmaturity are listed in **Box 2**. In particular, musculoskeletal problems are common. The most significant complications include incomplete ossification of the cuboidal bones, decreased muscle tone, and flexor tendon laxity.[1]

Disclosure: The authors do not have any conflicts of interest to disclose.
Department of Large Animal Clinical Sciences, Texas A&M University College of Veterinary Medicine & Biomedical Sciences, TAMU 4475, College Station, TX 77845, USA
* Corresponding author.
E-mail address: mcoleman@cvm.tamu.edu

Vet Clin Equine 33 (2017) 289–297
http://dx.doi.org/10.1016/j.cveq.2017.03.001
0749-0739/17/© 2017 Elsevier Inc. All rights reserved.

vetequine.theclinics.com

Box 1
Causes of high-risk pregnancy

Maternal Causes	Fetal Causes
History of previously abnormal foal	Twins
Systemic disease/endotoxemia	Fescue toxicosis
Malnutrition	Umbilical abnormalities
Uterine abnormality or torsion	Congenital abnormality
Placentitis	
Hydrops	
Pelvic anatomic abnormality	
Mare reproductive loss syndrome	
Hyperlipemia	
Hypogalactia	
Dystocia	

PATHOPHYSIOLOGY

The skeletal structures of the developing fetus are initially cartilaginous and then ossify as the fetus develops in utero. Ossification begins as gestation progresses, with ossification of the carpal and tarsal bones being among the last bones to ossify, typically beginning in the last 60 to 90 days of gestation. Most of this ossification occurs in the last several weeks of gestation and continues with in the first month postpartum.[2–4] Ossification of the carpus begins at approximately 254 days' gestation and initiates

---

Box 2
Clinical characteristics of premature/dysmature foals

General Characteristics

Low birth weight

Small frame

Silky hair coat

Domed forehead

Poor cartilage development of ears

Weak suckle

High chest wall compliance

Low lung compliance

Poor thermoregulation

Gastrointestinal tract dysfunction

Poor renal function

Entropion

Poor glucose regulation

Musculoskeletal Characteristics

Incomplete ossification of cuboidal bones

Flexor tendon laxity

Decreased muscle tone

at the accessory carpal bone,[3] and ossification of the tarsus begins at approximately 125 days' gestation with the calcaneus (**Box 3**).[5] Ossification of the cartilaginous templates of the cuboidal bones initiates at the center and gradually extends to the periphery by the process of endochondral ossification. In a normal foal, the ossification process is completed and extends to the periphery of the cartilaginous template by birth. In the premature or dysmature foal, however, ossification can be delayed, which is most notable at the periphery of these bones because this is the last area to become ossified.

The cartilaginous precursors to the epiphysis and cuboidal bones of the carpus and tarsus are pliable. Articular loading forces are unequally distributed and not perpendicular to the long axis and an increased load on the poorly ossified bones causes thinning of the precursor cartilage. In the carpus, the cartilage is compressed between the ulnar and fourth carpal bones and the intermediate and third carpal bones. In the tarsus, delayed ossification is most problematic in the sagittal plane. Loading forces are transmitted between the long axis of the tibia to the long axis of the third metatarsal bone through the central and third tarsal bones. Atrophy of the center of the third and central tarsal bones may occur, resulting in collapse of the tarsus.[6] Osteochondral fractures and subsequent osteoarthritis also may occur. This is most common in the tarsi, especially the dorsal aspect of the small tarsal bones, in which weight-bearing forces change direction from cranioproximal-caudaldistal to vertical.

HYPOTHYROIDISM AND CUBOIDAL OSSIFICATION

Congenital hypothyroidism in foals also has been indicated as a cause of developmental orthopedic abnormalities, including tendon contracture or rupture or delayed development of the small cuboidal bones of the carpus and tarsus. Thyroid hormones influence bone development by stimulation of the pituitary gland to produce growth hormone. Thyroid hormones also influence the cartilage production and degeneration and promote ossification.[7,8] Low circulating thyroid hormone may result in a compensatory increase in thyroid-stimulating hormone (TSH). Increased TSH causes hypertrophy and hyperplasia of thyroid follicular cells and eventual goiter or enlargement of the thyroid gland.

Two different syndromes have been described. Foals with congenital goiters have been described. This has been associated with ingesting either too much[9,10] or not enough[11,12] iodine or of goitrogenic plants by a mare resulting in hypothyroidism of the foal. These foals have visible goiters, and are typically born weak, with a poor suckle, delayed reflexes, and hypothermia. Foals have delayed ossification of the cuboidal bones, especially the third and central tarsal bones. Severely affected foals

Box 3		
Dates of appearance of the sites of ossification of the carpal and tarsal bones		
	Structure	Days of Gestation
Carpal bones	Accessory carpal bone	254
	Radial carpal bone	274
	Intermediate carpal bone	264–278
	Ulnar carpal bone	310
	Second, third, and fourth carpal bones	280–310
Tarsal bones	Calcaneus	125
	Tuberosity calcaneus	305
	Central, third, fourth, first, and second tarsal bones	280–325

may survive with thyroid supplementation, although appropriate dosing recommendations are limited.

A second syndrome of congenital hypothyroidism has been described in foals in the western United States and Canada.[2] The cause of this syndrome is unknown, although dietary deficiency or toxicity of the mare during gestation is suspected. Clinical findings besides the aforementioned musculoskeletal abnormalities include hyperplasia of the thyroid gland, prolonged gestational length, and mandibular prognathia. Other signs of prematurity also may be present, including silky haircoat and domed head. Baseline serum concentrations at birth are typically normal; however, TSH response is decreased. Consequently, thyroid hormone supplementation is not suggested, as hormone levels are normal at birth.

In one study, records of 2946 equine abortuses, stillborns, and dead neonatal foals in Western Canada were reviewed.[11] Abnormal thyroid glands were identified in 154 (5.2%) of the foals. Of those, 79 (2.7%) had concurrent musculoskeletal abnormalities. In this study, most (91%) of the thyroid glands were described as being normal in size or only slightly enlarged. For this reason, diagnosis of this condition may be challenging without histology of the thyroid gland.

Cuboidal ossification of surgically thyroidectomized foals has been evaluated.[2] Ossification was delayed, but to a lesser extent than in foals with congenital hyperplastic goiters. For this reason, the effects of prenatal hypothyroidism on the development of the carpus and tarsus is thought to be significant.

CLINICAL EVALUATION AND DIAGNOSIS

Foals should be born with adequate ossification of the carpal and tarsal bones following a normal gestation. Incomplete ossification of the cuboidal bones should be suspected and evaluated in any premature or dysmature foal. Clinical signs of incomplete ossification include uneven loading of the skeleton, resulting in an angular limb deformity: carpal valgus of the forelimbs or hyperextension of the tarsus. Signs of lameness may or may not be apparent; however, foals with affected tarsi may appear sickle-hocked and have a characteristic "bunny-hopping" gait. Joints are not swollen or warm and painful on palpation.

Diagnosis of incomplete ossification of the cuboidal bones can be confirmed radiographically. It is suggested that radiographs are taken on all high-risk foals shortly after birth. The radiographic views that are most informative for assessing ossification are the dorsopalmar and lateromedial views of the carpus and tarsus.[13] A grading system based on radiographic findings, known as the skeletal ossification index (SOI), was developed to classify foals with incomplete ossification of the tarsal/carpal bones (**Table 1**).[14] This index is based on lateral-medial view and dorsal-palmer or dorsal-plantar views of the carpus and tarsus taken within 2 weeks of birth. Examples of normal ossification (**Fig. 1**) and incomplete ossification (**Figs. 2** and **3**) are provided. A significant relationship between SOI and gestational age and body weight has been shown, with low SOI correlated with shorter gestational ages and/or low birth weights.

Sonographic evaluation of the small tarsal bones has been evaluated. In a study by Ruohoniemi,[3] radiographic and ultrasonographic findings of 10 foals were compared. Ultrasonographic findings suggested that sonographic evaluation reliably identified poorly ossified bones and might be a useful method for evaluation of the carpus and tarsus in high-risk foals. Ultrasonographic evaluation is typically performed with the foal in lateral recumbency with the limb held straight. A 7.5-MHz linear transducer is placed longitudinally on the dorsomedial aspect of the tarsus. Using this technique,

Table 1
Skeletal ossification index for neonatal foals

Grade	Description
Grade 1	• Some cuboidal bones of the carpus and tarsus have no radiographic evidence of ossification
Grade 2	• All cuboidal bones of the carpus and tarsus have radiographic evidence of ossification • First carpal bone not included • First tarsal bone not included • Proximal epiphysis of either third metacarpal or metatarsal bones present and physis is open • Lateral styloid process of distal radius absent or barely visible • Malleoli of tibia absent or barely visible
Grade 3	• All cuboidal bones of carpus and tarsus ossified, but small and with rounded edges • Joint spaces are wide • Proximal physis of either third metacarpal or metatarsal are closed • Lateral styloid process of the distal radius and malleoli of the tibia distinct
Grade 4	• All cuboidal bones shaped like bones of mature horse • Joint spaces are of expected width

the surface of the central tarsal bone, the third tarsal bone, and the proximal third metatarsal bone can be evaluated.

In a foal with an enlarged thyroid gland, hormone assays should be performed. In normal neonatal foals, thyroid hormone levels are high at birth and rapidly decline over the first few months. Plasma thyroid levels are often normal when developmental lesions associated with hypothyroidism are observed.

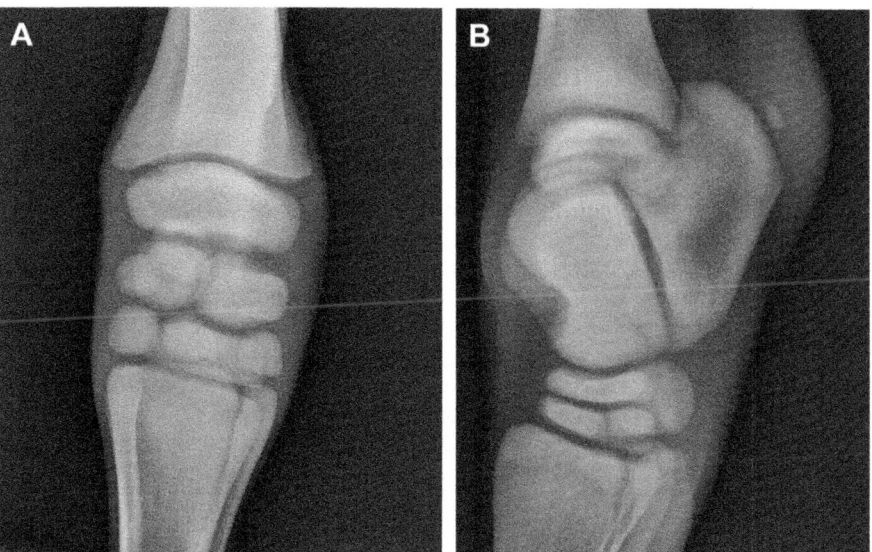

Fig. 1. (*A*) Dorsopalmar view of the left carpus of a 1-day-old Dutch warmblood colt born at 330 days' gestation. No evidence of incomplete ossification. (*B*) Lateromedial view of the left tarsus of a 1-day-old Dutch warmblood colt born at 330 days' gestation. No evidence of incomplete ossification.

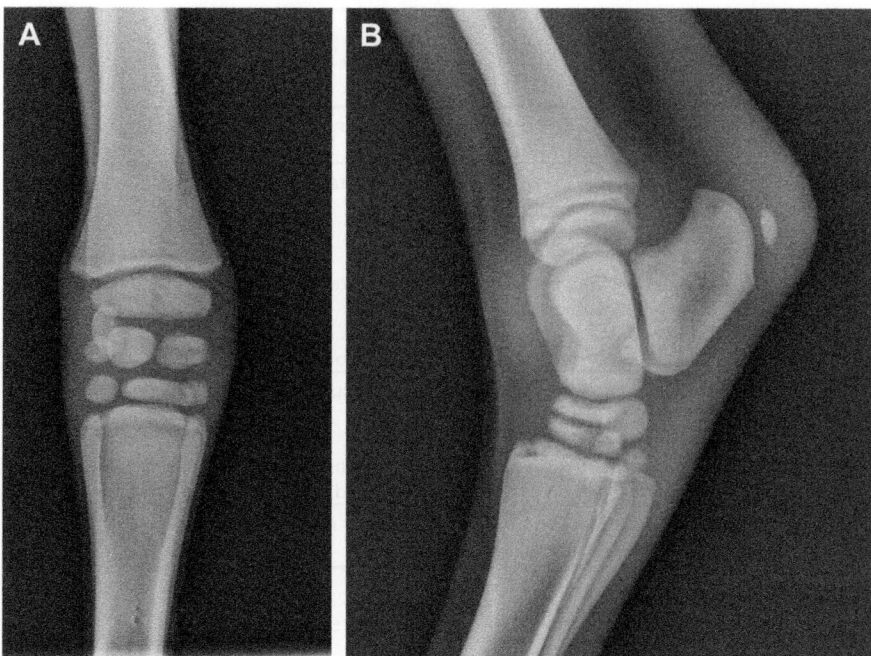

Fig. 2. (*A*) Dorsopalmar projection of the right carpus of a 5-hour-old quarter horse filly born at 300 days' gestation. Severe incomplete ossification of cuboidal bones, consistent with prematurity. A portion of the cuboidal bones of the carpus are mineralized, but remain small, rounded, and irregular. A portion of the proximal epiphysis of the third metacarpal bone is mineralized. (*B*) Lateromedial projection of the left tarsus of a 5-hour-old quarter horse filly born at 300 days' gestation. The cuboidal bones of the tarsus are severely hypoplastic. Within the tarsi, only a small portion of the third tarsal bone is mineralized. The remainder of the tarsal cuboidal bones and the proximal epiphysis of the third metatarsal bone is completely nonmineralized.

SEQUELAE TO INCOMPLETE OSSIFICATION

Incomplete ossification of the cuboidal bones may predispose the foal to angular limb deformities (ADL), degenerative joint disease, or osteochondrosis dissecans (OCD), all of which can have a negative impact on athletic performance and even quality of life, depending on severity.[2] Deformation of the cartilaginous cuboidal precursors from weight bearing and exercise and subsequent ossification of deformed cartilage results in ALD.[15] In the carpus, the third, fourth, and ulnar bones are the last to ossify. Deformation of these structures in the carpus results in carpal valgus. In the tarsus, the central and third tarsal bones are last to ossify, resulting in tarsal valgus and/or tarsal flexural deformities of the pelvic limbs. OCD of the cuboidal bones may occur as a result of shear stress on the cuboidal structures, creating separation of the cartilaginous and ossified portions of each bone.[2]

TREATMENT

Treatment of incomplete ossification of the cuboidal bones should be aimed at maintaining the longitudinal axis, allowing ossification to occur without further distortion of the cartilage. Conservative treatment includes stall confinement, limited weight

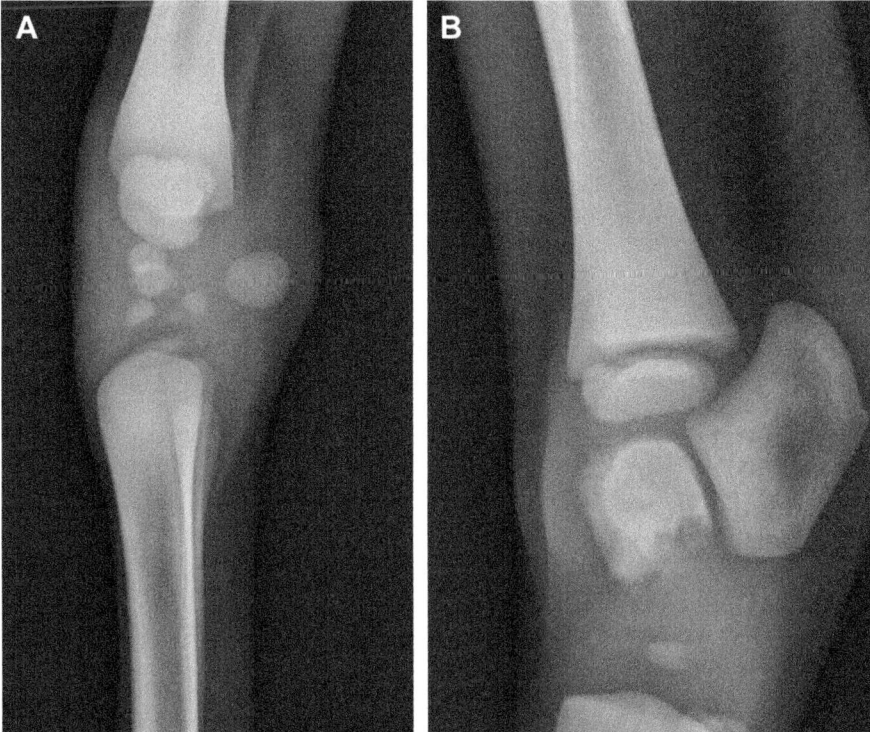

Fig. 3. (*A*) Lateromedial projection of the right carpus of a 2-day-old quarter horse colt born at 315 days' gestation. Partial ossification of the cuboidal bones of the carpus is observed. The cuboidal bones are small and round. The proximal physis of the third metatarsal bones is open. This is an SOI of grade 2. (*B*) Lateromedial projection of the left tarsus of a 2-day-old quarter horse colt born at 315 days' gestation. Partial ossification of the cuboidal bones of the tarsus is observed. The cuboidal bones are small and round. This is an SOI of grade 2.

bearing, and restriction of activity. Gradual increases in weight bearing and exercise may be introduced based on radiographic improvement. Alignment of the longitudinal axis can be maintained with splints or tube casts to support the limbs and reduce the compressive forces acting on the dorsal aspect of the limb.[15] If untreated, collapse of the cartilage template of the cuboidal bones may result in irreversible fusion of the small tarsal bones into a single irregularly shaped bone. Supportive care is important to prevent secondary complications, such as decubital ulcers and cast sores. Management of foals with ALD, OCD, or degenerative joint disease is discussed in other sections of this text.

EVALUATION OF OUTCOME AND LONG-TERM RECOMMENDATIONS

Follow-up radiographs should be performed at 2-week intervals until ossification is complete. Prognosis of foals with incomplete ossification is variable based on the degree of ossification and secondary complications. A guarded prognosis for a high-performance athlete should be given to any foal with incomplete ossification. Prognosis also depends on the presence of concurrent OCD or osteoarthritis. It has been suggested that foals may become clinically sound if fusion of the tarsal bones occurs, despite the development of osteoarthritis.[6]

A retrospective study of 22 foals with incomplete ossification of the tarsal bones was performed in foals ranging from 1 day to 10 months of age. In this study, radiographic lesions of the tarsal bones were classified into type I (incomplete ossification with <30% collapse of the affected bones) and type II (incomplete ossification with >30% collapse and pinching or fragmentation of the affected bones). Severity of radiographic lesions was associated with outcome. In total, 5 of 20 foals with incomplete ossification of the tarsal bones achieved athletic soundness. Only 3 of the 16 foals with a type II performed as intended, and 4 of the 6 foals with a type I lesion performed as intended.[16]

SUMMARY

Incomplete ossification of the cuboidal bones is a common finding in premature and dysmature foals, and possibly in foals with hypothyroidism. Radiographs of the carpus and tarsus should be performed in any high-risk foal to obtain a diagnosis. Goals of treatment include limiting weight bearing and exercise. The prognosis is guarded depending on the degree of incomplete ossification and secondary complications.

REFERENCES

1. Knottenbelt DC, Holdstock N, Madigan JE. Perinatal review. In: Equine neonatology medicine and surgery. 1st edition. London: Saunders; 2004. p. 1–27.
2. McLaughlin BG, Doige CE. A study of ossification of carpal and tarsal bones in normal and hypothyroid foals. Can Vet J 1982;23(5):164–8.
3. Ruohoniemi M. Use of ultrasonography to evaluate the degree of ossification of the small tarsal bones in 10 foals. Equine Vet J 1993;25(6):539–43.
4. McLaughlin BG, Doige CE, Fretz PB, et al. Carpal bone lesions associated with angular limb deformities in foals. J Am Vet Med Assoc 1981;178(3):224–30.
5. Soana S, Gnudi G, Bertoni G, et al. Anatomo-radiographic study on the osteogenesis of carpal and tarsal bones in horse fetus. Anat Histol Embryol 1998;27(5): 301–5.
6. McIlwraith MC. Incomplete ossification of carpal and tarsal bones in foals. Eq Vet Educ 2003;15:79–81.
7. Vivrette SL, Reimers TJ, Krook L. Skeletal disease in a hypothyroid foal. Cornell Vet 1984;74(4):373–86.
8. Saunders HM, Jezyk PK. The radiographic appearance of canine congenital hypothyroidism: skeletal changes with delayed treatment. Vet Rad 1991;32(4): 171–7.
9. Drew B, Barber WP, Williams DG. The effect of excess dietary iodine on pregnant mares and foals. Vet Rec 1975;97(5):93–5.
10. Eroksuz H, Eroksuz Y, Ozer H, et al. Equine goiter associated with excess dietary iodine. Vet Hum Toxicol 2004;46(3):147–9.
11. Allen AL, Doige CE, Fretz PB, et al. Hyperplasia of the thyroid gland and concurrent musculoskeletal deformities in western Canadian foals: reexamination of a previously described syndrome. Can Vet J 1994;35(1):31–8.
12. Baker JR, Wyn-Jones G, Eley JL. Case of equine goitre. Vet Rec 1983;112(17): 407–8.
13. Sedrish SA, Moore RM. Diagnosis and management of incomplete ossification of the cuboidal bones in foals. Equine Pract 1997;19:16–21.
14. Adams R, Poulos P. A skeletal ossification index for neonatal foals. Vet Rad 1988; 29(5):217–22.

15. Bramlage LR, Auer JA. Diagnosis, assessment and treatment strategies for angular limb deformities in the foal. Clin Tech Eq Pract 2006;5:259–69.
16. Dutton DM, Watkins JP, Walker MA, et al. Incomplete ossification of the tarsal bones in foals: 22 cases (1988-1996). J Am Vet Med Assoc 1998;213(11):1590–4.

Septic Arthritis, Physitis, and Osteomyelitis in Foals

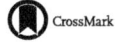

Kati Glass, DVM, Ashlee E. Watts, DVM, PhD*

KEYWORDS

- Septic synovitis • Arthritis • Physitis • Osteomyelitis • Foal

KEY POINTS

- Several features of musculoskeletal infections in the foal are different from the adult horse and the differences present diagnostic challenges and opportunities.
- Despite differences in etiology and diagnostics, the mainstay of therapy in the foal is similar to the adult: local lavage and/or debridement and local antimicrobial therapy.
- When there is physeal or bony involvement, more aggressive therapy and use of longer-term local antimicrobial therapy is indicated.
- When musculoskeletal infection is the primary problem, the prognosis appears to be fair to good for survival of synovial, bony, and physeal infections with appropriate and aggressive local therapy.
- Prognosticating future athleticism is difficult given current literature but most certainly varies with the disease state, comorbidities, and involvement of articular structures as well as the intended athletic use.

 Video content accompanies this article at http://www.vetequine.theclinics. com.

INTRODUCTION

Unlike the adult horse, infection of musculoskeletal structures in foals is most commonly hematogenous in origin. Failure of passive transfer, or respiratory, umbilical, or gastrointestinal infection are often concurrent or historical problems. These problems lead to hematogenous inoculation of the synovial membrane (type S infection), epiphyseal subchondral bone (type E infection), or metaphyseal side of the physis (type P infection). In the premature or dysmature foal, infection of the cuboidal bones of the carpus or tarsus (type T infection) also can occur. Bacterial

Disclosures: The authors have no commercial or financial disclosures related to this article.
Department of Large Animal Clinical Sciences, College of Veterinary Medicine & Biomedical Sciences, Texas A&M University, 4475 TAMU, College Station, TX 77843-4475, USA
* Corresponding author.
E-mail address: awatts@cvm.tamu.edu

vetequine.theclinics.com

isolates are commonly Enterobacteriaceae (especially *Escherichia coli*), *Salmonella*, *Actinobacillus equuli*, *Klebsiella* spp, *Staphylococcus*, *Streptococcus*, and *Rhodococcus equi*.

There are 2 separate groups of foals with musculoskeletal sepsis: the young foal (<3 weeks of age) with infection likely in multiple musculoskeletal sites, and the older foal (>3 weeks of age) with only 1 joint or physis affected. The younger group typically is affected by primary infections of the synovium or epiphyseal bone and the older group typically is affected by primary infections of the metaphyseal side of the physis.[1] This is because transphyseal vessels remain patent until 7 to 10 days of age, at which point slowed blood flow leads to enhanced bacterial adhesion and invasion of adjacent structures.[1] Extension of the infection from the primary site to the adjacent structures will occur when untreated. Clinical signs include lameness, synovial effusion, localized cellulitis, heat, and sensitivity to palpation. Unlike adult horses, fever is relatively common in the foal with a septic musculoskeletal structure.

DIAGNOSIS
Septic Synovitis/Arthritis

Clinical signs of septic arthritis can include effusion, peri-capsular swelling, lameness, heat over the joint, and pain on palpation of the affected joint. However, it is important to note that some foals show minimal to no lameness despite marked synovial sepsis or osteomyelitis (**Fig. 1**).

Like in the adult horse, clinical diagnosis of synovial sepsis is made by synovial fluid analysis. Synovial fluid from an infected joint will be serosanguinous, slightly cloudy to opaque, and will have decreased viscosity. Total nucleated cell counts of greater than 10,000 to 30,000 cells/μL, percentage of neutrophils of greater than 90%, and total protein of greater than 4 g/dL are strongly suggestive of joint sepsis. Neutrophils are usually nondegenerate and bacteria are not always seen despite confirmed sepsis. When there is a synovial effusion and signs of joint sepsis, but the neutrophils are 30% to 80%, one should suspect the effusion is sympathetic and there may be adjacent septic physitis or osteomyelitis or systemic inflammation leading to immune-mediated polysynovitis[2] (**Fig. 2**). Other synovial parameters also have been investigated to identify synovial sepsis, such as synovial lactate, glucose, and pH.[3] It appears that synovial lactate may be useful, but cutoff values have yet to be established.

Whenever synovial infection is suspected in the foal, a sample of synovial fluid for aerobic and anaerobic culture also should be collected. Ideally, the synovial fluid should be placed in a blood culture bottle. If there is a possibility of recent antimicrobial administration to the foal, the blood culture bottle should contain antimicrobial binding resins that will increase the chance of a positive culture, if bacteria are present. A multicenter retrospective study revealed growth from 85.7% of 70 antemortem synovial fluid samples from foals with septic arthritis that underwent bacterial culture.[4] Of the 72 bacterial isolates that were identified, 62.5% were gram negative and 37.5% were gram positive.[4] The addition of synovial biopsy for culture has failed to increase the expected yield of approximately 50% positive culture result from synovial fluid sample culture alone.[5] Additionally, blood culture should be performed, especially in the neonatal foal.

A complete radiographic examination is especially important in the foal with septic arthritis compared with the adult because of increased likelihood of adjacent bone involvement. This is also true when evaluating a foal with a septic digital flexor tendon sheath, as the proximal sesamoid bones may be affected. Although radiographic

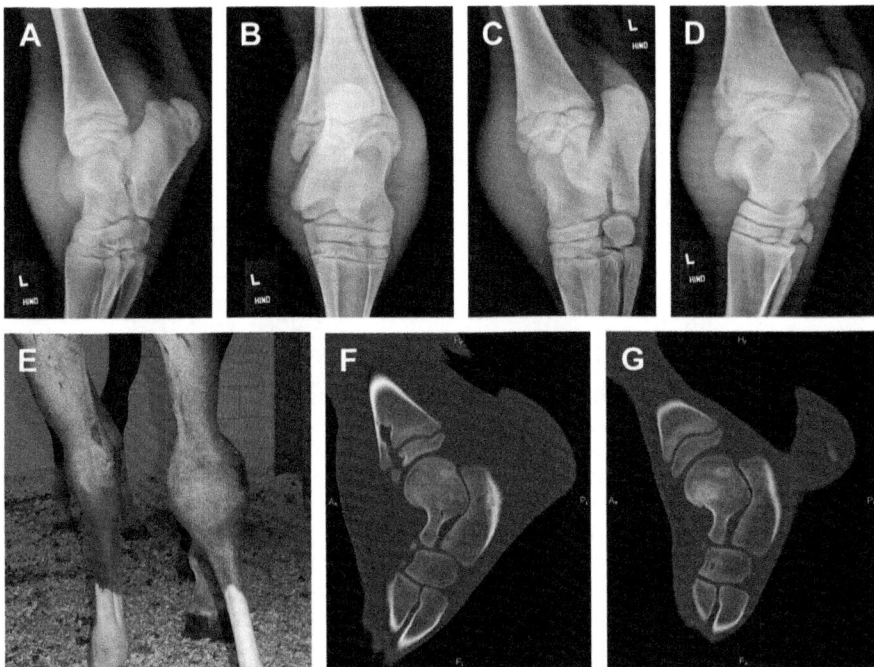

Fig. 1. Images from a 2-month-old Arabian colt that presented for 1 week of swelling of the left hock. No medications had been administered before presentation. (*A–D*) Radiographs revealed osteolysis of the distal medial tibial physis, metaphysis, and epiphysis (*E* and Video 1). There was no lameness and the physical examination was unremarkable other than marked left tarsocrural effusion, alopecia over the joint prominences, and heat over the joint. (*F*) Examination by CT confirmed osteolysis of the distal medial tibial physis, metaphysis, and epiphysis that communicated with the tarsocrural joint. (*G*) The normal right limb is provided for comparison. Cytologic analysis of synovial fluid confirmed septic arthritis (total nucleated cell count [TNCC] 40,270 cells/μL, total protein [TP] 4.1 g/dL, and 96% nondegenerate neutrophils). The colt was discharged to be euthanized at home due to the cost of therapy.

examination is easily performed and readily available in most practices, it is well established that radiographs may require 21 days before providing diagnostic images in most cases due to the lag between infection and osseous changes.[6] When the radiographic examination is unclear, but bone involvement is suspected, additional imaging modalities should be recommended.

Advanced diagnostic imaging modalities that have been useful in identification of septic osteomyelitis include computed tomography (CT), MRI, and less commonly nuclear scintigraphy. Cross-sectional imaging (CT or MRI) is particularly useful in the proximal limb where overlying soft tissues and incomplete ossification of subchondral bone limit complete evaluation of the joint surfaces, subchondral bone, and physes (**Fig. 3**). In our practice, CT is preferred to MRI because of the speed with which the foal can be imaged, reducing time under general anesthesia, the larger gantry allowing the entire body of larger foals to be imaged, and the superior contrast resolution for imaging bone.

Nuclear scintigraphy has been used to identify lesions in uncommon locations when CT was not available; however, the increased radiopharmaceutical uptake in the

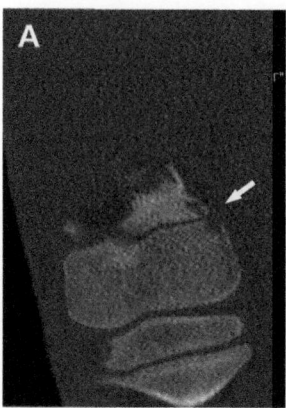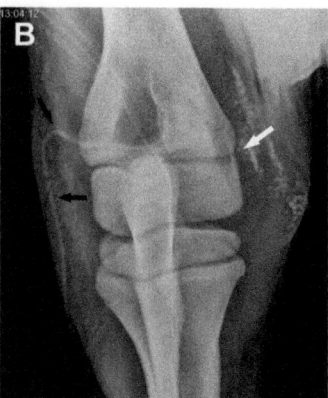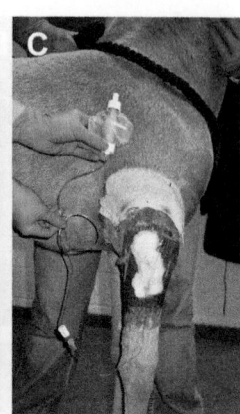

Fig. 2. Images from a 4-week-old quarter horse filly with septic osteomyelitis of the epiphyseal, physial, and metaphyseal bone of the right distal humerus. She was presented for moderate lameness of 3 days' duration, approximately 10 days after there was fever and diarrhea that resolved without treatment. The day of presentation there was no fever; however, flunixin had been administered by the owner. There was mild thickening of the soft tissues of the medial elbow and possible pain on palpation of the region. (*A*) CT examination of the elbow revealed osteolysis of the epiphyseal, physial, and metaphyseal bone of the right distal medial humerus (*white arrow*). Synovial fluid of the right elbow joint revealed what was considered sympathetic inflammation with a nucleated cell count of 3239 cells/μL and 45% neutrophils. The day of presentation bone biopsies were collected for microbial isolation, which were negative. (*B*) Postoperative radiograph reveals the radiopaque amikacin impregnated PMMA beads that were placed in the soft tissues adjacent to the bony lesion and the intra-articular pump (*black arrows*) that was placed in the elbow joint for the infusion of amikacin. The filly also was administered systemic ceftiofur. (*C*) An adhesive bandage was placed over the intra-articular catheter insertion site. A soft padded cotton bandage was placed over this for securing the pump reservoir. Microbiologic testing of the manure was positive for *Salmonella* and the filly was subsequently housed in the isolation unit. The lameness was nearly resolved 3 days after presentation, the pump was removed 5 days after presentation, and the filly was switched to oral chloramphenicol after 10 days of therapy for a further 4 weeks. The filly did not return to our hospital but the owner did with other horses throughout the remainder of the breeding season and he reported that the filly did well and did not develop additional lameness, limb deformity, or other complications.

active physes of young foals may result in confusion in cases of suspected septic physitis and is therefore rarely used.[6]

Ultrasound is a readily available modality that can provide additional information regarding peri-articular involvement of soft tissue and the presence and ultrasonographic character of joint effusion. The clinician should be aware of its limited ability to provide information regarding the amount of bone or cartilage involvement.[6]

Septic Physitis/Osteomyelitis

In foals with septic physitis or osteomyelitis, adjacent joints should be assessed by cytologic examination of collected synovial fluid. Some physeal infections nearly always involve the adjacent joint (distal femur, proximal humerus) and others involve only the adjacent joint when disease is very severe (distal radius). Joint involvement depends on the intra-articular or extra-articular location of the osteomyelitis and the severity of disease.

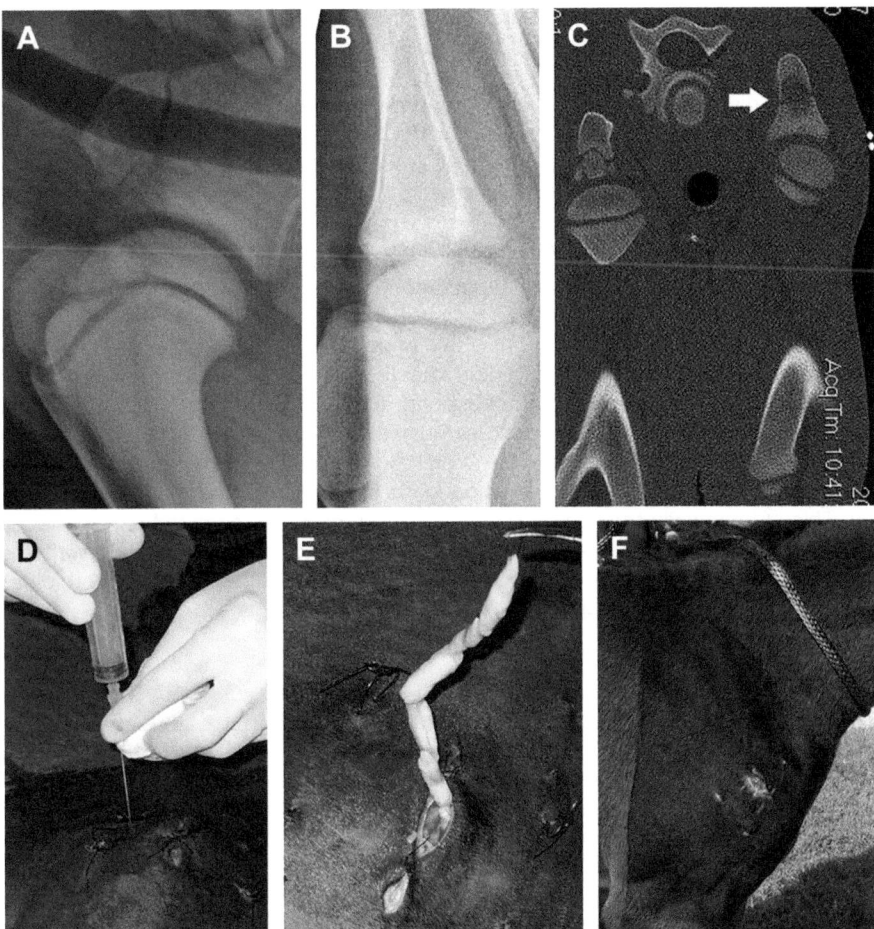

Fig. 3. Images from a 3-week-old Arabian filly with septic osteomyelitis of the supraglenoid tubercle physis that was presented for 2 days of very mild lameness. As a neonate, she had failure of passive transfer (immunoglobulin G was <400) and watery diarrhea that lasted 5 days. At presentation, there was a mild fever (102.1°F), a mild right forelimb lameness, no signs to allow localization of the cause of lameness, and mild pneumonia. Diagnostic anesthesia of the distal limb did not change the lameness. Radiographs of the proximal limb were unremarkable. Five days after presentation, the lameness became more severe and there was possible pain on palpation of the right shoulder joint, but no other abnormalities. (*A*, *B*) Repeated radiographs of the right shoulder were unremarkable. (*C*) CT of the right shoulder revealed supraglenoid tubercle physitis (*arrow*). The synovial cytology was consistent with sympathetic inflammation (TNCC of 3600 cells/μL, TP of 4.4 g/dL, and 37% neutrophils). Aspiration of physeal exudate and bone biopsies resulted in isolation of *Streptococcus equi* ssp *zooepidemicus*. Antibiotic-impregnated PMMA beads-on-a-string were placed. (*D*) The surgical wound to access the bone was partially closed to allow continued wound drainage. Daily intra-articular injection of antibiotic was performed. (*E*) The bead configuration was elected to facilitate complete bead removal after resolution of physitis. (*F*) Day of hospital discharge, 6 weeks after presentation: the filly was no longer on medications and there was no lameness. Two years later, the filly entered a training program and was sound without long-term complications.

As in cases of septic arthritis, aspirates of physeal exudate, physeal biopsies, or bone biopsies should be submitted for aerobic and anaerobic bacterial culture and sensitivity testing.

Similar to discussed previously, radiographic examination should be performed but often underestimates the presence and/or the severity of disease. CT provides the most sensitive evaluation when bony or physeal involvement is suspected, and is therefore recommended in almost all cases in our practice.

General Musculoskeletal Infection Diagnostics

In foals with identified or suspected septic arthritis, physitis, or osteomyelitis, the systemic condition of the foal also should be carefully investigated to identify any comorbidities. This is of paramount importance with ongoing evidence of failure of passive transfer, respiratory, umbilical, or gastrointestinal infection. Additional diagnostics that should be considered include ultrasound examination of the thorax, abdomen, and umbilical structures; radiographic examination of the thorax; fecal culture; and/or polymerase chain reaction. The foal should be continually monitored for the development of additional sites (newly affected joints or physes) during the course of therapy. This is especially true if the primary cause is ongoing (neonatal sepsis, septic omphalophlebitis, gastroenteritis, pneumonia) and should be discussed with the owner as a potential complication. Failure to identify and treat existing comorbidities negatively influences the prognosis.

THERAPY
Synovitis/Arthritis

Synovial infections in foals are always an emergency. The mainstay of treatment is local lavage and antimicrobial therapy. Antibiotics should be broad spectrum except in the rare case that the bacterial isolates and their sensitivities have already been identified. In the simple, acute septic joint without bony or physeal involvement, needle lavage(s) may be all that is required. When bony abnormalities are present, the condition is chronic, or is nonresponsive to needle lavage, arthroscopic lavage should be performed. Intra-articular bony lesions should be judiciously debrided, arthroscopically. When large amounts of fibrin and debris are present, the joint should be lavaged arthroscopically to allow thorough removal of all debris. In severe and/or chronic cases, arthrotomies are sometimes used as a salvage procedure. When there is adjacent physeal involvement, the duration of therapy is likely to be prolonged, and physeal debridement may be required.

Local antimicrobials can be applied in many ways. The simplest form of local antimicrobial therapy is by direct intra-articular injection of antibiotic. A single intra-articular injection of an antibiotic will result in synovial antibiotic concentrations above minimum inhibitory concentration (MIC) for at least 24 hours.[7,8] This is almost always performed at the completion of synovial lavage or after collection of synovial fluid. In some cases, daily direct synovial injection after collection of fluid for cytology to monitor progress may be all that is required. In complicated, severe, or chronic synovial sepsis, other routes of local antimicrobials are often used.

Local antimicrobial therapies, such as antimicrobial-containing beads made of bone cement (polymethyl methacrylate [PMMA]) or plaster of paris (POP) (**Fig. 4**), have been around for several decades. Although the technology has been available for quite some time, this is an often underused technique. Ten percent to 20% antibiotic (2–4 g antibiotic to 1 packet or 20 g bone cement) is added to the polymer (powder) and mixed thoroughly. The monomer (liquid) is added and mixed until the cement is

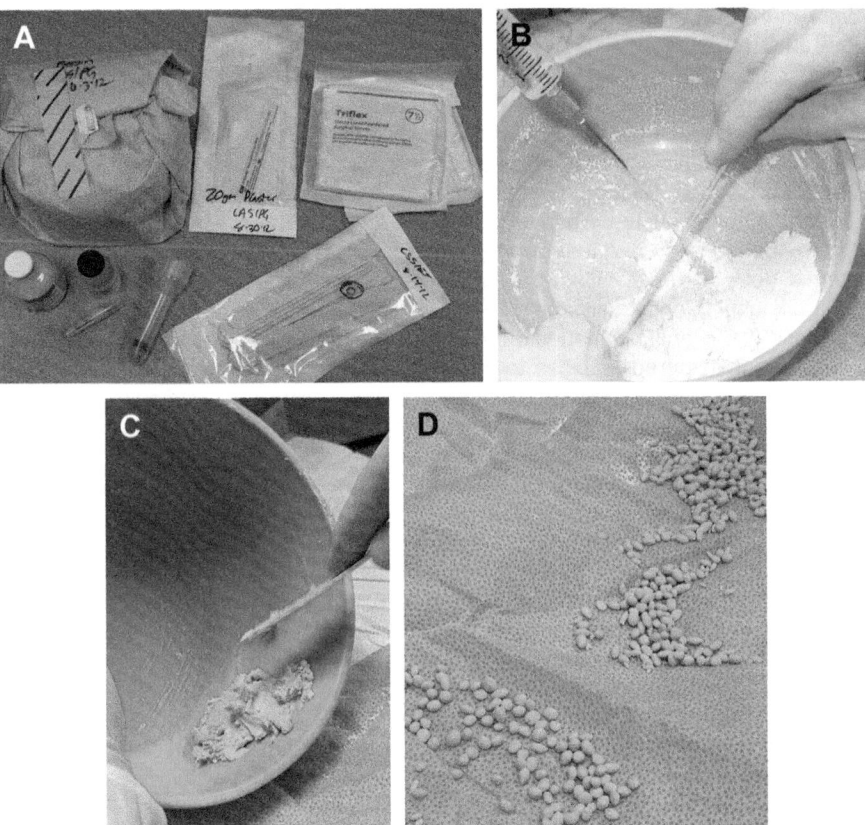

Fig. 4. (A) Supplies needed to make POP beads for local antimicrobial administration: bowl, POP (20 g), gloves, tongue depressor, antibiotic (2–4 g), and ~5 mL water. Beads should be made aseptically. If POP beads should require resterilization, a method other than steam sterilization should be used. (B) Antibiotic powder can be added to POP powder followed by addition of water or added to POP after being reconstituted in ~5 mL water and (C) mixed thoroughly. (D) Beads are made by rolling the material in the hand or against the table and will be adequately set-up for use approximately 20 to 120 minutes later dependent on ambient temperature and humidity. Bead molds also can be used.

the consistency of cake frosting, allowing it to be molded into beads or cylinders. The greater the surface area of each bead or cylinder (small beads and narrow cylinders) the greater the elution of antibiotic. Bead production can be performed aseptically immediately before implantation, or beads can be gas or steam sterilized (provided a heat-stabile antibiotic is used, such as an aminoglycoside) for later use. POP beads should not be steam sterilized.

A major drawback of bone cement beads is their permanence and need for surgical removal after resolution of infection. POP beads can be used as a bioabsorbable antibiotic depot for bone or subcutaneous implantation; however, not within the synovial environment, as they will very rapidly dissolve. Antimicrobial collagen sponges are a novel bioabsorbable local implant that obviates the need for surgical removal from within the synovial environment. Synovial implantation of gentamicin sponges results in very high gentamicin concentrations within the tarsocrural joint, but will remain above MIC for only 48 hours.[9] Because of this short duration, collagen sponges have not gained widespread favor. Hopefully the future will bring a bioabsorbable antimicrobial depot that does not induce inflammation within the joint and elutes antibiotic concentrations above MIC for 7 to 10 days.

Other local antimicrobial therapies, such as regional limb perfusion via intravenous (IV) or intraosseous injection, have been around for a couple of decades. The most important thing to consider when using regional limb perfusion in the foal as compared with the adult is to ensure that appropriate doses are used and subtracted from the systemic dose of drugs within the same class. For instance, if a foal is receiving 1.4 g amikacin, IV, once daily, the regional limb perfusion dose of one-third of the total body dose (0.5 g amikacin) should be subtracted from the systemic dose, and both should be administered as close to the same time as possible to avoid inadvertent overdosing. The clinician also should remember that antimicrobial synovial concentrations after regional limb perfusions are extremely variable. Intra-articular injection or constant-rate infusions are able to achieve higher antimicrobial concentrations much more reliably within the joint.

More recently, intrathecal catheters and constant-rate infusion pumps have been used for synovial, bone, and physeal infection in the foal (**Fig. 5**).[10–12] High synovial concentrations lead to very high bone and adjacent physeal antimicrobial concentrations. A kit is available from Mila International (Florence, KY, USA) that has a thick-walled intrasynovial catheter, flow control tubing, and an elastomeric pump. The thick wall and small diameter of the intrasynovial catheter prevent kinking. The catheter is usually placed arthroscopically, but can be placed without arthroscopic visualization. The elastomeric pump is 4 walled and the recoil from the balloon forces fluid from the pump. The flow control tubing allows the pump to deliver up to 0.8 mL/h, although when in a closed joint, the flow is often much slower due to the positive pressure within the joint.

In our hospital in a closed joint, we usually expect approximately 6 to 8 mL dispensed per 24 hours, although increased external pressure on the pump (ie, the foal laying down on the pump) can cause greater than the allotted 20 mL in 24 hours. This should be kept in mind, especially when using aminoglycosides or other potentially toxic antimicrobials in the small foal. To monitor the volume that has been dispensed, we weigh the pump at least daily (1 g is approximately 1 mL). The maximum volume that can be added to the balloon reservoir is 100 mL. Most often before microbial identification, we use an aminoglycoside within the pump and dilute it 1:1 or 1:2 with balanced polyionic solution. The use of lactated Ringers solution will result in elevated synovial lactate concentrations and should be avoided when using synovial lactate to monitor sepsis. When bacterial isolates are not sensitive to aminoglycosides, we have used other medications as directed by the sensitivity profile. It is important to keep in mind the duration of activity of many medications once reconstituted and maintained at room temperature. When the duration is only 24 hours, as in ceftazidime and other third-generation cephalosporins, we simply empty and refill the reservoir with a days' dose of freshly reconstituted drug, every 24 hours.

The use of local antimicrobial therapy does not negate the need for systemic antibiotics, joint lavage, and arthroscopic surgery when indicated, but it has been a very useful adjunct for synovial sepsis, osteomyelitis, and physitis. The intrasynovial pump has been especially helpful in proximal limb disease (elbow, shoulder, stifle, and hip) in which other local therapies, like regional limb perfusion, cannot be performed (**Fig. 6**). It should be maintained securely attached to the patient. The insertion site of the tubing should be maintained under a sterile bandage, and it should be monitored daily for dispensing volume, signs of leakage, or displacement.

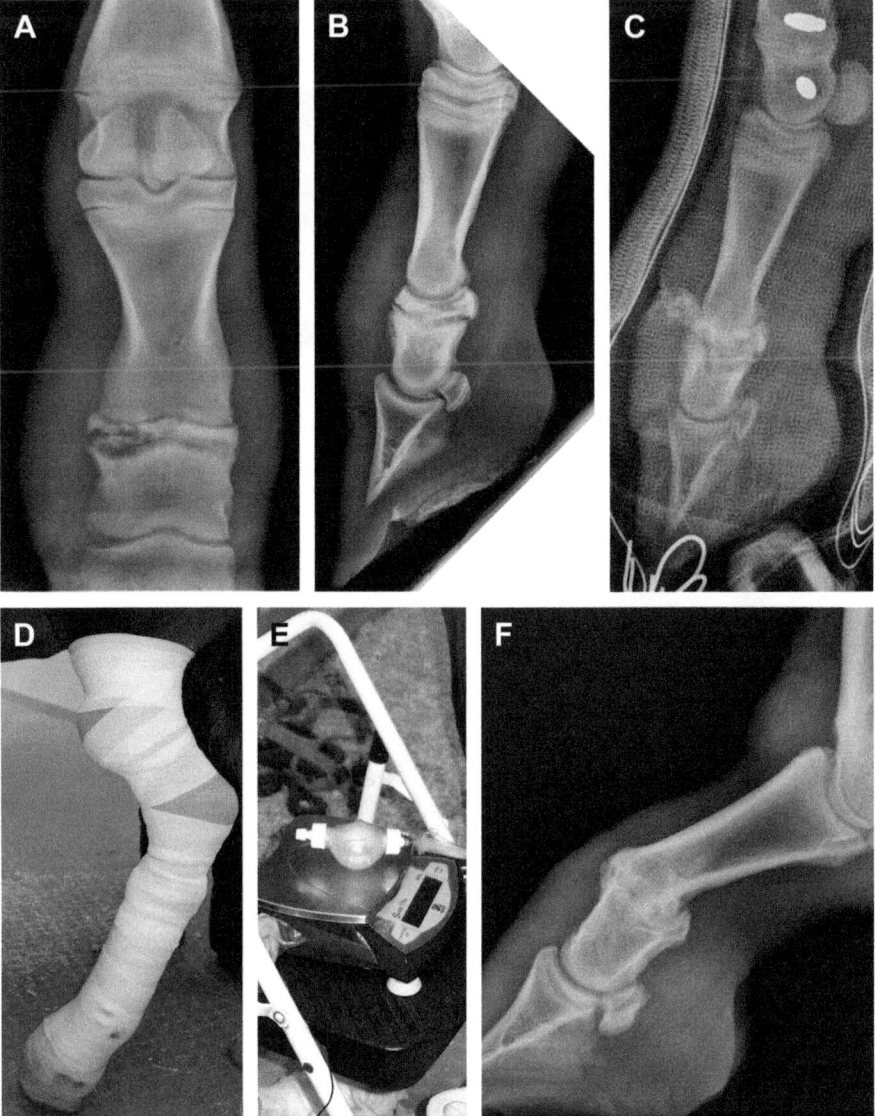

Fig. 5. Images from a 3.5-month old Arabian filly that was presented for fever and severe lameness presumed to be due to trauma of 2 weeks' duration. (*A, B*) Septic osteomyelitis of the proximal phalanx and septic arthritis of the pastern joint were diagnosed. She had been treated for pneumonia for 6 weeks before presentation. (*C*) The articular cartilage and abnormal subchondral and epiphyseal bone of the middle phalanx were debrided, an intra-articular catheter was placed in the pastern joint, cancellous bone graft and antibiotic-impregnated (gentamicin) POP beads were placed in the joint, and a pin cast was placed. The surgical wound was not closed to allow continued drainage. (*D*) The pump reservoir was contained within a bandage over the dorsal mid-tibia to prevent the foal from laying on the pump. (*E*) The pump was weighed daily to assess volume of administration in the previous 24 hours. *Streptococcus equi* ssp *zooepidemicus* sensitive to the antimicrobials with which she had been treated (amikacin, gentamicin and chloramphenicol) was isolated. Three weeks after presentation, the pump was removed after the surgical wound was fully granulated and soft tissue swelling around the pastern was resolved. Six weeks after presentation, oral antibiotics were discontinued. (*F*) Six-month recheck radiograph. There is bony fusion of the pastern joint in a dorsiflexed position and hyperextension of the fetlock joint. The filly was sound at a walk and there was mild lameness at a trot.

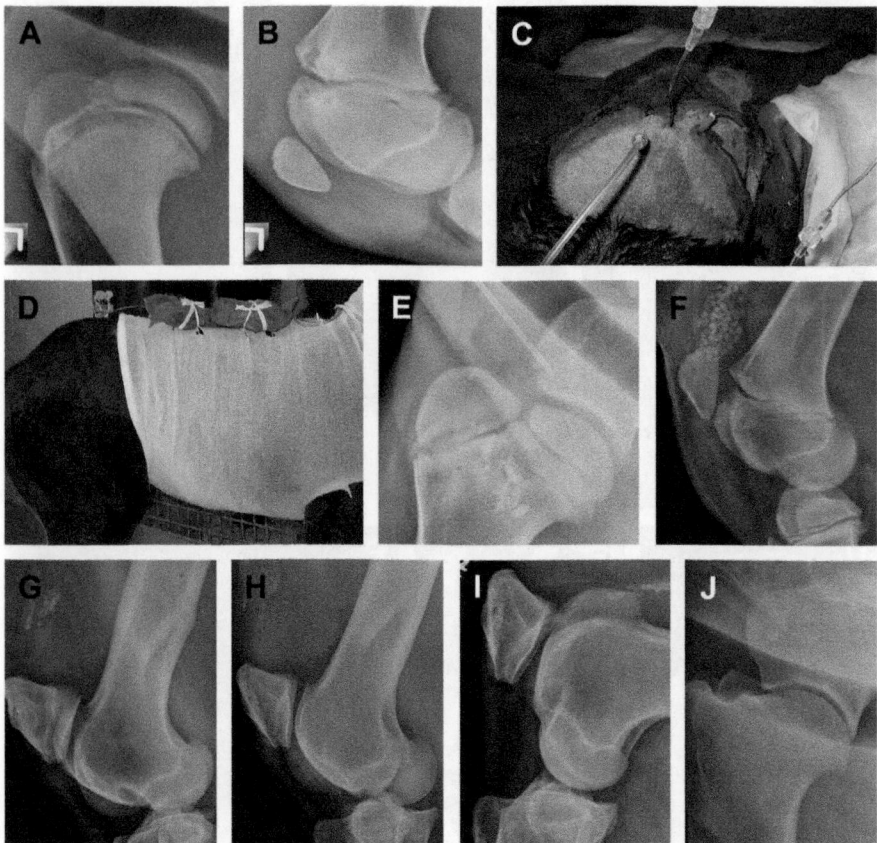

Fig. 6. Images from a 3-week-old quarter horse filly that was presented for fever and mild lameness of 3 days' duration. She had a history of failure of passive transfer and diarrhea. Septic arthritis of the shoulder joint with (A) septic osteomyelitis of the metaphysis and septic arthritis of the femoropatellar joint with (B) septic osteomyelitis of the metaphysis and epiphysis as well as septic omphalophlebitis were diagnosed. Omphalophlebectomy, joint lavage, collection of bone samples for culture, placement of intra-articular catheters, and placement PMMA beads in adjacent soft tissues was performed. Microbiologic testing of all samples resulted in no growth. (C) Daily needle lavage of the shoulder and stifle joints was performed until clinical signs of joint sepsis were resolved (1 week for the shoulder and 2.5 weeks for the stifle). (D) Intra-articular antibiotic administration via constant-rate infusion pumps that were secured to a "t-shirt" was continued for 2 to 4 days beyond discontinuation of daily lavage. Three weeks after presentation, daily lavage of the stifle was resumed and soft tissue PMMA beads adjacent to the stifle were replaced with beads containing a different antibiotic (ceftiofur) due to recurrence of lameness and neutrophilic synovitis of the left stifle. Three days later, daily lavage was discontinued. (E, F) Radiographs 6 weeks after presentation before hospital discharge: there is resolution of osteolytic lesions and PMMA beads are visible in the soft tissues. (G–J) Radiographs 4 years later: beads remain in the soft tissues and other than abnormal shape of the distal femoral physeal scar, there are no bony abnormalities. At a recheck examination at our hospital 4 years later, there was no lameness, joint effusion, or response to joint flexion.

The duration of local antimicrobial therapies is dictated by resolution of joint swelling, lameness, and synovial cytology. We generally treat the joint until the percentage of neutrophils on synovial cytology has dropped below 80%. Judicious use of anti-inflammatories, gastroprotectants, and probiotics should be considered mainstays of therapy for any hospitalized foal. Concurrent systemic antimicrobial administration is generally continued for a minimum of 2 weeks beyond the resolution of clinical signs.

Physitis/Osteomyelitis

Similar to cases of septic arthritis, use of local antimicrobials is a key feature of successful therapy. Antimicrobial-containing beads made of bone cement or POP, as discussed previously for septic arthritis, are especially useful in bone and physeal infection. This is because the physical presence of beads and bead permanence is less likely to be a problem in the extra-articular environment.

The affected bone or physis should be addressed surgically; however, overly aggressive debridement of bony or physeal lesions could increase the chance for disruption of normal physeal growth or collapse of the adjacent bone (**Fig. 7**). To avoid this, debridement is performed only as necessary to allow collection of samples for bacterial identification, removal of sequestrae and drainage of exudate from the physis to the surrounding soft tissues or surgical wound. In severe cases requiring extensive debridement, autologous bone grafting and external coaptation may be required (**Fig. 5**).[13]

Although the adjacent joint is not always affected, it is an excellent route for administration of local antimicrobials when treating bone or physeal infection. This is because intra-articular injection of antibiotics results in antimicrobial concentrations in the adjacent bone similar to those obtained by regional limb perfusion.[14] As discussed previously for septic arthritis, direct injection, local antimicrobial depots, and intrathecal pumps can be used to achieve high antimicrobial concentrations in the adjacent bone over several days to weeks.

The duration of antimicrobial therapy for physitis and osteomyelitis is longer than for septic synovitis. Resolution of lameness often will occur before the infection has been fully resolved. We generally like to have 1 week without signs of local sepsis (eg, neutrophilic synovitis, pain on palpation) or lameness before discontinuing local antimicrobials. Lack of continued bony lysis confirmed by radiography or repeated CT is ideal before discontinuation of local antimicrobials. Oral antimicrobials are generally continued for 2 to 4 weeks beyond the discontinuation of local antimicrobial therapies.

PROGNOSIS

Survival in foals treated for acute septic arthritis without significant comorbidities is generally good, although a broad range of survival has been reported: from 42% to 84%, and up to 89% when continuous intrasynovial infusion of antimicrobial was included in the treatment regimen.[4,12,15–18] The broad range covered in these reports probably reflects differences due to the rapidity of diagnosis and initiation of appropriate therapy as well as comorbidities. Additionally, it is common for financial considerations to affect survival, and this information is not always available in retrospective reports. In one study, 58 (84%) of 69 foals treated for septic arthritis survived to discharge and among these cases, signs were present for less than 24 hours in 74% of foals, only 5 had more than 1 joint involved, and only 1 foal had evidence of osteomyelitis.[18] In the same study, disease in systems other than the musculoskeletal system in addition to septic arthritis had a decreased likelihood of survival.[18] Similarly,

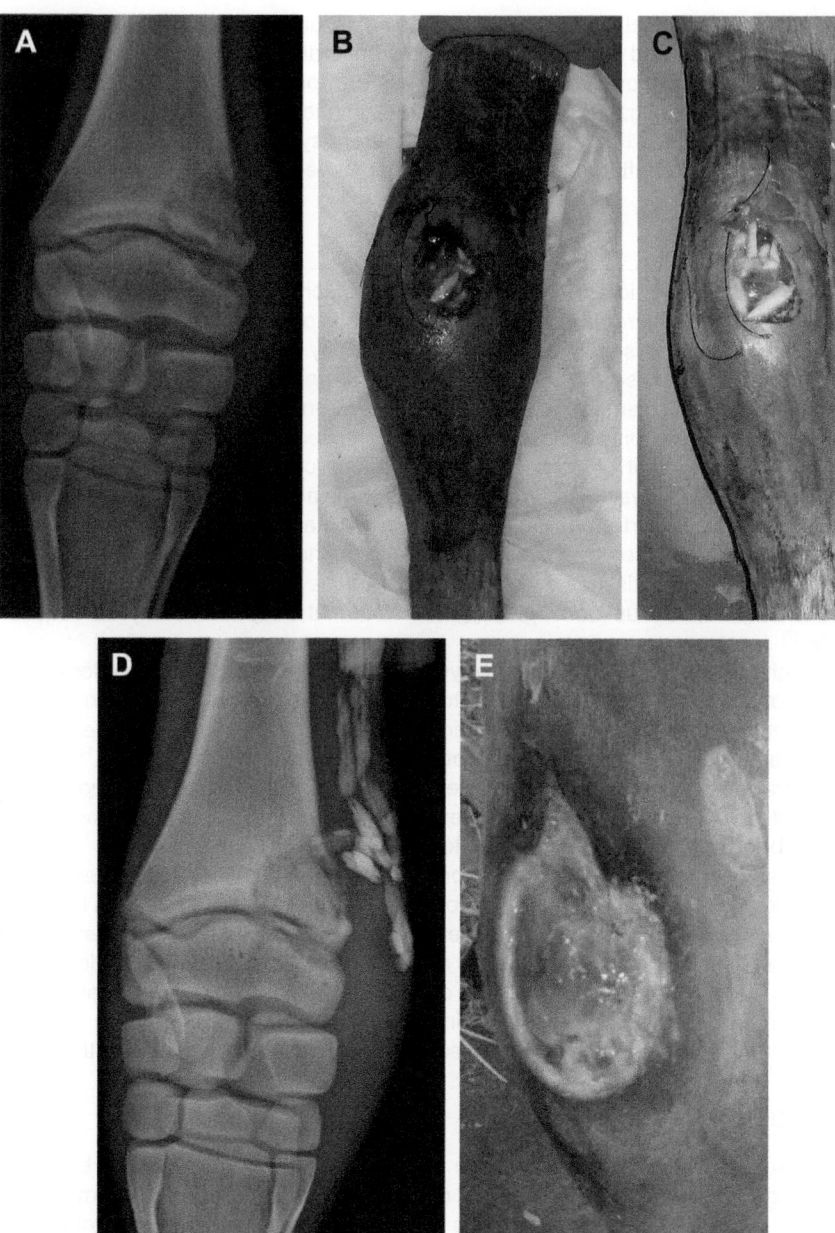

Fig. 7. Images from a 5-week-old thoroughbred filly that was presented for suspected septic physitis of the right radius. Radiographs of the distal radius 5 days before presentation were unremarkable. (*A*) The day of presentation, there was osteolysis of the metaphyseal side of the distal radial physis. There was diffuse cellulitis and a draining wound over the osteomyelitis. Ultrasound revealed the absence of radiocarpal or middle carpal effusion and anechoic synovial fluid. The cortical surface of the bone over the osteomyelitis was debrided to allow collection of samples for microbiologic identification and drainage. Gentamicin-impregnated PMMA beads were placed in the soft tissues via the wound, and regional limb perfusion with amikacin was performed daily for 10 days. *Salmonella* was identified

among a population of 1065 neonatal foals admitted to an intensive care unit from 1982 to 2008, the presence of musculoskeletal infection was significantly associated with nonsurvival.[19] The prognosis has been reported to be most favorable following aggressive and multimodal therapy and is reduced by multisystemic disease and the isolation of *Salmonella* sp from synovial fluid of affected joints.[16,20] It would appear that a septic joint with concurrent disease in other systems is a bad prognostic indicator, but a septic joint without epiphyseal bone involvement in an otherwise healthy foal should have a relatively good prognosis for survival given appropriate therapy.

In cases of osteomyelitis, the prognosis for survival is also fair to good with appropriate therapy. It should be kept in mind that when bony involvement is epiphyseal, the prognosis can be grave due to disruption of the subchondral bone (see **Fig. 8**).[21] In a report of 108 foals with osteomyelitis, 81% (87/108) survived to discharge.[22] Approximately 70% of these foals also had septic arthritis. In a report focusing on the outcome of septic arthritis, 52% (34/66) had concurrent osteomyelitis. In this report, only 45% of foals with septic arthritis survived to discharge from the hospital, but survival among those with osteomyelitis was not specifically stated.[15] In another report focused on the outcome of septic arthritis, the incidence of osteomyelitis of the epiphyseal bone or the physis was significantly higher (53%) in the nonsurvivors when compared with survivors (13%) among 81 foals with septic joints.[20] In summary, bony involvement when treating septic arthritis increases the importance of local therapy and probably reduces the prognosis for survival, especially if multimodal local therapy is not used.

The longer-term prognosis for full athletic function after musculoskeletal infection in the foal is less clear. Although septic synovitis, arthritis, physitis, and osteomyelitis are relatively prevalent diseases treated by equine practitioners, reports with sufficient case numbers and reports on nonracehorse populations are lacking. When infection is successfully eliminated before irreversible cartilage damage occurs, foals can become sound for athletic performance. The prognosis is influenced by the presence of systemic sepsis, number of joints involved, and presence of more than 95% neutrophils in the synovial fluid, prompt detection and initiation of treatment, and the presence of osteomyelitis.[16,23] Among a population of thoroughbred foals treated before 125 days of age and presented to public auction at weanling, yearling, or 2-year-old sales, there was no difference in the mean sales price or percentage of animals sold when compared with a control population.[24] However, in another study, thoroughbred horses discharged after treatment for septic arthritis were less likely to start on a racecourse and took significantly longer to start in their first race compared with siblings on the dam's side.[18] Of the affected foals that survived to discharge, only 48.3% started in a race compared with 66.2% of sibling controls.[18] Similarly, in a report of 93 standardbred and thoroughbred foals, of the 78.5% that survived to discharge, approximately one-third raced.[16] Interestingly, in the report of 108 thoroughbred foals with septic osteomyelitis of which approximately 70% had joint sepsis,

---

from bone cultures and fecal cultures. (*B*) The lameness improved 2 days after presentation, but there was continued soft tissue swelling. (*C*) Five days after presentation, the swelling was improved and there was no lameness. (*D*) PMMA beads are present in the wound and removal of beads was begun. Two weeks after presentation, the wound was granulated and most beads had been removed. The filly was discharged on intramuscular ceftiofur for 2 additional weeks. (*E*) One week later, the wound had started to contract and there was no recurrence of swelling or lameness.

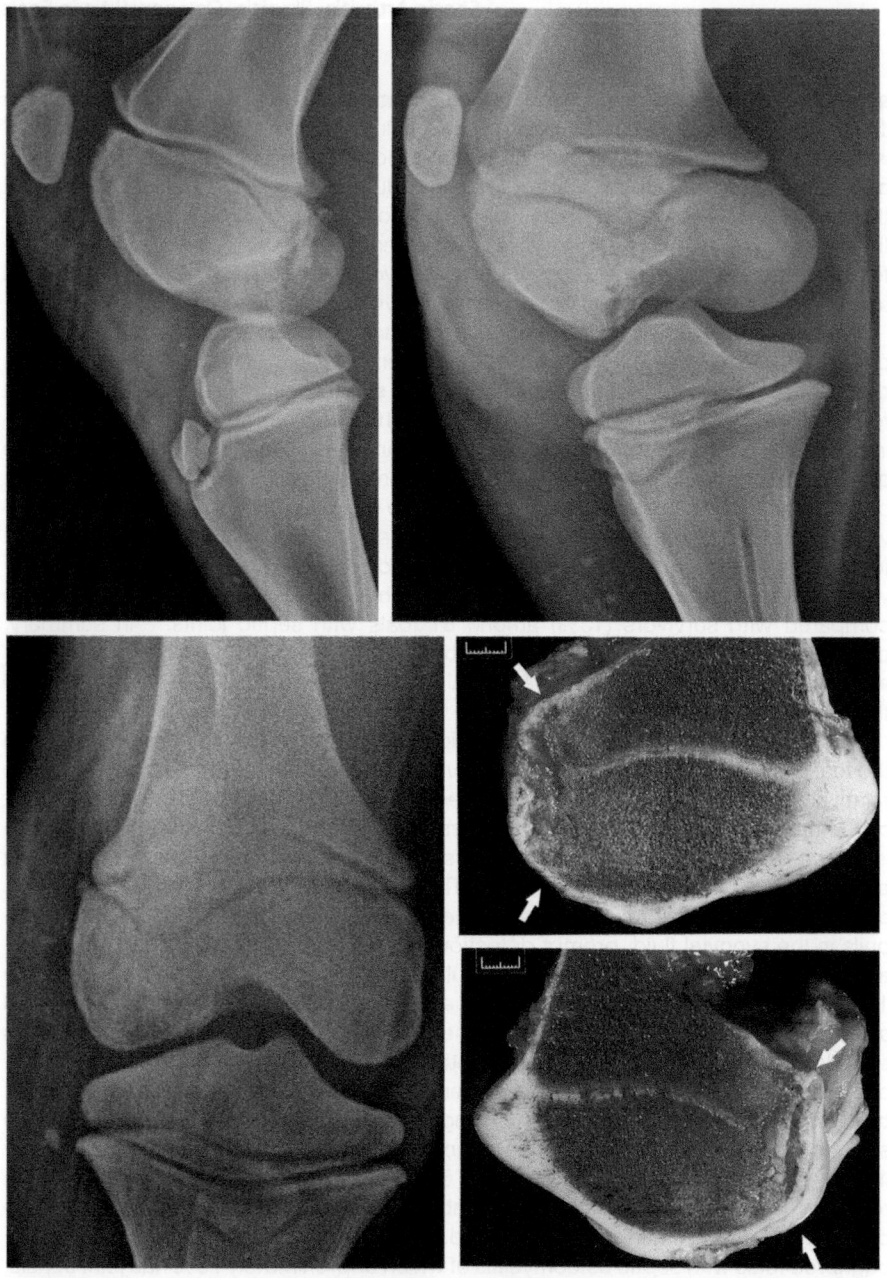

Fig. 8. Radiographs of the right stifle from a 4-week-old quarter horse filly that was presented for severe hind limb lameness of almost 3 weeks' duration. Bilateral septic arthritis of the stifle joints and osteomyelitis of the caudal lateral femoral condyles was diagnosed. The filly was euthanized due to severity of epiphyseal bone involvement, poor prognosis, and cost of treatment. Radiographically, there are multifocal ill-defined radiolucent regions within the caudal lateral femoral condyle with multiple round to amorphous mineral opaque foci, presumed to be debris and severe distention of the stifle joint and thickening of the soft tissues at the level of the stifle. The appearance of the patella and medial and lateral trochlear ridges are normal for a foal of this age. Sagittal section through the lateral femur demonstrates loss of epiphyseal bone and overlying articular cartilage (*arrows*). (*Courtesy of* Dr Jose Delgado and Dr Brian Porter, Texas A&M University; with permission.)

48% (52/108) raced.[22] Unfortunately, comparison with a control population was not performed.

SUMMARY

Recent literature may indicate that prognosis for survival and potential athleticism in foals that are treated expediently with local therapies and are without comorbidities may be more favorable than has been previously indicated.

SUPPLEMENTARY DATA

Supplementary video related to this article can be found at http://dx.doi.org/10.1016/j. cveq.2017.03.002.

REFERENCES

1. Firth EC. Current concepts of infectious polyarthritis in foals. Equine Vet J 1983; 15(1):5–9.
2. Madison JB, Scarratt WK. Immune-mediated polysynovitis in four foals. J Am Vet Med Assoc 1988;192(11):1581–4.
3. Dechant JE, Symm WA, Nieto JE. Comparison of pH, lactate, and glucose analysis of equine synovial fluid using a portable clinical analyzer with a bench-top blood gas analyzer. Vet Surg 2011;40(7):811–6.
4. Hepworth-Warren KL, Wong DM, Fulkerson CV, et al. Bacterial isolates, antimicrobial susceptibility patterns, and factors associated with infection and outcome in foals with septic arthritis: 83 cases (1998-2013). J Am Vet Med Assoc 2015; 246(7):785–93.
5. Madison JB, Sommer M, Spencer PA. Relations among synovial membrane histopathologic findings, synovial fluid cytologic findings, and bacterial culture results in horses with suspected infectious arthritis: 64 cases (1979-1987). J Am Vet Med Assoc 1991;198(9):1655–61.
6. Paradis MR. Septic arthritis in the foal: What is the best imaging modality? Equine Vet Education 2010;27:334–5.
7. Lloyd KC, Stover SM, Pascoe JR, et al. Plasma and synovial fluid concentrations of gentamicin in horses after intra-articular administration of buffered and unbuffered gentamicin. Am J Vet Res 1988;49(5):644–9.
8. Mills ML, Rush BR, St Jean G, et al. Determination of synovial fluid and serum concentrations, and morphologic effects of intraarticular ceftiofur sodium in horses. Vet Surg 2000;29(5):398–406.
9. Ivester KM, Adams SB, Moore GE, et al. Gentamicin concentrations in synovial fluid obtained from the tarsocrural joints of horses after implantation of gentamicin-impregnated collagen sponges. Am J Vet Res 2006;67(9):1519–26.
10. Lescun TB, Adams SB, Wu CC, et al. Continuous infusion of gentamicin into the tarsocrural joint of horses. Am J Vet Res 2000;61(4):407–12.
11. Lescun TB, Adams SB, Wu CC, et al. Effects of continuous intra-articular infusion of gentamicin on synovial membrane and articular cartilage in the tarsocrural joint of horses. Am J Vet Res 2002;63(5):683–7.
12. Lescun TB, Vasey JR, Ward MP, et al. Treatment with continuous intrasynovial antimicrobial infusion for septic synovitis in horses: 31 cases (2000-2003). J Am Vet Med Assoc 2006;228(12):1922–9.
13. Baird AN, Taylor JR, Watkins JP. Debridement of septic physeal lesions in 3 foals. Cornell Vet 1990;80(1):85–95.

14. Werner LA, Hardy J, Bertone AL. Bone gentamicin concentration after intra-articular injection or regional intravenous perfusion in the horse. Vet Surg 2003; 32(6):559–65.
15. Schneider RK, Bramlage LR, Moore RM, et al. A retrospective study of 192 horses affected with septic arthritis/tenosynovitis. Equine Vet J 1992;24(6):436–42.
16. Steel CM, Hunt AR, Adams PL, et al. Factors associated with prognosis for survival and athletic use in foals with septic arthritis: 93 cases (1987-1994). J Am Vet Med Assoc 1999;215(7):973–7.
17. Meijer MC, van Weeren PR, Rijkenhuizen AB. Clinical experiences of treating septic arthritis in the equine by repeated joint lavage: a series of 39 cases. J Vet Med A Physiol Pathol Clin Med 2000;47(6):351–65.
18. Smith LJ, Marr CM, Payne RJ, et al. What is the likelihood that thoroughbred foals treated for septic arthritis will race? Equine Vet J 2004;36(5):452–6.
19. Giguere S, Weber EJ, Sanchez LC. Factors associated with outcome and gradual improvement in survival over time in 1065 equine neonates admitted to an intensive care unit. Equine Vet J 2015;49(1):45–50.
20. Vos NJ, Ducharme NG. Analysis of factors influencing prognosis in foals with septic arthritis. Ir Vet J 2008;61(2):102–6.
21. Hance SR, Schneider RK, Embertson RM, et al. Lesions of the caudal aspect of the femoral condyles in foals: 20 cases (1980-1990). J Am Vet Med Assoc 1993; 202(4):637–46.
22. Neil KM, Axon JE, Begg AP, et al. Retrospective study of 108 foals with septic osteomyelitis. Aust Vet J 2010;88(1–2):4–12.
23. Wright IM, Smith MR, Humphrey DJ, et al. Endoscopic surgery in the treatment of contaminated and infected synovial cavities. Equine Vet J 2003;35(6):613–9.
24. Corley KT, Corley MM. Hospital treatment as a foal does not adversely affect future sales performance in thoroughbred horses. Equine Vet J Suppl 2012;(41):87–90.

Flexural Deformity of the Distal Interphalangeal Joint

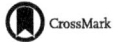

Fred J. Caldwell, DVM, MS

KEYWORDS

- Club foot • Contracted tendon • Flexural deformity
- Accessory ligament of the deep digital flexor desmotomy
- Inferior check ligament desmotomy • Distal interphalangeal joint • Foal

KEY POINTS

- Flexural deformity of the distal interphalangeal joint can be either congenital or acquired, which are commonly managed differently.
- Early recognition and treatment are essential to prevent hoof capsule abnormalities that can lead to poor performance and/or chronic lameness as adults.
- Identification of contributing factors and their appropriate management are important to ensure successful resolution.
- Surgical intervention should be considered in severe cases or those refractory to conservative therapy efforts.

 Video content accompanies this article at http://www.vetequine.theclinics.com.

INTRODUCTION

Flexural deformity of the distal interphalangeal joint, or "club foot," in young horses can be caused by a multitude of factors and can have a negative impact on the animal's future soundness if not recognized early and successfully managed. These cases are commonly presented to equine veterinarians, especially those whose practices include a fairly large broodmare population. Flexural deformities of the distal interphalangeal joint are characterized by a shortening of the deep flexor muscle-tendon unit, which results in flexion of the distal interphalangeal joint due to its close proximity to the insertion of the deep digital flexor tendon (DDFT).[1] The persistent flexion of the distal interphalangeal joint results in a broken forward hoof pastern axis with the foal walking on the toe. Depending on the cause, one or both forelimbs

Department of Clinical Sciences, JT Vaughan Large Animal Teaching Hospital, 1500 Wire Road, College of Veterinary Medicine, Auburn University, Auburn, AL 36849, USA
E-mail address: caldwfj@auburn.edu

Vet Clin Equine 33 (2017) 315–330
http://dx.doi.org/10.1016/j.cveq.2017.03.003
vetequine.theclinics.com

can be affected (**Fig. 1**). Flexural deformities in young horses are erroneously referred to as "contracted tendons," which implies a pathologic process of the tendon. This is technically not correct in cases other than those involving a primary injury to the tendon, leading to a true contracted state upon healing, which is unusual in foals.[2,3]

Flexural deformities are classified as either congenital (present at birth) or acquired (occur during a later stage of development). The pathogenesis, clinical presentation, management, and response to treatment can vary depending on the time of onset, but there are similarities in the methodology with how each form is handled.[4] The approach to these cases depends greatly on when the deformity developed, and the severity, duration, complicating factors, and owner expectations.[4,5] The prognosis for future athleticism is typically good for mild to moderate cases that are identified early and managed aggressively. Severe cases and those unresponsive to therapy can lead to secondary complications, such as significant hoof capsule distortion, changes in P3, and early onset degenerative joint disease that results in a guarded prognosis for long-term soundness.

CONGENITAL FORM
Pathogenesis

Foals are rarely born perfectly conformed, and most have some degree of flexor tendon laxity, flexural deformity, and/or angular limb deformity. In mild cases, this is considered a normal finding, and the vast majority self-correct over time with exercise.[6] Medical and/or surgical treatment is usually required in moderate flexural limb deformity cases or mild cases that do not resolve on their own. Foals with severe flexural limb deformities bordering on arthrogryposis warrant euthanasia.

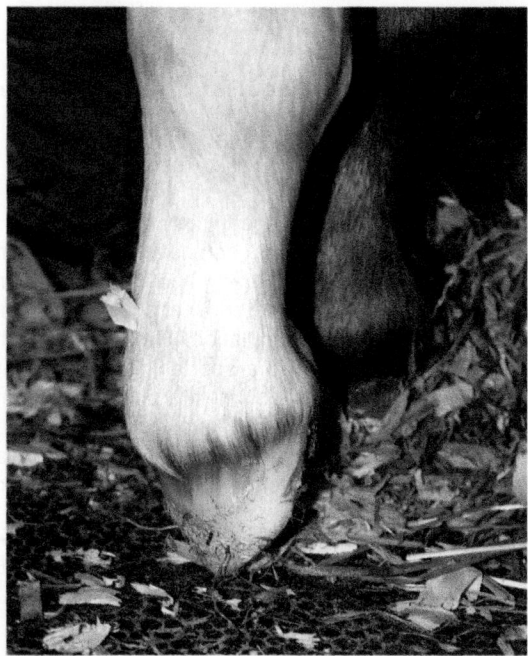

Fig. 1. Foal with bilateral severe (stage II) flexural deformity of the distal interphalangeal joint.

Causes of congenital flexural deformities are not often clearly determined but have been theorized to be associated with factors such as the following[5,7,8]:

- Uterine malposition
- Bone or joint malformations
- Ingestion of toxic plants of other teratogens by the mare
- Specific diseases of the mare during foal development
- Genetic factors
- Other minor associations

Clinical Signs and Patient Evaluation

Although congenital flexural deformities can involve the distal interphalangeal joint, the metacarpo/tarsophalangeal joint, and/or carpus, is more commonly affected.[3,6,9] Chronic cases of flexural deformity develop more permanent states of contracture of the musculotendinous unit and concomitant contracture and fibrosis of the flexor joint capsule. This results in maintenance of the contracture and emphasizes the importance of early recognition and treatment.[3,5]

Nonsurgical Management

Medical treatment
Flexural deformity of the distal interphalangeal joint can be caused by and/or result in pain and lameness in the limb. In addition, techniques such as passive stretching and physical therapy combined with splinting can cause discomfort for the foal. The use of analgesics, most commonly nonsteroidal anti-inflammatory drugs (NSAIDs), can be useful in the management and ultimate improvement or correction of deformities. The practitioner should always be cognizant of the potential side effects of their use in young animals. It is prudent to prescribe gastro-protectants concurrently with NSAID administration to prevent gastric ulceration in these young patients. The stress and discomfort associated with the treatment of flexural deformity of the distal inter-phalangeal joint in foals justify the use of gastric protectants even without the use of NSAIDs.[8] Periodic monitoring of serum creatinine and total protein should be performed with prolonged NSAID administration.

Traditionally, it has been recognized that oxytetracycline can be useful for the treatment of foals with flexural deformities.[10,11] Positive results were originally thought to be mediated through the calcium chelation properties of the drug on inhibiting muscle contraction. This mechanism does not fully explain its effects in flexural deformities of the distal limb, such as flexural deformity of the distal interphalangeal joint, where there is no muscle tissue between the origin of the accessory ligament of the DDFT and insertion of the DDFT on P3.

It has been shown that most cells in foals' accessory ligament of the DDFT and DDFT are myofibroblasts through positive immunohistochemical staining for alpha-smooth muscle actin.[12] Eloquent work by Arnoczky and coworkers[13] later demonstrated that oxytetracycline induced a dose-dependent inhibition of gel contraction by equine myofibroblasts cultured from the accessory ligament of the DDFT of foals. They also observed a decrease in matrix metalloproteinase 1 (MMP-1) messenger RNA (mRNA) expression by equine myofibroblasts.[13] The proposed mode of action is through inhibition of tractional structuring of collagen fibrils by equine myofibroblasts through a downregulation of interstitial collagenase (MMP-1) mRNA expression.[13] Later work evaluating tail tendon fasicules in rats administered oxytetracycline demonstrated significantly decreased viscoelastic properties of 1-month-old, but not 6-month-old, rats. This is a similar finding to that in foals where greater effects are observed in younger versus older foals, which is thought to be related to the increased collagen cross-linking and tendon stiffness in mature animals.[14]

The recommended oxytetracycline dose varies among practitioners, but typically is 44 mg/kg intravenously (IV; 2–4 g) diluted in 1 L saline. If the desired effect is not achieved, it can be repeated daily or every other day for 3 treatments. Complications with oxytetracycline administration are uncommon, but transient carpal hyperextension, sudden collapse, and renal failure have been reported.[9,15]

In the author's experience, administration of oxytetracycline results in temporary improvement, and the author has had limited success in the utilization of this therapy specifically for the treatment of flexural deformity of the distal interphalangeal joint, with many foals failing to respond or returning to their previous conformation shortly after treatment. It is a therapy that seems to be more effective in flexural deformities of the carpus and metacarpo/tarsophalangeal joints, providing enough relaxation for other therapies to have time to take effect. Madison and coworkers[16] found that a single dose of 44 mg/kg oxytetracycline IV in foals with flexural deformity of the distal interphalangeal joint had no effect on distal interphalangeal joint angle and concluded that it might have limited usefulness for club foot.

Bandaging, splints, and casting

Application of rigid coaptation in the form of splints or casts, or dynamic articulating bracing systems (Dynasplint, Dynasplint Systems, Inc., Severna Park, MD, USA), is frequently combined with other therapies such as IV oxytetracycline and controlled exercise. Casting can also be very effective, but will require frequent recasting as improvement in joint angle occurs. These techniques are directed at loading the muscle-tendon unit, resulting in flexor relaxation through the inverse myotactic reflex.[17] It is critically important to appropriately pad the limbs under these devices and change them frequently because foals are highly susceptible to pressure sores and skin excoriation. Unfortunately, these methods do not work as well with flexural deformities of the distal interphalangeal joint as they do elsewhere. In very young foals with mild flexural deformity of the distal interphalangeal joint, the application of a simple padded bandage can induce enough laxity through the deep flexor muscle-tendon unit to allow exercise to further resolve the flexural deformity.

Physical therapy and exercise

Repetitive passive extension of the distal phalanx in 10-minute sessions 4 to 6 times daily can be beneficial in fatiguing the deep flexor muscle-tendon unit in congenital cases.[18] This is most easily performed with the foal recumbent immediately following nursing or controlled exercise. The foal is usually more tolerant of the physical therapy at this point due to its exhaustion. Benefits of passive stretching techniques also work best when coupled with oxytetracycline administration.

It is the author's opinion that controlled exercise on a firm surface is helpful in cases of flexural deformity of the distal interphalangeal joint. It is best performed with the mare led in hand on a good firm surface to allow the foal to follow for short periods of time to gain the most benefit from loading and stretching of the deep digital flexor musculotendinous unit. Foals that do not respond to conservative management, or that demonstrate pain in the DDFT, can benefit from the application of temporary heel wedge cuffs.[19] In cases with lameness as the underlying cause, analgesics should be used judiciously and exercise should be more restricted.

Surgical Management

Surgical management is generally not required for the congenital form other than in severe cases. Surgical intervention is more commonly elected for the management of acquired flexural deformity of the distal interphalangeal joint, and the procedures described for surgical correction are discussed later in detail in the acquired section.

ACQUIRED FORM
Pathogenesis

Acquired deformities develop after birth, and their cause is likely multifactorial. Some of the proposed theories related to their development are excessive nutrition contributing to longitudinal bone growth that outpaces the elongation of the musculotendinous unit, chronic disproportionate limb loading related to lameness, forelimb grazing posture preferences that influence limb loading discrepancies and hoof wear patterns (forward foot vs rearward foot), or a neuromuscular dysfunction. Acquired deformities have been suggested to be part of the developmental orthopedic disease complex along with osteochondrosis, angular limb deformities, physitis, and cervical vertebral malarticulations/malformations.[3,5] Conditions that result in pain or lameness can contribute to contraction of the muscular portion of the musculotendinous unit because tendons and ligaments have a limited ability to contract.[3] Debate continues among investigators regarding the cause of flexural deformity of the distal interphalangeal joint, but the 2 predominate causes seem to involve painful conditions leading to uneven limb loading and disproportionate growth between bone and the musculotendinous unit.

Clinical Signs and Patient Evaluation

Flexural deformity of the distal interphalangeal joint is frequently acquired and typically develops during periods of rapid growth most commonly between 1 and 6 months of age. The condition nearly exclusively affects the forelimbs and is commonly bilateral, although one limb is typically more severely affected. Horses presenting with flexural deformity of the distal interphalangeal joint are classically young; however, mature horses can develop flexural deformity of the distal interphalangeal joint. The causes between these 2 types are not always similar and therefore may require different management approaches.

Foals with flexural deformity of the distal interphalangeal joint are typically fast growing and can present with varying degrees of lameness, which can be quite severe in some cases. These foals can have concurrent physitis in addition to the flexural deformity of the distal interphalangeal joint, and both conditions are interrelated and require consideration. Initially the author examines these foals by merely observing them from a distance as they move about the stall. It may be necessary to watch them on a firm flat surface to appreciate the severity of the deformity.

Following the initial anamnesis and observation, the foal should undergo a thorough physical examination, paying particular attention to any evidence of enlargement, heat, or pain on palpation of the physes indicating possible physitis. If lameness is perceived, it should be thoroughly investigated with diagnostic analgesia techniques in order to isolate and treat before implementing therapy for the flexural deformity, as continued lameness postoperatively would negatively affect the response to flexural deformity treatment.[1,4] With the foal weight-bearing, it is a useful exercise to palpate the flexor tendons individually to determine tension versus laxity. The degree of flexural deformity of the distal interphalangeal joint in the acute phase is categorically divided into the following 2 stages:

- Stage I flexural deformity of the distal interphalangeal joint is described as the dorsal hoof wall being ≤90° with respect to the ground (**Fig. 2**A).
- Stage II resulting in the dorsal hoof wall being greater than 90° to the ground (**Fig. 2**B).

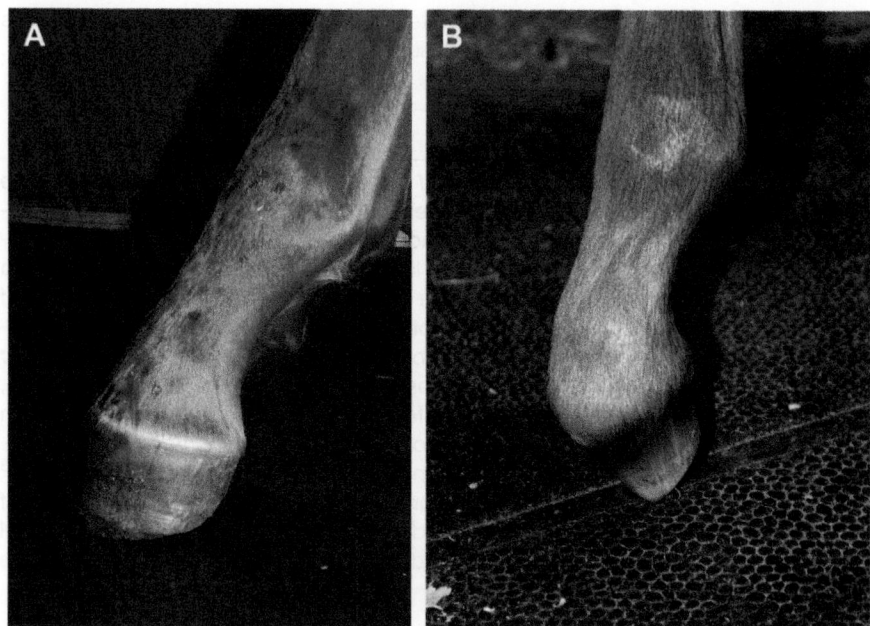

Fig. 2. Stage I (*A*) and stage II (*B*) flexural deformities of the distal interphalangeal joint in young foals.

The stage does not necessarily influence the approach to treatment but can have an effect on prognosis for resolution and resulting athleticism. Once flexural deformity of the distal interphalangeal joint becomes chronic, the sequela can be significant hoof capsule distortion. A grading system has been previously described in order to classify the degree of distortion and monitor response to therapies (**Table 1**).[1,19,20]

Palpation of the foot and attempts at manual extension of the distal limb is also a useful exercise to determine the reaction of the foal. Chronic flexural deformity of the distal interphalangeal joint can result in deep digital flexor tendonitis, which may also influence the treatment approach. These foals will be very resistant to extension of the distal interphalangeal joint. The toe should be examined closely because, depending on the chronicity and the foal's environment, it can have varying degrees of damage, separation at the white line, and flaring of the hoof wall. Many foals will be sensitive to digital pressure on the sole region at the toe due to focused weight-bearing and bruising of this area.

Radiographs are generally unnecessary in the diagnosis of flexural deformity of the distal interphalangeal joint but are frequently indicated in chronic or severe cases. Foals should be lightly sedated, and both forelimbs placed on wooden blocks of equal height for even loading.[1] Good-quality weight-bearing lateral, 45° dorsopalmar, and horizontal dorsopalmar radiographic projections should be obtained to evaluate the distal phalanx and distal interphalangeal joint. Chronic cases of flexural deformity of the distal interphalangeal joint can have significant radiographic evidence of rotational displacement of the distal phalanx with hoof capsule distortion, degenerative joint disease in the distal interphalangeal joint, osseous remodeling or demineralization of P3, and septic osteitis of P3, which can greatly reduce the long-term prognosis (**Fig. 3**).

Table 1
Club foot grading system according to Redden

Grade	Description
I	Dorsal hoof wall angle is 3°–5° greater than the opposing foot angle, fullness through coronary band as a result of partial luxation of P2-P3
II	Dorsal hoof wall angle is 5°–8° greater than the opposing foot angle, growth rings compressed dorsally, heel does not contact the ground when normally trimmed to the plane of the frog
III	Dorsal hoof wall is dished; growth rings at the heel are twice the width of those at the dorsal hoof wall, radiographic evidence of flaring and/or osseous resorption at tip of P3
IV	Pronounced dished appearance with ≥80° angle of the dorsal hoof wall, the coronary band distance from the ground at the heel the same as at the toe, radiographic changes include extensive P3 demineralization and possible rotation

From Redden RF. Hoof capsule distortion: understanding the mechanisms as a basis for rational management. Vet Clin Equine 2003;19:443–62.

Nonsurgical Management

Nutrition

A common cause involves excessive energy intake, contributing to rapid growth in these foals. Physitis is usually also present, which can contribute to reduced limb loading due to pain. Excessive intake may occur through a heavy lactating mare or via concentrate supplementation. In these situations, it is crucial to reduce the caloric intake and provide a balanced ration based on the daily nutritional requirements. It is not uncommon to see these conditions develop in foals that have a sudden change in their intake (increase after a period of deficiency such as postweaning or change in

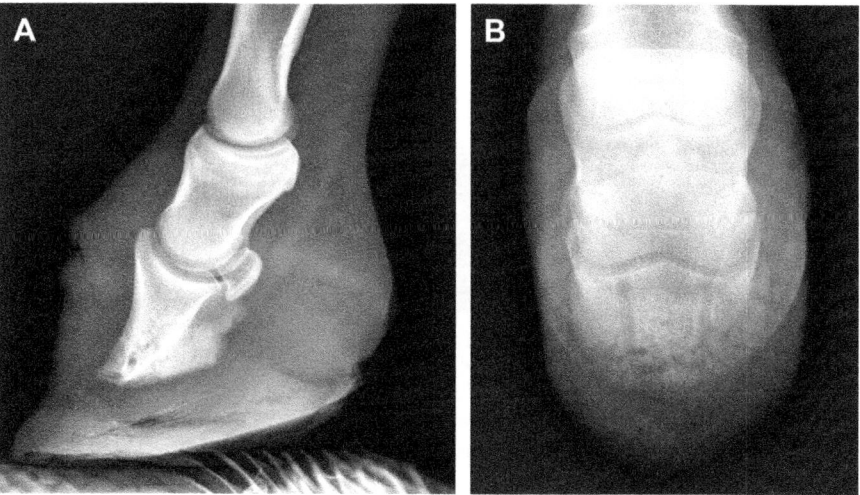

Fig. 3. Lateral (*A*) and dorsopalmar (*B*) radiographs of a 5-month-old foal with a chronic history of flexural deformity of the distal interphalangeal joint. Note the hoof capsule distortion and gas lucency along the dorsal laminae consistent with abscessation (lateral), and significant remodeling of the distal border of P3 (DP).

management). Affected foals of heavy lactating mares should be weaned early or the mare's ration reduced. Older foals should have their diet reduced and be maintained on good-quality hay or pasture and a balanced mineral supplement.

Medical treatment

In many cases, the acquired form of flexural deformities in young horses is secondary to painful conditions and subsequent reduced limb loading, and therefore, it is imperative that the primary cause of lameness be addressed. Exercise should be limited and controlled closely in these cases as well as using judicious use of NSAIDs.

Oxytetracycline does not seem to have the same effects in older patients as it does in younger foals and likely is associated with the age-related effects of extracellular matrix maturation in developing tendons.[14] For this reason, oxytetracycline is not generally used in foals greater than 30 days of age.[6]

Corrective trimming and shoeing

Trimming of the heels is an important component of the management of flexural deformity of the distal interphalangeal joint, but only in cases where the heels are in contact with the ground. In longstanding cases, the heels are typically overgrown, whereas the toe has worn excessively. This contributes to the upright appearance of the hoof capsule or "boxy" conformation (**Fig. 4**). Any evidence of wall separation dorsally or seedy toe should be addressed appropriately. Rasping the heels in cases where they are not in contact with the ground will further reduce solar contact area, which can exacerbate loading through the toe and contribute to dorsal laminar separation, inflammation, and pain.

In cases where the heel is in contact with the ground, a balance exists in trimming the heels where it contributes to stretching the DDFT and to the point of causing pain and lameness, leading to reduced limb loading. The author recommends rasping the foot from the quarters back to the heels to lower them just to the point that there is a slight gap under them when the foal is standing squarely. This can be performed as frequently as every 7 to 10 days depending on the age of the foal and the severity of the deformity and continue until correct hoof pastern axis alignment is achieved. A technique of using a wedge pad placed in reverse orientation under the toe to

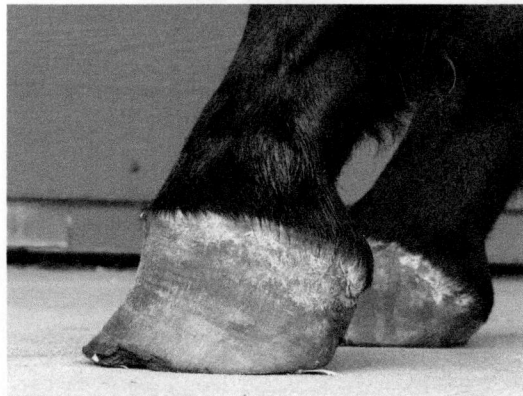

Fig. 4. Classic appearance of a chronic flexural deformity of the distal interphalangeal joint with distortion of the dorsal hoof wall, separation of the wall at the toe, broken forward hoof-pastern axis, overly long heel height, widened hoof wall rings at the heel, and a nearly parallel orientation of the coronary band to the solar surface.

determine how much the heels can be safely lowered before causing discomfort can also be a useful technique.[21] If improvement is not observed, or the foal demonstrates discomfort and relapses, then surgical intervention should be considered.[4]

Toe extensions can also increase load and stretching of the deep flexor muscle-tendon unit while walking, but should be used cautiously because their risks can outweigh any benefits. In mild stage I cases, but not in severe cases, the author commonly fashions toe extensions with acrylic (Equilox, Equilox International, Inc., Pine Island, MN, USA) in young foals up to 3 to 4 months of age. This also serves to protect further damage to the toe region of the hoof as the foal is exercised. It is imperative that a conservative amount of material is used to create the toe extension (target of one-quarter of a 2-ounce container per extension) because these materials harden through an exothermic reaction and application of an excess amount of material to the sole and hoof capsule can lead to thermal necrosis of the sensitive lamina and potentially deeper structures. Application of ice packs during the acrylic's curing phase is recommended. Caution should be exercised in applying toe extensions to hoof capsules with a more upright angle or those with already compromised integrity, because this can contribute to laminar separation and hoof capsule damage by increasing mechanical forces dorsally (**Fig. 5**). Toe extensions should not be used in cases where there is no heel contact with the ground when the foal is standing squarely on a non-deformable surface.

In older foals and weanlings, the application of a toe shoe can achieve the same goals of improving the hoof pastern axis, protecting the toe region of the hoof capsule,

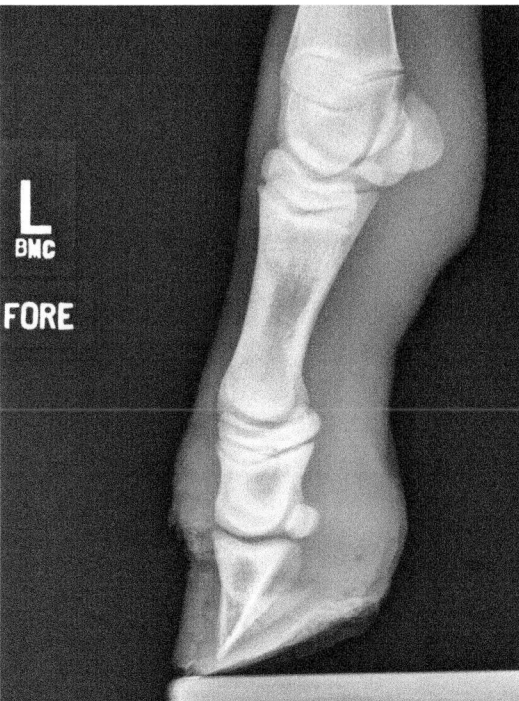

Fig. 5. Lateral radiograph of a 5-week-old foal with stage I flexural deformity of the distal interphalangeal joint that was treated initially with a toe extension. There is evidence of rotational displacement of P3 and osteitis. Note the lack of heel contact with the ground.

and loading the muscle tendon unit to promote stretching and elongation while avoiding the risks of laminar separation and hoof capsule distortion that can occur with acrylic toe extensions.[1,22] The shoe is thicker at the toe and then gradually thins as it progresses back toward the quarters, ending at approximately the widest part of the solar surface of the foot (**Fig. 6**). The shoe can either be glued on with composite materials in younger horses or nailed in older foals. It is preferable to glue the shoe in place if possible to avoid further compromising hoof capsule integrity with using nails.

Surgical Management

Accessory ligament of the deep digital flexor tendon desmotomy

Surgical intervention is indicated in foals unresponsive to conservative methods of treatment. Desmotomy of the accessory ligament of the DDFT is a commonly performed procedure for horses that requires correction of flexural deformity of the distal interphalangeal joint.[23–26] Although when choosing a surgical treatment, many different factors must be taken into account and each case must be considered independently, there are general recommendations depending on severity of the flexural deformity of the distal interphalangeal joint in young foals (**Table 2**).[27,28]

Traditional techniques

Surgical approaches for the traditional open technique of desmotomy of the accessory ligament of the DDFT are directly over the accessory ligament of the DDFT on the medial or lateral aspect of the metacarpus with the horse positioned in lateral recumbency for a unilateral procedure, or dorsal recumbency for bilateral cases. A 5-cm incision is created over the DDFT, centered at the junction of the proximal and middle thirds of the metacarpus.[29] The subcutaneous tissue is separated bluntly to identify the separation between the DDFT and its accessory ligament. An incision through fibers covering the confluence of the ligament and tendon may be required to identify the separation. A curved hemostat is used to isolate the ligament by passing it between the ligament and tendon, and thereby entering the distal aspect of the carpal flexor sheath, and then dorsally between the accessory ligament and suspensory ligament. The accessory ligament is then positively identified and exteriorized from the incision. The ligament is then sharply divided taking care to not damage the adjacent

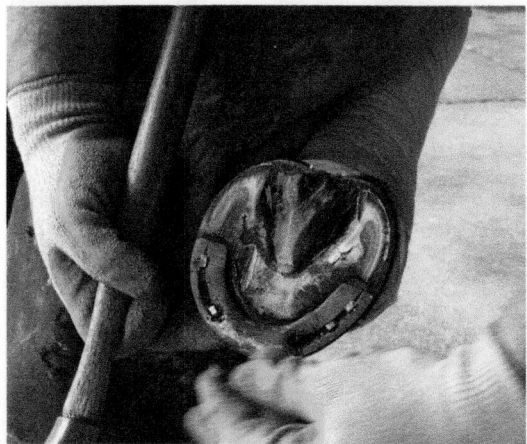

Fig. 6. A toe shoe being applied to a weanling. The horse had an accessory ligament of the DDFT desmotomy the previous day.

Table 2
Recommendations for the surgical treatment of flexural deformity of the distal interphalangeal joint according to hoof-ground angle

Hoof-Ground Angle	Surgical Treatment
Higher than normal but <90° (stage I)	Accessory ligament of the DDFT desmotomy
90°–115° (stage II)	Accessory ligament of the DDFT desmotomy or DDFT tenotomy
>115° (severe stage II)	DDFT tenotomy

neurovascular bundle. Extension of the digit should produce a gap within the cut ends of the ligament. Some surgeons prefer to remove a segment of the ligament, but the author finds this difficult to perform precisely and is unnecessary. The incision is closed routinely in 2 layers (absorbable continuous pattern in the paratenon/subcutaneous layer, and intradermal in the skin).

Good surgical principles and delicate instrument dissection are essential to maximize the cosmetic result, especially in young foals. The author additionally routinely recommends bandaging for 4 to 6 weeks to help minimize surgical site blemishes. Significant improvement is typically immediate, but the full benefit of the procedure might not be recognized for 2 to 3 days postoperatively. Foals are provided controlled exercise for 2 weeks, after which they are allowed free pasture exercise, assuming normal postoperative surgical site healing and no evidence of deep digital flexor tendonitis.

Complications of this procedure include inadvertent transection of structures other than the accessory ligament of the DDFT, excessive swelling, infection, and incisional dehiscence, which can result in the development of an unsightly scar and poor cosmetic results. An ultrasound-guided technique for desmotomy of the accessory ligament of the DDFT has been previously described.[30,31] This technique has been reported to minimize the incisional size and reduce postoperative scarring when compared with the traditional open technique.

Minimally invasive technique

A minimally invasive tenoscopic approach for desmotomy of the accessory ligament of the DDFT through the distal aspect of the carpal flexor sheath has been described.[32] The horse is positioned in dorsal recumbency and the affected limb or limbs are suspended by a hoist. Toe extension is essential to place maximal tension in the accessory ligament of the DDFT to facilitate division and is accomplished by supporting the limbs from the palmar aspect. The carpal sheath is distended routinely, and the arthroscope is placed into the medial aspect of the sheath over the accessory ligament of the DDFT, where fluid distention can be appreciated. The arthroscope and cannula are initially advanced proximally into the sheath, but then gradually withdrawn into the distal aspect of the sheath to visualize the DDFT palmarly and accessory ligament of the DDFT dorsally. An instrument portal is created into the lateral aspect of the sheath directly across from the arthroscopic portal in a horizontal plane with respect to the limb in order to visualize division of the ligament (**Fig. 7**). Once triangulation is established, desmotomy is performed while visualizing the division of the fibers transversely (Video 1). Once the lateral aspect of the accessory ligament of the DDFT has been divided, the arthroscope is moved to the lateral portal in order to visualize insertion of the blade through the medial portal for transection of the remaining medial fibers of the accessory ligament of the DDFT. The area between the accessory ligament of the DDFT and the suspensory ligament is identified as loose areolar tissue

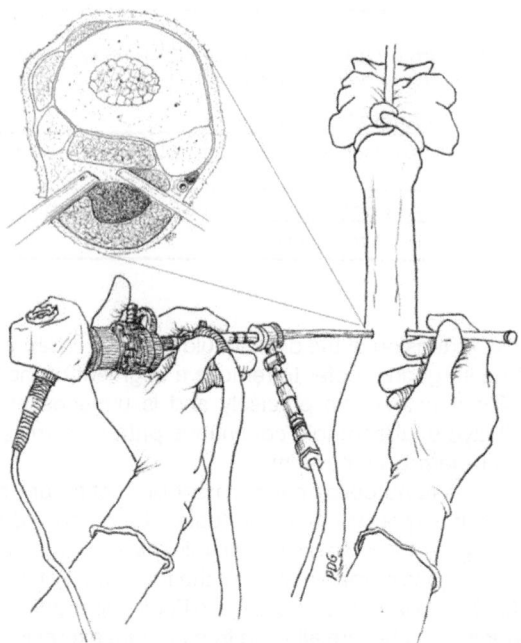

Fig. 7. Procedure being performed in the right forelimb of a horse in dorsal recumbency. The lateral portion of the AL-DDFT has been divided, and the arthroscope is now in the lateral aspect of the distal carpal flexor sheath with the tenoscopic blade in the medial aspect of the distal carpal flexor sheath in order to visualize and divide the remaining medial intact fibers. (*inset*) Cross-section illustration at the surgical site showing the remaining intact medial fibers of the AL-DDFT being divided. Note support rope positioned palmarly with towel padding between the rope and heel bulbs to maximize toe extension.

and can be visualized once the accessory ligament of the DDFT is fully divided (Video 2). The tenoscopic portals are closed routinely.

The advantages of this approach are that it is minimally invasive and results in less surgical dissection than the traditional open approach. Because of the smaller incisions, horses are able to return to earlier exercise without the risk of incisional complications. In the author's opinion, the cosmetic result is superior compared with the traditional open approach because of the smaller incisions required with the tenoscopic technique. In addition, the ability to transect the accessory ligament of the DDFT in situ with tenoscopic visualization avoids the need to dissect and exteriorize the ligament to ensure that all fibers of the accessory ligament of the DDFT are transected. This can potentially reduce postoperative scar tissue formation at the surgical site. Disadvantages compared with the traditional open approach include prerequisite experience with arthroscopic/tenoscopic procedures, need for advanced instrumentation and therefore increased cost of the procedure, and the potential for iatrogenic damage to surrounding tissues, such as the medial neurovascular bundle, DDFT, or the suspensory ligament.

The technique has been performed in a total of 17 horses that presented for the surgical treatment of flexural deformity of the distal interphalangeal joint (abstract presented at the 2016 Veterinary Orthopedic Society meeting). Mean age of horses was 6.7 months (range 4–16 months) at the time of presentation. The accessory ligament of the DDFT was successfully transected using the tenoscopic approach to the distal carpal flexor sheath in 20 forelimbs of 17 horses. Surgery time from incision to suture placement was approximately 30 minutes per limb. No surgical complications occurred, and all surgical incisions healed primarily. On follow-up, the flexural deformity of the distal phalangeal joint was completely corrected or greatly improved in all horses, and an excellent cosmetic result at the surgical site was observed in all cases (**Fig. 8**). All owners were pleased with the cosmetic result of the procedure and indicated that they would request the same technique in future cases if indicated. The author has successfully performed the minimally invasive tenoscopic approach for desmotomy of the accessory ligament of the DDFT of foals as young as 2 weeks of age; however, it is considerably more difficult than in older foals and weanlings.

Clinical improvement generally occurs immediately following surgery regardless of the technique, and support bandaging should be continued for an additional 30 days following suture removal. The author feels that this is beneficial in minimizing the surgical site scar tissue formation, especially with the traditional open technique. Corrective trimming/shoeing should also be implemented at this time, especially in older horses.

Deep digital flexor tendon tenotomy

In severe and/or chronic cases, a DDFT tenotomy may be required because changes in the joint capsule and peritendinous soft tissue attachments "locks" the digit in its flexed state and is refractory to the effects of accessory ligament of the DDFT desmotomy.[26] Techniques for DDFT tenotomy have been previously described.[33–36] Performing the tenotomy at the pastern level results in more extension through the distal interphalangeal joint.

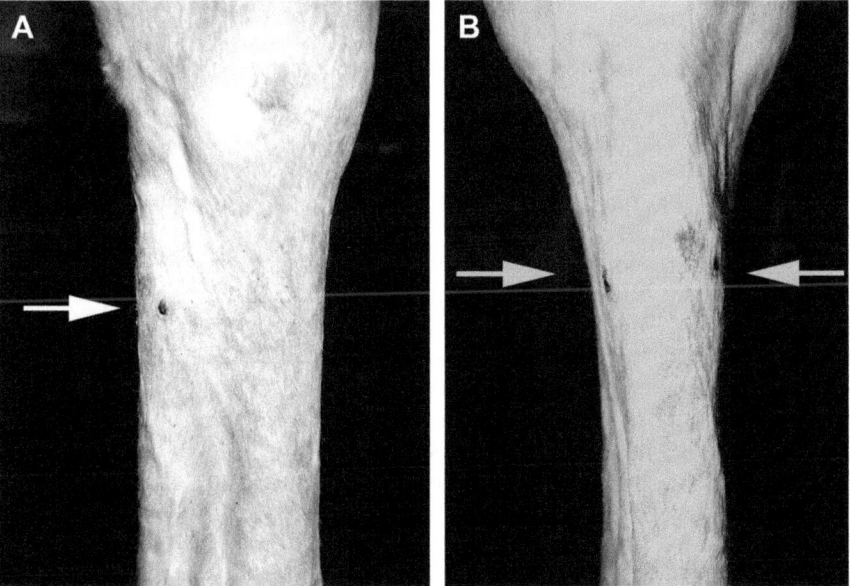

Fig. 8. Lateral (*A*) and palmar (*B*) images of typical surgical site appearance (*arrows*) 30 days following minimally invasive tenoscopic approach for desmotomy of the accessory ligament of the DDFT.

OUTCOME

Previous reports suggest that the prognosis for success in horses treated after 1 year of age were not as good when compared with horses treated at a younger age.[30,37,38] It was generally thought that surgical intervention in horses greater than 1 year of age did not have as good an outcome as that of younger horses. A recent retrospective study in 15 horses with ages between 2 and 6 years with flexural deformity of the distal interphalangeal joint that underwent desmotomy of the accessory ligament of the DDFT had a similar prognosis as that reported in horses less than 1 year of age when treated.[39] Horses that require DDFT tenotomy are unable to withstand the rigors of performance; however, some have been able to be used for light riding.

SUMMARY

Flexural deformities are classified as congenital or acquired, and their cause is complex and commonly multifactorial. Flexural deformity of the distal interphalangeal joint is frequently acquired, typically develops during periods of rapid growth in young horses, and is commonly bilateral with one limb often more severely affected. Flexural deformities are readily observable; however, a thorough physical examination is important in order to identify causative factors.

Flexural deformity of the distal interphalangeal joint is seen during a predictable window of development in foals, but can develop or worsen in any age of horse.[19] This condition is classified as stage I and II, with stage II being more severe and subsequently having a worse prognosis for long-term resolution. Because flexural deformity of the distal interphalangeal joint can develop quickly in rapidly growing foals and can be difficult to treat, early recognition is critical for successful resolution. Minimally invasive tenoscopic accessory ligament of the DDFT desmotomy can result in an earlier return to exercise and improved cosmetic result.

SUPPLEMENTARY DATA

Supplementary data related to this article can be found at http://dx.doi.org/10.1016/j.cveq.2017.03.003.

REFERENCES

1. O'Grady SE. Flexural deformities of the distal interphalangeal joint (clubfeet). Equine Vet Educ 2012;24(5):260–8.
2. Fackelman GE. Deformities of the appendicular skeleton. In: Jennings Paul BJ, editor. The practice of large animal surgery. Philadelphia: Saunders; 1984. p. 950–82.
3. Kidd J, Barr A. Flexural deformities in foals. Equine Vet Educ 2002;14:311–21.
4. Hunt RJ, Acvs D. Management of Clubfoot in Horses: Foals to Adults. Available at: http://www.ivis.org. Accessed June 13, 2016.
5. Auer JA. Flexural limb deformities. In: Auer JA, Stick JA, editors. Equine surgery. Philadelphia: Saunders; 2006. p. 1150–65.
6. Ruggles AJ, McIlwraith CW. Management of angular and flexural disorders in foals. Proc AAEP Focus Meeting: First Year Life 2008;2008:60–7.
7. Schramme MC, Labens R. Diseases of the foot and distal limbs. In: Mair TS, Love S, Schumacher J, et al, editors. Equine medicine, surgery and reproduction. 2nd edition. St Louis (MO): Saunders Elsevier; 2013. p. 329–68.
8. Trumble TN. Orthopedic disorders in neonatal foals. Vet Clin North Am Equine Pract 2005;21(2):357–85, vi.

9. Embertson RM. Congenital abnormalities of tendons and ligaments. Vet Clin North Am Equine Pract 1994;10(2):351–64.

10. Lokai MD, Meyer RJ. Preliminary observations on oxytetracycline treatment of congenital flexural deformities in foals. Mod Vet Pract 1985;66:237–9.

11. Lokai MD. Case selection for medical management of congenital flexural deformities in foals. Equine Pract 1992;14:23–5.

12. Hartzel DK, Arnoczky SP, Kilfoyle SJ, et al. Myofibroblasts in the accessory ligament (distal check ligament) and the deep digital flexor tendon of foals. Am J Vet Res 2001;62(6):823–7.

13. Arnoczky SP, Lavagnino M, Gardner KL, et al. In vitro effects of oxytetracycline on matrix metalloproteinase-1 mRNA expression and on collagen gel contraction by cultured myofibroblast obtained from the accessory ligament of foals. Am J Vet Res 2004;65(4):491–6.

14. Wintz LR, Lavagnino M, Gardner KL, et al. Age-dependent effects of systemic administration of oxytetracycline on the viscoelastic properties of rat tail tendons as a mechanistic basis for pharmacological treatment of flexural limb deformities in foals. Am J Vet Res 2012;73(12):1951–6.

15. Vivrette S, Cowgill LD, Pascoe J, et al. Hemodialysis for treatment of oxytetracycline-induced acute renal failure in a neonatal foal. J Am Vet Med Assoc 1993;203(1):105–7.

16. Madison JB, Garber JL, Rice B, et al. Effect of oxytetracycline on metacarpophalangeal and distal interphalangeal joint angles in newborn foals. J Am Vet Med Assoc 1994;204(2):246–9. Available at: http://www.ncbi.nlm.nih.gov/pubmed/8144385. Accessed June 14, 2016.

17. Mc Ilwraith CW. Diseases and problems of tendons, ligaments and tendon sheaths. In: Stashak T, editor. Adams' lameness in horses. 4th edition. Philadelphia: Lea & Febiger; 1987. p. 447–81.

18. Levine DG. The normal and abnormal equine neonatal musculoskeletal system. Vet Clin North Am Equine Pract 2015;31(3):601–13.

19. Floyd A. Deformities of the limb and their relevance to the foot. In: Floyd AE, Mansmann RA, editors. Equine podiatry. 1st edition. St Louis (MO): Saunders Elsevier; 2007. p. 205–23.

20. Redden RF. Hoof capsule distortion: understanding the mechanisms as a basis for rational management. Vet Clin Equine 2003;19:443–62.

21. O'Grady SE. How to manage the club foot - birth to maturity. Proc AAEP 2014;60: 62–72.

22. Watts AE. Treatment of angular and flexural limb. Proc AAEP Focus Meeting: First Year Life 2014;25–8.

23. Lose MP, Hopkins EJ. Correction of contracted tendon in a filly foal by desmotomy of the inferior check ligament. Vet Med Small Anim Clin 1977;72(8): 1349–53. Available at: http://www.ncbi.nlm.nih.gov/pubmed/242885. Accessed June 5, 2016.

24. McIlwraith CW, Fessler JF. Evaluation of inferior check ligament desmotomy for treatment of acquired flexor tendon contracture in the horse. J Am Vet Med Assoc 1978;172(3):293–8.

25. Sønnichsen HV. Subcarpal check ligament desmotomy for the treatment of contracted deep flexor tendon in foals. Equine Vet J 1982;14(3):256–7.

26. Fackelman GE, Auer JA, Orsini J, et al. Surgical treatment of severe flexural deformity of the distal interphalangeal joint in young horses. J Am Vet Med Assoc 1983;182(9):949–52.

27. Baxter GM. Flexural deformities. In: Baxter GM, editor. Adams and Stashak's lameness in horses. 6th edition. West Sussex (United Kingdom): Wiley-Blackwell; 2011. p. 1145–54.

28. Adams S, Santschi E. Management of congenital and acquired flexural limb deformities. Proc AAEP 2000;46:117–25.

29. Kidd JA. Flexural limb deformities. In: Auer JA, Stick JA, editors. Equine surgery. 4th edition. St Louis (MO): Elsevier Inc; 2012. p. 1221–39.

30. White NA 2nd. Ultrasound-guided transection of the accessory ligament of the deep digital flexor muscle (distal check ligament desmotomy) in Horses. Vet Surg 1995;24(5):373–8.

31. Tnibar A, Christophersen MT, Lindegaard C. Minimally invasive desmotomy of the accessory ligament of the deep digital flexor tendon in horses. Equine Vet Educ 2010;22(3):141–5.

32. Caldwell FJ, Waguespack RW. Evaluation of a tenoscopic approach for desmotomy of the accessory ligament of the deep digital flexor tendon in horses. Vet Surg 2011;40(3):266–71.

33. Allen D, White NA, Foerner JF, et al. Surgical management of chronic laminitis in horses: 13 cases (1983-1985). J Am Vet Med Assoc 1986;189(12):1604–6.

34. Hunt RJ, Allen D, Baxter GM, et al. Mid-metacarpal deep digital flexor tenotomy in the management of refractory laminitis in horses. Vet Surg 1991;20(1):15–20.

35. Eastman TG, Honnas CM, Hague BA, et al. Deep digital flexor tenotomy as a treatment for chronic laminitis in horses: 35 cases (1988-1997). J Am Vet Med Assoc 1999;214(4):517–9.

36. Waguespack RW, Caldwell F, Vaughan JT. How to Perform a Modified Standing Deep Digital Flexor Tenotomy at the Level of the Proximal Interphalangeal Joint. 2009. Available at: www.ivis.org. Accessed June 9, 2016.

37. Wagner PC, Grant BD, Kaneps AJ, et al. Long-term results of desmotomy of the accessory ligament of the deep digital flexor tendon (distal check ligament) in horses. J Am Vet Med Assoc 1985;187(12):1351–3.

38. Stick JA, Nickels FA, Williams MA. Long-term effects of desmotomy of the accessory ligament of the deep digital flexor muscle in standardbreds: 23 cases (1979-1989). J Am Vet Med Assoc 1992;200(8):1131–2.

39. Yiannikouris S, Schneider RK, Acvs D, et al. Desmotomy of the accessory ligament of the deep digital flexor tendon in the forelimb of 24 horses 2 years and older. Vet Surg 2011;40:272–6.

Flexural Limb Deformities of the Carpus and Fetlock in Foals

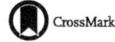 CrossMark

Earl M. Gaughan, DVM

KEYWORDS

- Flexural deformity • Foal • Carpus • Fetlock

KEY POINTS

- Flexural deformities of the carpus and fetlock can be present at birth or develop with growth, or secondary to injury or disease.
- Medical and physical treatment directed at stretching the limb deformities to correct conformation is usually successful.
- In chronic or very severe cases, surgery may be required.
- Failure to respond to treatment carries a poor prognosis for future soundness and athleticism.

INTRODUCTION

Flexural limb deformities in foals can be characterized as congenital, present at birth, or acquired, implying that an affected foal had normal limb conformation at birth and the flexural deformity developed with time and growth.[1] A misnomer that has been associated with flexural deformity of equine limbs at any age is "contracted tendon(s)." The term "contracted tendons" is misdirected, because tendon tissue does not have contractile properties; any active "contracture" must be initiated by muscle tissue proximal to the tendon and tendinous insertion. Congenital flexural deformities in foals most likely originate from uterine position during fetal development, abnormal development of the fetus, or a disease or malnutrition state in the mare. Acquired flexural limb deformities in foals, before weaning, can occur from postural changes due to pain in the affected limb (physitis) or developmental orthopedic disease resulting in pain or abnormal skeletal development. Flexural deformities also can occur secondary to injury and subsequent disuse of the affected limb. Age and breed-dependent variability in limb deformities may exist as well.[2] Close observation of an individual foal

There are no conflicts of interest or funding sources to report.
Merck Animal Health, 2 Giralda Farms, Madison, NJ 07940, USA
E-mail address: earl.gaughan@merck.com

Vet Clin Equine 33 (2017) 331–342
http://dx.doi.org/10.1016/j.cveq.2017.03.004
vetequine.theclinics.com

from birth to weaning and on through final skeletal development is important to adult musculoskeletal health and potential athletic ability.[3]

Flexural deformities with joint hyperextension also can occur, resulting in back-at-knee conformation and/or dropped fetlocks. These deformities are nearly always congenital and are unlikely to be acquired except in the cases of prolonged contralateral limb lameness, which is discussed in the article (See Ashlee E. Watts article, "Septic Arthritis, Physitis and Osteomyelitis in Foals," elsewhere in this issue). When congenital laxity is present, it is most commonly the fetlocks and can be only the hind fetlocks or all 4 fetlocks. When the carpi are affected, the fetlocks commonly are affected as well. Farriery and methods to protect the musculoskeletal structures while the foal "outgrows" joint laxity are discussed in the article (See Michelle C. Coleman article, "Orthopedic Conditions of the Premature and Dysmature Foal," elsewhere in this issue).

PATIENT EVALUATION OVERVIEW

Diagnosis of a flexural limb deformity of the carpus or fetlock is usually straightforward and based mostly on visual and physical examination determinations. Congenital flexural deformities may offer some challenges to full understanding, as the degree of deformity may not be readily apparent if an affected foal cannot stand at an expected time after birth. Therefore, it is important to complete a thorough physical examination on a neonatal foal, including limb palpation; range of motion assessments for carpus, fetlock, and digital joints; and observe for standing conformation.

A complete understanding of the systemic status of a foal affected with a flexural limb deformity is essential for a final positive outcome.[1] It is important to understand that the physical and medical treatments of a flexural limb deformity are not without repercussions for the foal. Immunocompromise of a neonate can be complicated by the imposition of the added stresses of manipulation and medication that may be required to address limb deformities. Parallel to understanding and monitoring systemic health, care of affected foals should ensure normal nursing or nutritional behaviors, as well as avoidance of the complications associated with prolonged recumbency. Failure of an affected foal to respond to treatment, improve conformation, and to thrive, is often an indication of continued poor likelihood of a successful outcome.

Congenital flexural limb deformities of the carpi are quite common and are often self-limiting. However, veterinary evaluation of severity and any need for intervention are important at the time of postfoaling neonatal examination (**Fig. 1**). Normal carpal conformation should be noted as a vertical, continuous association of the antebrachium, carpus, and metacarpus. Any cranial deviation or flexing forward of the carpus, therefore creating an angulation centered at the carpus, should be considered abnormal. (Any caudally directed abnormal position of the carpus is probably due to laxity on the flexor surface and should be carefully observed and managed as well.) Similar to the physical examination of an angular limb deformity centered at the carpus, the reducibility of a carpal flexural deformity should be determined at first examination. With a foal standing or recumbent, the metacarpus can be held in the palm of one hand while the other hand is used to gently place caudally oriented pressure from the dorsum of the carpus. Palpation of the flexor surface may indicate which tissues tighten. This has been described as a means of determining which tissues are responsible for the flexural deformity.[1] However, specificity may not be obvious from palpation alone. If the carpal and limb confirmation can be readily reduced to normal, the flexural deformity is reducible and may be corrected with a conservative treatment plan. If the attempts to reduce the flexural deformity are not successful, or a foal cannot stand because of the magnitude of limb deformity, additional

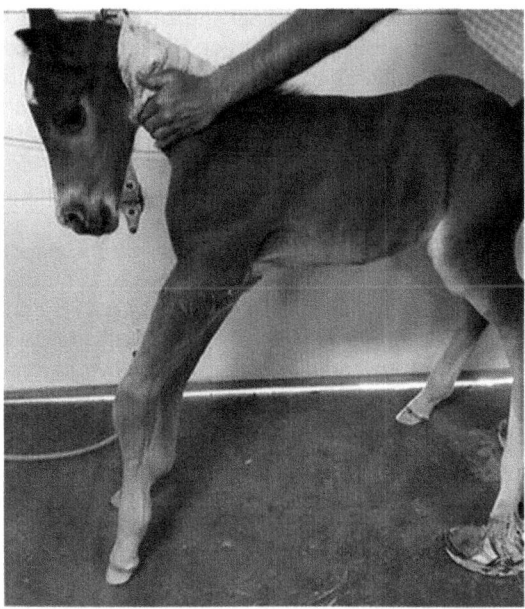

Fig. 1. A 3-day-old foal affected with flexural deformity of the carpus. The deformity is not manually reducible and will require medical and physical treatment.

diagnostic measures and a more aggressive therapeutic plan, which usually includes splinting, are likely required.

Acquired flexural deformities of the carpal region of young, growing horses are not as common as deformities in the more distal limb. This appears to particularly be the case for foals after the first month of life, through weaning, and beyond. Development of flexural deformity of the carpus, after a foal was noted to have normal carpal conformation at birth, can be the result of weight-bearing adjustment after injury or a reduction in normal limb "engagement." Reduced weight bearing can be secondary to the presence of a painful site in the limb, often in the form of physitis. However, this painful origin of a flexural limb deformity is much more commonly observed in the fetlock and distal interphalangeal joint regions than in the carpus.

A structural fault that can create a flexural deformity in the carpal region of young foals is rupture of the common digital extensor tendon (CDET). Rupture of the CDET can occur unilaterally or bilaterally. The characteristic observations are a dorsally flexed carpus accompanied by lateral longitudinal swelling over the dorsal surface of the affected carpus. The swelling is typically nonpainful and effusive, as excess fluid is contained in the tendon sheath. Rupture of the CDET appears to occur at the musculotendinous junction, which can be palpated percutaneously and visualized with ultrasound. Required treatment is usually minimal and as described. Prognosis for return to normal is favorable.[1] When there is rupture of the CDET secondary to moderate to severe carpal flexural deformity, more aggressive therapy (ie, splinting) might be required.

Flexural deformities centered at the fetlock can be classified as type 1 or type 2, depending on severity. Type 1 deformities indicate that the limb at the fetlock is postured between normal angulation and up to vertical alignment of the metacarpus to the phalanges. Type 2 flexural deformity of the fetlock indicates that the fetlock is cranially displaced past vertical and is "over" at the fetlock. This classification system has been helpful in description as well as for prognosis, as type 2 deformities are much more difficult to correct than type 1.[4] Flexural deformities at the fetlock have been described as the result of "contraction of the superficial digital flexor tendon," but as previously described, this is an inaccurate understanding of the pathogenesis of this type of limb deformity, because tendon tissue does not contract, and it is more appropriately termed shortening of the musculotendinous unit.

Congenital flexural deformities of the fetlock are often associated with similar abnormal conformation in the carpal region. Occasionally, a fetlock deformity will be observed as a sole entity, but examination of complete limb conformation, in and out of weight bearing, is important to understand current skeletal status. If a fetlock flexural deformity can be manually reduced, a conservative treatment plan will likely be successful gaining normal conformation. If not reducible, the fetlock region will likely require aggressive physical and medical management, including splinting and potentially surgical intervention. The conformation of the distal interphalangeal joint and foot should be carefully noted at this time, as often fetlock and foot flexural deformities can occur in concert.

Acquired flexural deformities of the fetlock in foals between birth and weaning may not be as common as deformities noted to occur after weaning, during the substantial and rapid growth phases that occur between months 4 and 14 of a young horse's life. Acquired fetlock deformities can occur secondarily to prolonged lack of normal weight bearing and engagement of the flexural surface tissues in the affected limb (**Fig. 2**). This is most often due to pain from the physeal region of the distal radius. This

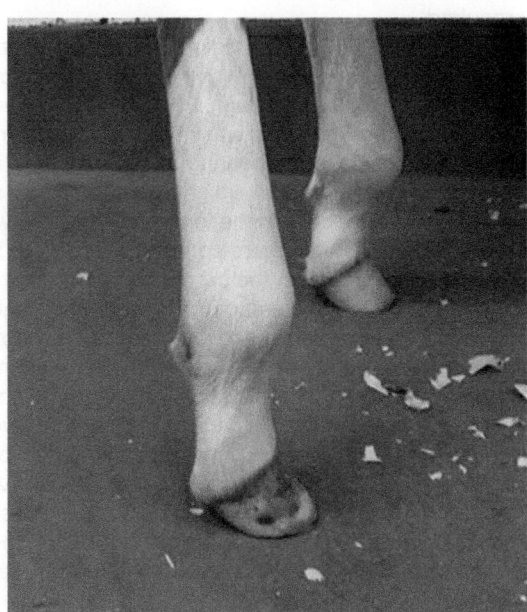

Fig. 2. A young foal with a flexural deformity of the fetlock. The deformity was acquired after normal conformation was noted at birth. Medical and physical treatment will be required for conformation correction and surgical treatment may be required if more conservative efforts fail.

same phenomenon can occur after an injury or other local, regional, or systemic orthopedic disease.

DIAGNOSIS

Diagnosis of congenital flexural limb deformities is most often defined by physical examination observations.[1] Physical impressions can be augmented by imaging, and further assessments of an individual foal's maturity and immune status. Radiographic assessment of the carpus and fetlock may be indicated if skeletal immaturity is suspected. Radiographic identification of incompletely developed carpal cuboidal, metacarpal, phalangeal, or sesamoid bones are covered in the article (See Michelle C. Coleman article, "Orthopedic Conditions of the Premature and Dysmature Foal," elsewhere in this issue).

Acquired fetlock and carpal deformities may require similar diagnostic efforts to fully understand the current status of affected limbs and to make the best therapeutic plan. Radiography, and possibly other imaging modalities, can help understand skeletal structure and potential sources of the developing flexural deformity. It is important to not limit the imaging target to the site of the deformity. For instance, flexural deformity of a fetlock, may have its origin from pain at the distal radial physis. Therefore, complete imaging studies may include the affected fetlock as well as the distal radial physeal region of the same limb. Similar consideration should be taken if a septic nidus in the affected limb is suspected, as pain can certainly originate in such a site, yet it may be distant from the flexurally deformed portion of the limb. Blood chemistry and cellular analysis also can be helpful when indicated by physical and imaging examination findings.

PHARMACOLOGIC TREATMENT OPTIONS

The obvious treatment goal for foals with carpal and flexural deformities is to correct the abnormalities and develop normal and functional limb conformation. Several pharmacologic treatment options can be considered for a foal with a fetlock or carpal flexural deformity. Perhaps the most common first consideration is directed at creating relaxation of potential tension forces on the flexor surface of the limb. Intravenous oxytetracycline (44 mg/kg or 1–3 g in 250–500 mL saline, 1 to 3 times in the first week of life) has been associated with the chelation of circulating calcium, which in turn reduces muscle contractility.[1,3] The result is less muscular tension on the flexor tendons and an increased opportunity to stretch the flexor surface and create or return to normal, correct limb conformation.[5] Oxytetracycline also has been associated with a dose-dependent reduction in matrix metalloproteinase mRNA expression in equine myofibroblasts, allowing tissue elongation.[6,7] Diazepam (0.05–0.44 mg/kg intravenous [IV])[8] also has been administered to reduce anxiety in an affected foal and to secondarily produce some relaxation in the affected limb. Alfa-2 agonist agents (xylazine 0.1–0.5 mg/kg IV, 0.25–1.0 mg/kg intramuscular [IM][8]; detomidine 10–40 μg/kg IV; 1–5 μg/kg IM[8]) can be administered to sedate a foal and therefore achieve some short-term musculoskeletal relaxation that can facilitate other, physical manipulations. Butorphanol tartrate (0.01–0.04 mg/kg)[8] can enhance sedation and provide some short-term analgesia during limb manipulation.

Another pharmacologic consideration is the judicious administration of nonsteroidal anti-inflammatory drugs (NSAIDs) in an attempt to reduce inflammation and pain that may be inhibiting a foal from assuming normal conformation.[6] The use of systemic NSAIDs is probably best used in older foals, out of the first month of life; however, when determined to be appropriate, NSAIDs can be administered safely to neonatal foals. The use of NSAIDs for foals affected with carpal or fetlock flexural deformity can assist other treatment modalities by helping to maintain comfort and counter some of the expected pain that can accompany the physical therapy aspects of treatment. All cautions, of minimal dosing and duration, should be observed to avoid the potential complications associated with NSAID use in foals. Both intravenous and oral administration can be performed with success. Ketoprofen (1.1–2.2 mg/kg IV),[8] phenylbutazone (1.1 mg/kg, once to twice per day),[8] flunixin meglumine (1 mg/kg once to twice per day),[8] and firocoxib (0.1 mg/kg by mouth, after 2.0 mg/kg loading dose)[8] have all produced the desirable effects of reducing inflammation and pain while addressing flexural limb deformities in foals.[1] Gastrointestinal mucosal protectants should be considered parallel to NSAID administration in foals.[1]

NONPHARMACOLOGIC TREATMENT OPTIONS
Shoeing and Trimming Considerations

Fundamental practices of protecting the toes, and providing variations of heel elevation and or toe extension can provide support to efforts to correct conformation in foals affected with flexural deformities of the carpus and fetlock. The specific indications and techniques are discussed in the article (See Fred J. Caldwell article, "Flexural Deformity of the Distal Interphalangeal Joint," elsewhere in this issue).

Physical Therapy

Mild and reducible flexural deformities of the fetlock and carpus may be amenable to physical stretching exercises. With a recumbent or standing foal, the affected joint location can be stretched to, or toward, normal conformation by holding the limb distal to the affected site and pushing against the affected joint. Several recommendations have been made for how to stretch, but the most effective techniques appear to apply slowly increasing stretch pressures over extended periods. Stretch to the point of resistance or resentment by the foal and holding that position for 15 to 30 seconds, followed by relaxation, and then repetition for 10 to 15 minutes 3 to 6 times per day has been successful in correcting mild carpal and fetlock flexural deformities in neonatal and very young foals.[3] Simultaneous massage of the caudal surface antebrachial musculature may help some foals relax while performing stretching exercises.

Exercise Management

Normal mare and foal behavior determines that the foal follow the mare, and therefore the foal may control its own exercise only when it simply cannot keep up with the mare or stand at all. Therefore, controlling the exercise allowed to the mare, and the foal, is an important consideration when working to correct flexural limb deformities. Excessive movement and weight bearing on limbs that are painful, or cannot structurally support body weight, can compound the excessively flexed conformation, and the cycle can become very difficult to reverse. A serviceable rule is to confine a mare and foal if the foal is made more painful or the flexural limb deformity made worse, with anything more than stall rest.

The converse to rest is certainly a viable option and a successful tool in the correction of flexural limb deformities. If a foal is determined to be comfortable enough, and able to tolerate some exercise, then regular, controlled walking can apply the strain of weight bearing to the flexor surfaces and help stretch a limb toward more normal conformation. Exercise, when well controlled and tolerated by the foal, can be a substantial component of flexural limb deformity treatment. When not controlled and poorly tolerated, exercising an affected foal, can have very negative results.

Complementary/Integrative Therapies

Acupuncture may have a serviceable role in the treatment of flexural limb deformities. If acupuncture can result in local, regional, and systemic analgesia and possibly tranquilization, perhaps the benefits of these results can be obtained without the concerns for pharmaceutical administration. Consultation with a regular practitioner of complementary/integrative therapies may add another dimension to the treatment approaches to carpal and fetlock flexural deformities.

External Coaptation

External coaptation in the form of a well-padded splint is the most common and reliable means of reducing and maintaining complete, or progressive, correction of carpal and fetlock flexural deformities in foals. Fiberglass casts also can be applied for rigid coaptation, and can be helpful in the management of flexural deformities, but the need for removal and replacement typically makes the use of casts cumbersome and expensive. Splints applied over bandages are simple to produce and place on the affected limb and control costs when rigid support is desired.

Splints can be made out of various materials. PVC pipe can be cut to length to customize fit. PVC pipe of 4-inch to 8-inch diameter works for most foals. The author prefers to cut the determined length of PVC pipe in half, lengthwise, to achieve better fit of the limb within the interior of a splint; making 2 splints from 1 tube of PVC pipe. It is recommended to select a diameter of PVC pipe that will allow good fit over adequate padded bandage material. Although more than 2 splints can be cut from a single length of PVC pipe, the narrower splints are more difficult to maintain in desired position and are also prone to bending.

Fiberglass cast tape also can be used to make a custom splint. Appropriate bandage material should be applied first, typically in Modified Robert Jones fashion. Cast tape can then be applied in a lengthwise manner to establish the rigid component of the bandage-splint. Enough cast tape (7–8 layers) needs to be applied such that the foal is supported, the extension pressures on the limb maintained, and splint breakage can be avoided. Allowing the cast material to cure, or harden, for at least 20 minutes before final application to the affected limb can minimize the chances of inappropriate bending or breakage of the newly formed splint.

GENERAL GUIDELINES FOR SPLINT APPLICATION

Splints should be considered when an affected foal has difficulty standing and moving normally. Rigid support for a foal that spends excessive time in recumbency can allow more consistent standing, nursing behavior, ambulation, and better stretch of the abnormal limb(s).

Splints over bandages are used for mild, moderate, or severe deformities, and the duration of splinting will be somewhat dictated by the severity of the deformity and the age of the foal. Many times, the deformity can be corrected with or without the use of splints, and the use of splints is determined by the individual experiences of the treating veterinarian and the owner. However, splints are absolutely required when the foal either cannot or will not stand to nurse with normal frequency and duration.

Best results from splint application are achieved when rigid support is placed on the flexor surface. The splint should bridge the site of flexural deformity with as much rigid support proximal and distal as possible, which can assist in gaining mechanical advantage. Placing the splint on the flexor surface allows for "pulling" the abnormally flexed site into the rigid column of the splint. This also appears to help the foal adjust to the rigid, fixed position of the limb and maintain the ability to be ambulatory.

HOW OFTEN SHOULD SPLINTS BE REMOVED OR ADJUSTED?

Several recommendations for splint application and management have been made through the years. This is likely due to individual experiences and several factors, such as severity of the problem, age of the foal, and the ability of the person responsible for splint application. An early recommendation was to have splints in place for 6 to 12 hours and then removed for 6 to 12 hours. This would in turn be repeated until an affected limb achieves conformational correction.[3] Others have recommended 24-hour splint placement followed by a splint and bandage change to evaluate limb health and flexural deformity correction. The key point is that recommendations for removing or adjusting splints are made to prevent decubital erosion of the skin at splint-induced pressure points. The other key point in determining the splinting duration is to avoid inducing overrelaxation and laxity of the splinted joints. For the most common carpal and fetlock flexural deformities, splints placed on the flexor surface for up to 5 days have been successful.[1] The success of the prolonged splint placement is predicated on adequate padding, placed to avoid movement or slippage and securely fit to the limb and splint. This appears to help avoid skin erosion and compression wounds induced by a splint.

Bandage-Splint Layers

1 Primary layer: roll cotton or cast padding. Thickness adequate to fill the interior lumen of the chosen splint material (**Fig. 3**)
2 Secondary layer: Cotton roll gauze

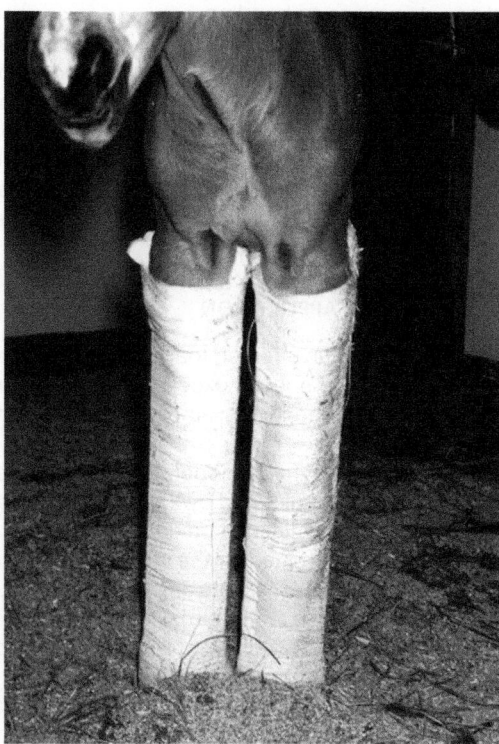

Fig. 3. Adequate, properly applied cotton padding placed to support PVC splints to address bilateral carpal flexural deformity.

3 Elastic tape: Evenly applied to avoid irregular compression and distal bandage slippage
4 Splint
5 Elastic tape to secure splint to the bandage material
6 Wear-resistant tape (duct tape): optional, but can help improve the duration of the bandage-splint and produce a moisture barrier

Padded bandage should extend proximal and distal to the extent of the splint. This can help reduce splint migration and potential skin injury from the splint.

Splint for a carpal flexural deformity:
1. Splint length should reach from the elbow to the proximal sesamoid bones at the fetlock. Leaving the digit free to move and bear weight can assist the splint in application of extension forces. The splint must be well secured to avoid distal migration and need for adjustment or replacement.

Splint for fetlock flexural deformities:
1. Splint length may be variable. Often a full limb splint (from elbow to ground surface) can be best for rapid correction. An alternative is a splint that reaches from proximal metacarpus to the ground.
2. The foot should be exposed for weight bearing.
3. Additional padding should be placed between the splint and the palmar surface of the pastern. This will help push the digit dorsally and maintain extension strain. With the assistance of the foot in weight bearing, this splint support will have better success than full splint coverage of the fetlock and digit.

Dynamic Splints

Dynamic splints are designed to place forces that act to stretch the limb such that correction of flexural deformities can be corrected. These splints have been applied to angular limb deformities and some veterinarians also use them for flexural deformities in young foals. The splints are designed to place contact and pressure in minimized fashion on specific locations on the limb depending on the deformity being addressed. Adequate padding on compressed sites is vital to avoid decubital lesion development.[3]

COMBINATION THERAPIES

Best results in correction of flexural limb deformities of the carpus and fetlock are likely obtained using external coaptation, physical therapy, and pharmacologic treatments in combination. The administration of oxytetracycline and an analgesic agent can enhance the ability of a bandage-splint to place an affected limb in more normal conformation. This treatment combination can maintain limb position while the desired flexor surface "stretch" occurs and also enhance the foal's discomfort. Close attention to the systemic health of the foal is crucial for overall success, as this is a stressful time for an affected foal at a life stage that can be negatively affected by these imposed stresses.

SURGICAL TREATMENT OPTIONS

Surgical treatment of flexural deformities of the carpus and fetlock is not commonly indicated or required in young foals. Most affected individuals respond to analgesic medication, muscle relaxation, physical therapy, splint application, or combination therapy. Young foals appear readily responsive to more conservative measures directed at stretching affected limbs to achieve conformation correction.

Rarely, flexural deformities of the fetlock may require surgical treatment. Proximal check desmotomy can allow some improved ability to improve fetlock angulation toward normal. With increasing severity, fetlock flexural deformities may benefit from also performing a distal check desmotomy at the same time as transection of the proximal check ligament.[9] Typically, continued utilization of an external splint will be required to correct fetlock conformation after surgery.

Flexural deformities of the carpus require surgical treatment even less frequently than those of the fetlock. Transection of accessory ligament to the superficial digital flexor tendon and/or the tendons of the ulnaris lateralis and the flexor carpi ulnaris may release the restrictive forces on the flexor surface of the carpus and allow limb straightening.[1,10] Transection, or release, of the retinaculum that forms the carpal canal may allow some improved response to rigid external splintage. As a sole treatment procedure, carpal canal release is not likely to result in correction of carpal flexural deformity.

TREATMENT RESISTANCE/COMPLICATIONS

Persistence with physical therapies, including splintage, supported by appropriate pharmaceutical utilization, is typically met with good results. Readily establishing corrected limb conformation can result in a favorable expectation for an affected foal to return to its expected athletic future. Decubital pressure erosion of the skin is the most common complication of splint application in foals; therefore, careful splinting and appropriate and well-padded bandage management is very important. If correction is not obtained with conservative therapies, surgical treatment can be attempted and may improve the opportunities for successful resolution of flexural conformation faults. Failure to correct carpal and fetlock flexural deformities should be an indication to reevaluate diagnostic observations. Congenital abnormalities, like arthrogryposis, can be difficult to correct and can mimic simple flexural deformities.

Severe, irreducible congenital flexural deformities may not respond to physical, medical, or surgical treatment and can be difficult to correct. Staged treatment is often required, as rigid splint application or cast utilization may not be possible in the early stages. Foals with severely deformed limbs often are coincidently affected with systemic weakness, immunocompromise, and potentially other concurrent disease. It is essential to address these systemic challenges as a priority while the flexural limb deformities are treated. Weakness may assist limb conformation correction with physical therapy (stretching). If an affected limb cannot be placed in external supports, the frequency of physical therapy may need to be increased to 4 or more times per day. A foal that responds to both systemic medical treatment and to physical therapy may allow splint placement and more typical therapies for flexural limb deformities. A foal that does not respond to treatment, such that splint placement cannot be accomplished, and maintains severe limb deformity, carries a poor prognosis for limb correction and perhaps survival. Secondary musculoskeletal injury can occur as well when the primary flexural deformity does not improve (**Fig. 4**). Protracted incomplete response to treatment, or complete failure of affected limbs to respond, is likely a poor indicator for survival as well.

EVALUATION OF OUTCOME AND LONG-TERM RECOMMENDATIONS

It is uncommon for a young horse to experience recurrence or complications of flexural deformities of the carpus or fetlock once correction has been obtained. When

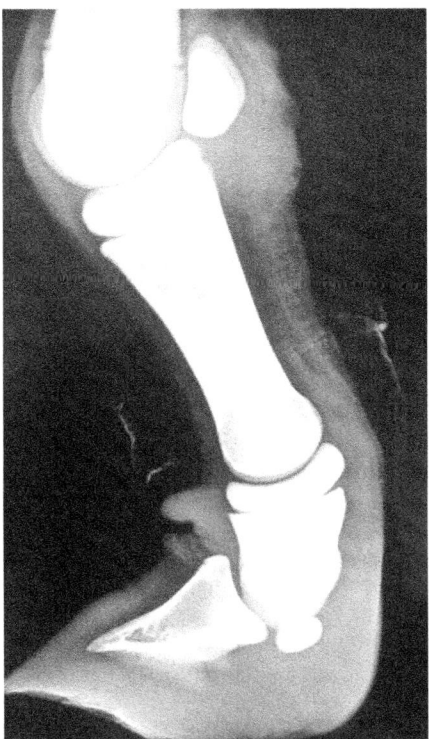

Fig. 4. A lateral radiographic projection of the distal limb of a foal. The film indicates sub-luxation of the distal interphalangeal joint after a fetlock flexural deformity failed to respond to treatment.

these deformities are corrected by the time of weaning, long-term recommendations essentially become those of typical management of a young horse with a continually developing musculoskeletal system. As the rapid phases of skeletal growth begin, and a foal ages toward and after weaning, the discomfort of physitis can occasionally cause the carpal region to bow forward and some "carpal shaking" can be observed. If unaddressed, this postural change can result in recurrence of carpal flexural deformity. Careful observation, timely administration of NSAIDs, and control of exercise usually prevent this conformational change from becoming a persistent problem. Generally, the prognosis for foals affected with carpal and fetlock flexural deformities is favorable for a return to athletic expectations when limb conformation is initially corrected.

SUMMARY

Foals can experience congenital flexural deformity of the carpus and/or fetlock. Foals also can acquire these deformities between birth and weaning as consequences of abnormal skeletal development, rapid growth, and/or pain, which can affect weight bearing. Early recognition and accurate diagnostic understanding can lead to timely and successful treatment. Physical therapies, both "in hand" and with bandages and splintage can support affected limbs while conformation correction occurs. Medical assistance to reduce muscle strain, and reduce pain and anxiety can assist the physical management tools. Foals that respond well and develop normal conformation are considered likely to have normal expectations for future use and athleticism. Foals that do not respond, or incompletely respond to treatment, will not likely have a normal future due to conformational constraints that can be complicated by continued growth and use.

REFERENCES

1. Auer JA, Stick JA. Flexural deformities. In: Auer JA, Stick JA, editors. Equine surgery. 2nd edition. Philadelphia: Saunders; 1999. p. 752–65.
2. Robert C, Valette JP, Denoix JM. Longitudinal development of equine forelimb conformation from birth to weaning in three different horse breeds. Vet J 2013; 198:75–80.
3. Levine DG. The normal and abnormal equine neonatal musculoskeletal system. Vet Clin Equine 2015;31:601–13.
4. Wagner PC, Shires GM, Watrous BJ, et al. Management of acquired flexural deformities of the metacarpophalangeal joint in Equidae. J Am Vet Med Assoc 1985; 187(9):915–8.
5. Wintz LR, Lavagnino M, Gardner KL, et al. Age-dependent effects of systemic administration of oxytetracycline on viscoelastic properties of rat tail tendons as a mechanistic basis for pharmacologic treatment of flexural deformities in foals. Am J Vet Res 2012;73(12):1951–6.
6. Auer JA. Diagnosis and treatment of flexural deformities in foals. In: Auer JA, editor. Clinical techniques in equine practice. St Louis (MO): Elsevier, Inc; 2006. p. 282–95.
7. Arnoczky SP, Lavagnino M, Gardner KL, et al. In vitro effects of oxytetracycline on matrix metalloproteinase-1 mRNA expression and on collagen gel contraction by cultured myofibroblasts obtained from the accessory ligament of foals. Am J Vet Res 2004;65:491–6.
8. Orsini JA, Divers TJ. Appendix 9: equine emergency drugs. In: Orsini JA, Divers TJ, editors. Equine emergencies. St Louis (MO): Elsevier; 2014. p. 835–60.
9. Stick JA, Nickels FA, Williams MA. Long-term effects of desmotomy of the accessory ligament of the deep digital flexor muscle in standardbreds: 23 cases (1979-1989). J Am Vet Med Assoc 1992;200(8):1131–2.
10. Charman RE, Vasey JR. Surgical treatment of carpal flexural deformity in 72 horses. Aust Vet J 2008;86(5):195–9.

Angular Limb Deformities
Growth Augmentation

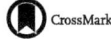

José M. García-López, VMD

KEYWORDS

- Foal • Growth plate • Valgus • Varus • Periosteal transection • Elevation

KEY POINTS

- The most common angular limb deviation seen in the foal include carpal or tarsal valgus and fetlock varus.
- Angular limb deformities (ALDs) or deviations are common in young foals, with most deviations able to self-correct with minimal intervention, including modifications in exercise.
- Trimming of the hoof can be highly effective in cases of mild deviations; for valgus or varus deviations, the lateral or medial aspect of the hoof is trimmed, respectively.
- Hemicircumferential transection and elevation (periosteal stripping procedure) are performed on the concave aspect of the deviation.

ALDs are commonly seen in young foals and are defined as lateral or medial axial deviations of the limb in the frontal plane distal to a particular joint. A carpus valgus deformity refers to a lateral deviation of the limb distal to the carpus in relation to the limb proximal to this joint (**Fig. 1**). On the other hand, a fetlock varus deformity refers to a medial deviation distal to the fetlock in relation to the rest of the limb proximal to the fetlock (**Fig. 2**). Foals affected by a valgus deformity commonly exhibit a toed-out conformation and those affected with varus deformity exhibit a toed-in conformation.

RISK FACTORS

Risk factors commonly associated with ALD include perinatal factors, such as premature birth, twin pregnancy, placentitis, perinatal soft tissue trauma, and flaccidity of the soft tissue structures surrounding the joints.[1-4] These factors can potentially lead to incomplete ossification of the cuboidal bones of the carpi and tarsi (**Fig. 3**) and excessive laxity of the joints. Normally, most foals are born with some degree of limb deviation, mostly due to ligament laxity and muscle weakness, which usually corrects itself

Disclosure Statement: No conflicts or commercial affiliations to disclose.
Department of Clinical Sciences, Cummings School of Veterinary Medicine, Tufts University, 200 Westboro Road, North Grafton, MA 01536, USA
E-mail address: jose.garcia-lopez@tufts.edu

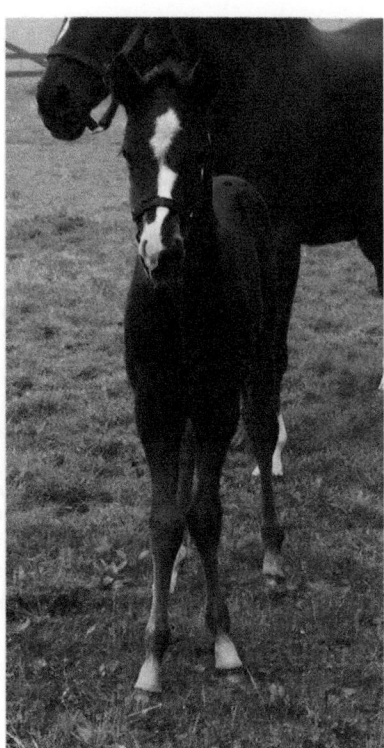

Fig. 1. Frontal view of a foal with bilateral carpus valgus deformity. (*Courtesy of* Dr Gustavo Abuja, LV, DACVS, Rhinebeck Equine Hospital, Rhinebeck, NY.)

as the foal matures and exercises.[1,2,4] If incomplete ossification of the cuboidal bones is present and not adequately recognized, however, affected foals run the risk of having these small bones crushed from exercise and the uneven load that is placed on the joint due to laxity. Once ossification occurs, an ALD results due to the crushing and resulting abnormally shaped cuboidal bones. To minimize this risk, limited and strictly controlled exercise encourages appropriate ossification. If a foal's activity cannot be strictly managed and the foal has moderate strength, sleeve casts are recommended to prevent cuboidal bone crush. Sleeve casts should be changed or removed in 10 days to 14 days in a growing foal. Radiographic re-evaluation every 2 weeks helps determine the length of time a cast is required.[2] Incomplete ossification is discussed by Michelle C. Coleman and Canaan Whitfield-Cargile's article, "Orthopedic Conditions of the Premature and Dysmature Foal," in this issue.

In addition, developmental and acquired factors, such as unbalanced nutrition, excessive growth rate, and excessive exercise and/or trauma, can result in ALD in older foals.[1–3] Crib feeding of foals may lead to excessive grain intake by the dominant foals, creating an imbalance in their diet, in particular, an excess of carbohydrates and protein intake. Nutritional imbalance may cause disproportionate growth across the growth plate, thus causing the deviation. Exercise is an important element in the proper development and growth of foals. If the amount of exercise is excessive, however, this trauma can lead to microfractures and crushing of the growth plate, which cause the development of ALD.[1,2]

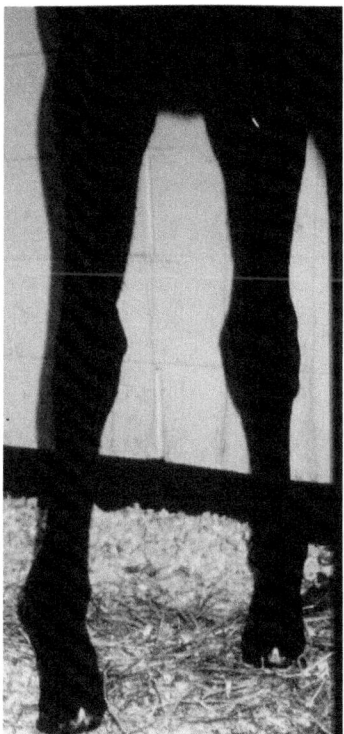

Fig. 2. Frontal view of a foal with marked right front fetlock varus deformity.

CLINICAL EXAMINATION AND RADIOGRAPHY

Deformities can be assessed subjectively by visual examination. The foal should stand as squarely as possible, with the foot directly below the proximal part of the limb. Deviations from this stance exacerbate any deformities that truly present. Repositioning foals several times to evaluate each limb independently is often necessary because they often only stand still for short periods of time. This allows observation of how a foal stands most frequently in a relaxed position. The clinician stands directly in front of the dorsum of the long bones for evaluation of the forelimbs, not necessarily at the front of the toe. The forelimbs can also be evaluated by standing shoulder to shoulder with the foal, looking down the limb toward the ground. The orientation of the toe may be affected by a concurrent rotational deformity, which confounds interpretation. Hind limbs should be evaluated similarly but directly from behind.[2] All limbs also should be evaluated with the foal walking away from and toward the clinician. Breakover is determined for each foot, which may be helpful in deciding the most appropriate way to manage the foal. The entire assessment of a foal should be graded and recorded on video or on paper for future reference.

Radiography provides an objective assessment of angular deformity (**Fig. 4**), but sequential radiography may be unreliable if the obliquity varies. Differences in radiographic projection can result in a misinterpretation of worsening or improvement, which is particularly true when trying to quantify small differences in the angle. Radiography is essential to identify cuboidal injury or malformation (see **Fig. 3**). Such a deformity dramatically worsens a foal's prognosis. Foals with angular deformity

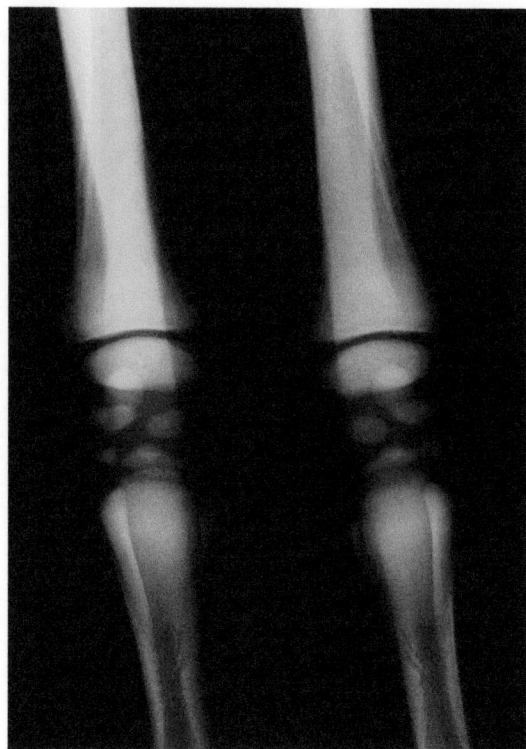

Fig. 3. Dorsopalmar radiographic view of a carpus with mild incomplete ossification of the carpal bones and valgus deformity.

resulting from cuboidal bone abnormalities usually have compromised range of motion, but this often is detected best with a foal in lateral recumbency.[2]

Growth rates are most rapid in the neonate and slow considerably within the first year. Most of the growth from the distal radial and tibial physes is within the first 6 months of age. Most of the growth from the distal third metacarpal (McIII) and third metatarsal (MtIII) bones is within the first 3 months of age. Minimal changes take place beyond this age. Radiography alone cannot be used to determine the end of bone growth, because the physis is radiographically apparent long after clinically relevant growth has abated. A normal foal should correct a carpus valgus to within 5° to 7° of normal by 4 months of age and should be almost straight by 8 months to 10 months of age.[2]

MEDICAL MANAGEMENT

Periarticular laxity is the major cause of congenital ALDs and often improves dramatically within the first 4 weeks of life, without any intervention, because the periarticular tissues become less elastic. The improvement is most dramatic in a windswept foal, which has a tarsus valgus of one limb and a concurrent varus of the other. Limited exercise is all that is required for these foals to become normal.[2,4]

Infrequently the deformity can be so severe, particularly in the fetlock, that a foal is unable to bear weight on the sole of its foot. Immediate treatment is required to establish normal weight bearing. Custom-made glue-on shoes are particularly useful to

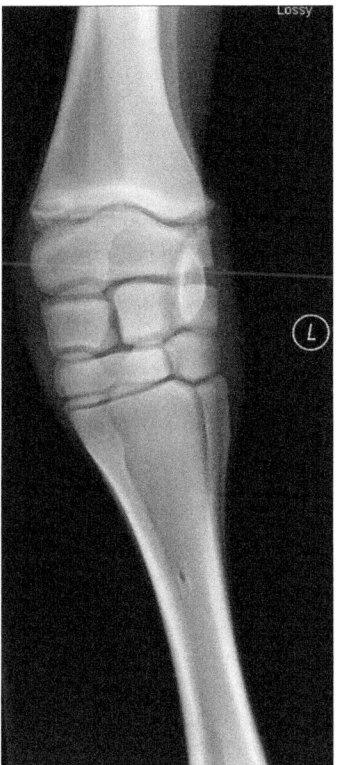

Fig. 4. Dorsopalmar radiographic view of a carpus with valgus deformity. Lateral is to the right.

prevent abnormal breakover and to keep the foot flat on the ground. If a foal has excessive laxity of the lateral collateral ligaments and a tendency to break over on the lateral side of the foot, a lateral extension shoe is used to maintain appropriate alignment of the limb.[2] The foal should initially be restricted to a stall before turnout in a small paddock or round pen with just the mare. Soft tissues become progressively stronger, and normal activity can be permitted within a short time. Allowing premature excessive exercise can lead to proximal sesamoid bone fractures and other injuries. Glue-on shoes are usually required for several weeks, but they then should be removed to avoid contracture of the foot. External coaptation also should be avoided if possible. Splints are used only to maintain joint alignment if absolutely necessary. Splints are contraindicated to try to pull or push a limb straight. Rigid support from a splint or cast usually leads to greater soft tissue laxity.[2] Trying to support a limb results in continued laxity and soft tissue wounds from bandaging. Every foal must be managed on an individual basis with the goal of achieving normal weight bearing and function while providing the minimal amount of support necessary.

Asymmetric growth of a distal physis is a cause of ALD. Greater growth from the distal physis of the radius medially compared with growth laterally results in carpus valgus.[2] Continued asymmetric growth precludes the normal correction anticipated with resolution of periarticular laxity. Greater growth from the lateral distal physes of the McIII or MtIII bones results in fetlock varus. With time and limited exercise (stall or small paddock turnout, alone with the mare) substantial self-correction occurs for most foals with angular deformities. Radiography can be used to evaluate objectively the degree of deformity and the difference in physeal growth, but it is not always required.[2]

In most situations, judicious minimal intervention is all that is required to ALDs.[2,4] Surgical intervention should be reserved for those foals that are not improving fast enough for the amount of growth potential remaining or have a severe deformity.[2,4] Therefore, it is critical for frequent re-evaluation of a foal with an ALD to monitor progress. Surgical intervention has a greater effect on a young foal because of the more rapid growth; thus, early surgical intervention should be considered for a foal with a severe deformity.[2]

SURGICAL MANAGEMENT

A high proportion of foals with ALDs are treated successfully conservatively, but surgical intervention is warranted if a deviation is severe or if deformity persists despite adequate management, including restriction of exercise and corrective farriery.[2] A variety of surgical techniques aimed at accelerating or decreasing the growth on a particular side of the growth plate have been described.[1–8] Surgical technique, whether aimed at accelerated or restricted growth, depends on the age of the horse, the degree of ALD, the anatomic site, and whether the deformity is varus or valgus.[1–8] This article focuses on growth augmentation techniques.

Before surgery, all the limbs should be assessed from the front and back and while standing next to the limbs. Good-quality radiographs, which include a substantial length of the bones proximal and distal to the deviation, should be obtained to assess bone structure (see **Fig. 4**) and to determine the pivot point and pivot point angle of the deviation.[2] The pivot point is the intersection of 2 lines drawn parallel to the long axis of the bones proximal and distal to the articulation in question. The pivot point indicates the origin of the deviation and helps determine whether the cuboidal bones, in cases of the carpus and tarsus, are involved in the deviation, or if deviation is caused by disproportionate physeal growth only (**Fig. 5**).[2] Abnormalities in the structure of these bones can have a substantial influence on the effect of the procedure and the future athletic potential of the horse. The pivot point angle is the angle formed by the intersection of these 2 lines and indicates the severity of the condition.[9]

Hemicircumferential periosteal transection and elevation, or periosteal stripping, aim to accelerate growth on the concave side of the limb, laterally for valgus and medially for varus deformities.[1–4] Previous work on chicken radii had shown that a circumferential division of the periosteum, rather than a longitudinal one, resulted in increased bone growth. The proposal was that the periosteum functioned as a fibroelastic tube, which spanned the diaphysis and provided an even tension between both epiphyses, that was responsible for the regulation of growth.[1,10] A horizontal or circumferential division of the periosteum would result in a release of tension at the level of the growth plate, resulting in the induction of new bone production on the side of the division.[10]

Hemicircumferential periosteal transection and elevation (aka Periosteal Stripping) has been thoroughly described in the literature[1–8,11] and can be performed alone or in combination with growth retardation techniques described by Taralyn M. McCarrel's article, "ALD: Growth Retardation," in this issue. To summarize, hemicircumferential periosteal transection and elevation are performed with the foal in lateral recumbency under general anesthesia, with the concave side of the affected limb uppermost. If the procedure is going to be performed bilaterally, dorsal recumbency is recommended. The position of the physis, which in carpal deviations can be generally

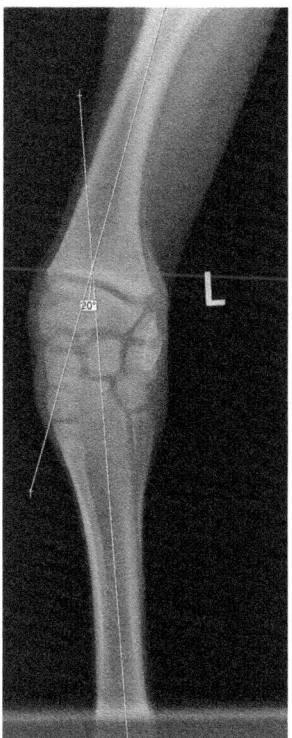

Fig. 5. Dorsopalmar radiographic view of a carpus with severe valgus deformity in a 17-day-old quarter horse colt. Lines are drawn parallel to the long axis of the radius and McIII. The point where these lines intersect is known as the pivot point. (*Courtesy of* Dr Ashlee Watts.)

palpated as the widest region in the distal radial metaphysis, is identified using a 20-gauge needle. For a carpus valgus deformity, a 4-cm to 6-cm longitudinal incision is made between the common and lateral digital extensor tendons starting just proximal to the physis. The incision is extended through to the periosteum. Using a curved scalpel blade (no. 12), a horizontal incision is made 1 cm to 2 cm proximal and parallel to the physis, at the distal end of the initial incision (parallel to the skin incision) forming an inverted T. The periosteal flaps are elevated with the aid of a periosteal elevator and then allowed to return to the normal position. It is important to transect the remnant of the ulna, or, if the ulna is ossified, it should be removed with the aid of rongeurs.[1,2] In foals with hind limb tarsus valgus the veterinarian should bear in mind that a fibular remnant may be present. The incision is closed routinely and the area is bandaged for 10 days to 14 days. The foal is kept in a large stall or small paddock until the deformity has been corrected.

Hemicircumferential periosteal transection and elevation have been reported to exert effects for up to 2 months, but the procedure can be repeated if further correction is needed.[1,2] There are no reports of overcorrection of the deformity. Early reports suggested approximately an 80% success rate[1,2,7]; however, more recent work indicates less favorable results.[11–13] A large retrospective study in Thoroughbred racehorses investigated racing performance after hemicircumferential periosteal transection and elevation.[11] A lower percentage of treated horses were able to start a race and had a lower starts percentile ranking number compared with half-siblings. Most of the foals seemed to respond favorably to hemicircumferential periosteal transection and elevation based on external appearance of the limbs, but preexisting conditions, such as abnormal cuboidal bone formation from incomplete ossification or osteoarthritis secondary to abnormal loading of the limb before correction, may have influenced subsequent performance.[11]

ALDs are probably the most common orthopedic problem affecting Thoroughbred foals.[11,14] Early surgical intervention was previously recommended to take maximum advantage of the growth potential of the physis, to try to provide foals with excellent conformation, and to enhance sale value and possibly potential performance. Based on current knowledge, it seems likely that many foals with mild ALDs underwent unnecessary surgery. The reported success for correction of ALDs, particularly in the carpus, after hemicircumferential periosteal transection and elevation, has recently been challenged. Foals suffering from carpus valgus that underwent hemicircumferential periosteal transection and elevation were no more likely to improve compared with those managed with stall rest and corrective farriery.[12,13] Although the efficacy or need to perform hemicircumferential periosteal transection and elevation when treating foals with mild to moderate carpus valgus deviations is a matter of constant debate, the same cannot be said necessarily in other regions of the limb, such as the tarsus and fetlocks, without further investigation.

Tarsus valgus deformities frequently are unrecognized by both owners and veterinarians, possibly from lack of observation of foals from behind and the inherent offset position of the tarsus.[2,15,16] Early recognition and sometimes more aggressive surgical management of tarsal ALDs are critical to achieve satisfactory results. Although the distal tibial physis has a tremendous growth rate until 4 months of age, foals younger than 2 months of age responded more favorably to hemicircumferential periosteal transection and elevation than older foals. Transphyseal bridging (Taralyn M. McCarrel's article, "ALD: Growth Retardation," in this issue) was more effective than hemicircumferential periosteal transection and elevation, especially in foals older than 2 months of age.[15] This is a significant change from the previous perception that hemicircumferential periosteal transection and elevation alone were adequate when managing most tarsus valgus deformities in foals 4 months to 6 months of age. Early recognition of incomplete ossification of the tarsal bones is crucial, because the condition, if unrecognized, leads to collapse of the third or central tarsal bones, resulting in osteoarthritis.[15,16] Of 22 foals with incomplete ossification of the tarsal bones, 73% had tarsus valgus deformities. Only 32% of the foals were able to reach the intended use.[16]

REFERENCES

1. Auer JA. Angular limb deformities. In: Auer JA, Stick JA, editors. Equine surgery. 4th edition. St Louis (MO): Elsevier; 2012. p. 1201–21.

2. García-López JM, Parente EJ. Angular limb deformities. In: Ross MW, Dyson SJ, editors. Diagnosis and management of lameness in the horse. 2nd edition. St Louis (MO): Elsevier; 2011. p. 640–5.

3. Hunt RJ. Angular limb deviation. In: White NA, Moore JN, editors. Current techniques in equine surgery and lameness. 2nd edition. Philadelphia: Saunders; 1998. p. 323–6.

4. Trumble TN. Orthopedic disorders in neonatal foals. Vet Clin North Am 2005;21: 357–86.

5. Auer JA, Martens RJ, Williams EH. Periosteal transection for correction of angular limb deformities in foals. J Am Vet Med Assoc 1982;181:459–66.

6. Fretz PB, Donecker JM. Surgical correction of angular limb deformities in foals: a retrospective study. J Am Vet Med Assoc 1983;183:529–32.
7. Bertone AL, Turner AS, Park RD. Periosteal transection and stripping for treatment of angular limb deformities in foals: clinical observations. J Am Vet Med Assoc 1985;187:145–51.
8. Adams SB, Fessler JF. Surgical treatment of angular limb deformities. In: Adams SB, Fessler JF, editors. Atlas of equine surgery. Philadelphia: WB Saunders; 2000. p. 363–70.
9. Brauer TS, Booth TS, Riedesel E. Physeal growth retardation leads to correction of intracarpal angular deviations as well as physeal valgus deformity. Equine Vet J 1999;31:193–6.
10. Crilly RG. Longitudinal overgrowth of chicken radius. J Anat 1972;112:11–8.
11. Mitten LA, Bramlage LR, Embertson RM. Racing performance after hemicircumferential periosteal transection for angular limb deformities in thoroughbreds: 199 cases (1987-1989). J Am Vet Med Assoc 1995;207:746–50.
12. Slone DE, Roberts CT, Hughes FE. Restricted exercise and transphyseal bridging for correction of angular limb deformities (abstract). Proc Am Assoc Equine Pract 2000;46:126.
13. Read EK, Read MR, Townsend HG. Effect of hemi-circumferential periosteal transection and elevation in foals with experimentally induced angular limb deformities. J Am Vet Med Assoc 2002;221:536–40.
14. O'Donohue DD, Smith FH, Strickland KL. The incidence of abnormal limb development in the Irish thoroughbred from birth to 18 months. Equine Vet J 1992;24:305–9.
15. Dutton DM, Watkins JP, Honnas CM, et al. Treatment response and athletic outcome of foals with tarsal valgus deformities: 39 cases (1988-1997). J Am Vet Med Assoc 1999;215:1481–4.
16. Dutton DM, Watkins JP, Walker MA, et al. Incomplete ossification of the tarsal bones in foals: 22 cases (1988-1996). J Am Vet Med Assoc 1998;213:1590–4.

Angular Limb Deformities
Growth Retardation

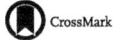

Taralyn M. McCarrel, DVM

KEYWORDS

- Foal • Angular limb deformity • Transphyseal bridge • Transphyseal screw

KEY POINTS

- Familiarity with normal growth of the young horse is critical for appropriate case selection of foals that require surgical retardation of physeal growth to correct an angular deformity that would not correct by other means.
- Preoperative radiographic evaluation is critical to confirm that the deformity has the potential to respond to physeal growth retardation.
- Growth retardation procedures are performed on the convex side of the physis of interest and may be combined with growth-promoting procedures on the concave side of the limb.
- The single transphyseal screw has become the preferred approach to surgical retardation in many cases; however, more knowledge on the use of this technique during the rapid growth phase and physitis is required to determine if significant complications will arise.

INTRODUCTION

Ideal musculoskeletal conformation, for reasons of both form and function, has long been a preoccupation of the equine enthusiast. The definition of perfect limb conformation remains elusive for several reasons, including[1–6]

- Differences in breed and discipline standards, with varying degrees of evidence to support those standards
- Challenges objectively and accurately measuring all aspects of the 3-D limb in clinical practice
- The presence of concurrent deformities further complicating subjective interpretation
- The range of expected normal deviations that correct spontaneously as the young horse grows
- The limited number of studies providing objective information on the precise effect of limb deformities on performance and the degree of severity associated with athletic injury

The author has nothing to disclose.
Large Animal Clinical Sciences, College of Veterinary Medicine, University of Florida, Box 100136, Gainesville, FL 32610-0001, USA
E-mail address: tmccarrel@ufl.edu

Vet Clin Equine 33 (2017) 353–366
http://dx.doi.org/10.1016/j.cveq.2017.03.006
0749-0739/17/© 2017 Elsevier Inc. All rights reserved.

Therefore, arguably the most critical skill that contributes to successful management of angular limb deformities in foals is mastering the art of monitoring development of the young horse and knowing which treatments to use and when and, just as important, when not to treat.

Angular limb deformity, defined as a deviation of the limb in the sagittal plane, is a common developmental orthopedic disease in the horse. The deformity is named based on the direction of deviation of the distal limb and the joint that appears to be deviated. The location of the deformity, however, is most commonly at the level of the metaphysis (also the physis and occasionally the epiphysis) of the long bone proximal to the joint (**Box 1**). The distal radial physis and distal third metacarpal/metatarsal physis are most commonly affected, with the distal tibial physis requiring treatment less often.[7] There are several options available for treatment of this disorder. This article focuses on surgical procedures that retard the growth of the physis on the convex (long) side of the affected long bone. The procedures discussed share the same fundamental principle, that is, static compression of the physis on the convex side to slow growth while allowing the opposite concave (short) side to continue to grow and straighten the limb.[8] Appropriate case selection, surgical options, and complications are discussed.

PATIENT EVALUATION
Foal Conformation Evaluation

The details of orthopedic examination of the foal are covered elsewhere in this issue. Briefly, a foal should be observed standing squarely from the front and behind (**Fig. 1**). Observers should align themselves with the dorsal or caudal face of each limb to evaluate for angular limb deformity. The foal should also be walked toward and away from the clinician to allow observation of foot flight and tracking. Dynamic evaluation is important because the limb does not travel in a straight line if an angular deformity is present (ie, fetlock varus causes the toe to deviate medially during the flight phase). Careful attention should be paid to note concurrent deformities (ie, carpal valgus and fetlock varus).

Knowledge of normal conformation for the age of the foal, growth stages for the physes of interest, and age at physiologic growth plate closure is essential for correct interpretation of the conformation examination and the most appropriate treatment strategies, if any. Foals are typically born with carpal valgus (<10°) and fetlock valgus or fetlock varus. The entire forelimb often appears outwardly rotated due to the narrow

---

Box 1
Angular limb deformity definitions

Valgus: lateral deviation of the limb distal to the origin of the deformity

Varus: medial deviation of the limb distal to the origin of the deformity

Fetlock angular limb deformity: common term referring to angular deformity originating from the distal third metacarpal/metatarsal physeal region

Carpal angular limb deformity: common term referring to angular deformity originating from the distal radial physeal region

Tarsal angular limb deformity: common term referring to angular deformity originating from the distal tibial physeal region

Offset knee: common term referring to lateral displacement of the carpus and third metacarpal bone relative to the radius at the level of the radiocarpal joint.[7] This is not a true angular deformity but can benefit from growth retardation procedures.

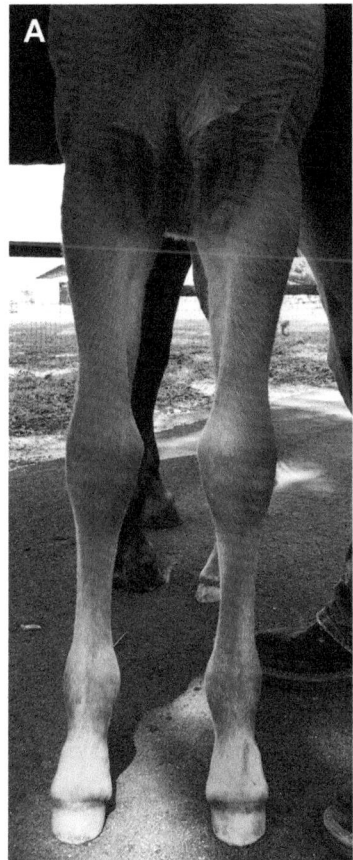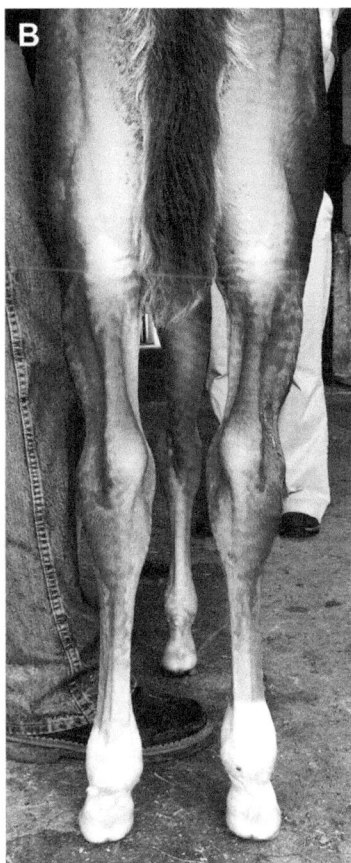

Fig. 1. A foal standing square observed from the (*A*) front and (*B*) behind for conformation evaluation. Due to the typical outward rotation of the forelimbs, it is important the observer align themselves with the face of the limb to accurately assess alignment.

chest of the foal; however, the carpus and fetlock should still align in the axial plane.[7] Foals should be examined every 2 weeks to monitor progression. The fetlock should improve to straight axial alignment from the metacarpus/metatarsus to the toe by 4 months of age, at which time the rapid linear growth phase of the limbs has ended and potential remaining growth in the distal metacarpal/metatarsal physes is minimal.[7,9] Carpal valgus (5°–7°) is expected at this age, with further correction during accelerated growth of the distal radial physis at 8 months to 10 months of age.[1,7,9] As the chest becomes broader, the forelimbs rotate inward (a normal outwardly rotated foal becomes straight; a straight foal develops inward rotation). Therapies are instituted when a foal is not developing as expected or when the initial deformity is severe (mild <5°, moderate 5°–10°, or severe >15°).[9] Indications for growth retardation surgery are outlined in **Box 2** (**Fig. 2**).[7]

Radiographs

Radiographic evaluation is always indicated when an abnormal angular deviation of the limb is severe, not improving as expected, or increasing in severity. The location

---

Box 2
Indications for growth retardation procedures

- Severe deformities that are unlikely to correct spontaneously before physiologic physeal closure

- Severe deformities that are either causing, or resulting in worsening of, concurrent angular deformities elsewhere in the limb

- Mild to moderate deformities that are increasing in severity over time or have remained static and no longer have sufficient time for physiologic correction before growth plate closure

- Deformity located at the level of the physeal region. Diaphyseal and intra-articular deformities do not benefit significantly from physeal manipulation.

Data from Bramlage LR, Embertson RM. Observations on the evaluation and selection of foal limb deformities for surgical treatment. AAEP 1990;36:273–9; and Auer JA. Angular limb deformities. In: Auer JA, Stick JA, editors. Equine surgery. 4th edition. St Louis (MO): Elsevier Saunders; 2012:1201–21.

---

and degree of angulation can be determined as well as complicating factors that may decrease prognosis or eliminate certain procedures as a viable option (**Fig. 3**). The presence of complete ulnas and fibulas in pony and miniature horse foals causing severe angular limb deformity has been reported.[10,11] Due to the severity of the deformity, treatment is not commonly attempted and there is little information on treatment strategies. If treatment were attempted, segmental ulnar or fibular ostectomy would be a necessary surgical procedure to allow physeal manipulation.

The dorsopalmar view of the carpus and front fetlock and dorsoplantar view of the tarsus and hind fetlock should be evaluated. Angulation of the distal tibia is difficult to assess radiographically because of the tibia angles away from the cassette; however, physeal pathology can be assessed. The lateral-medial radiographic projection of the tarsus is also important to evaluate the cuboidal bones for evidence of crushing. Crushing of the carpal or small tarsal bones decreases prognosis for future soundness and cannot be corrected by physeal manipulation.[8]

A study by Brauer and colleagues[12] compared limb deformity of the carpal region using the pivot point method (angle and location of deformity determined based on the intersection of line drawn through the radius and metacarpus) and the individual angle method (angle of deformity measured at the level of the distal radial physis and each joint of the carpus and summed to produce the final deviation). Radiographs were evaluated before and after growth retardation in young horses with carpal valgus. The physis was the predominant contributor to the overall deformity in the carpal region (82% of cases) and there was a high degree of correlation between the pivot point and individual angle methods. There was improvement in the deviations at the level of the carpal joints after physeal growth retardation. These minor changes, however, cannot be expected to overcome the deformities that occur with significant carpal bone crushing due to incomplete ossification of the cuboidal bones.

SURGICAL GROWTH RETARDATION PROCEDURES

Reported surgical techniques for physeal growth retardation include the transphyseal staple, screw and wire transphyseal bridge, and the single transphyseal screw. Equine limbs undergo an initial rapid linear increase in length for the first 10 weeks of life, after which the rate of growth decreases dramatically.[13] Several studies have evaluated

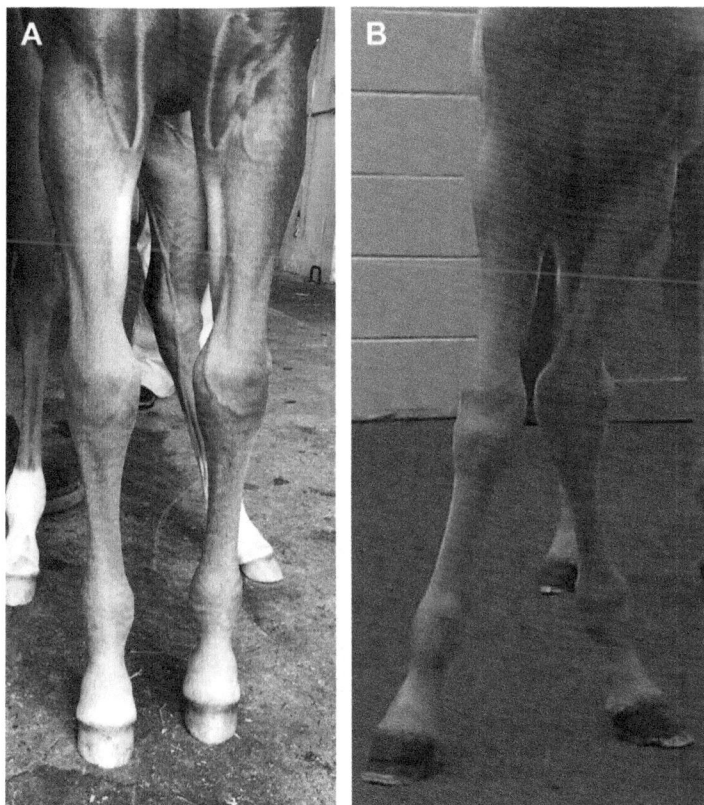

Fig. 2. (*A*) A 1-month-old foal with mild bilateral carpal varus. Although the deformity is mild, it is significant because a foal this age is expected to have mild carpal valgus and outward rotation of the limb. The deformity does not necessitate a growth retardation procedure but continued close monitoring and conservative measures and/or growth promoting procedures should be considered. (*B*) A 3-month-old foal with severe left carpal valgus and physeal inflammation of several physes. Given the degree of deformity, radiographic evaluation for bony abnormalities accompanying the physeal deformity should be performed before growth retardation surgery to determine prognosis. Note the large lateral flare on the left front foot and the medial to lateral imbalance of the foot. Management to balance the foot is essential after growth retardation surgery.

bone growth below the carpus and tarsus where cessation of growth is reported to occur between 140 days and 210 days (4.6–7 months); however, the earlier time point is more broadly accepted.[4,14–16] Growth of the distal radius is effectively complete after approximately 60 weeks of age.[13] Growth retardation procedures are typically performed after the rapid growth phase of the region of interest is complete, while leaving sufficient remaining time and growth to achieve correction (**Table 1**).

Transphyseal Staples

The transphyseal staple was the first technique developed to place an implant in the epiphysis and metaphysis to bridge the physis and thereby limit growth on the convex side of the limb.[8] The most recent study reporting the outcome of the technique used 7/64-inch Steinmann pins to make staples.[12] Horses between 1 week and 2 years of

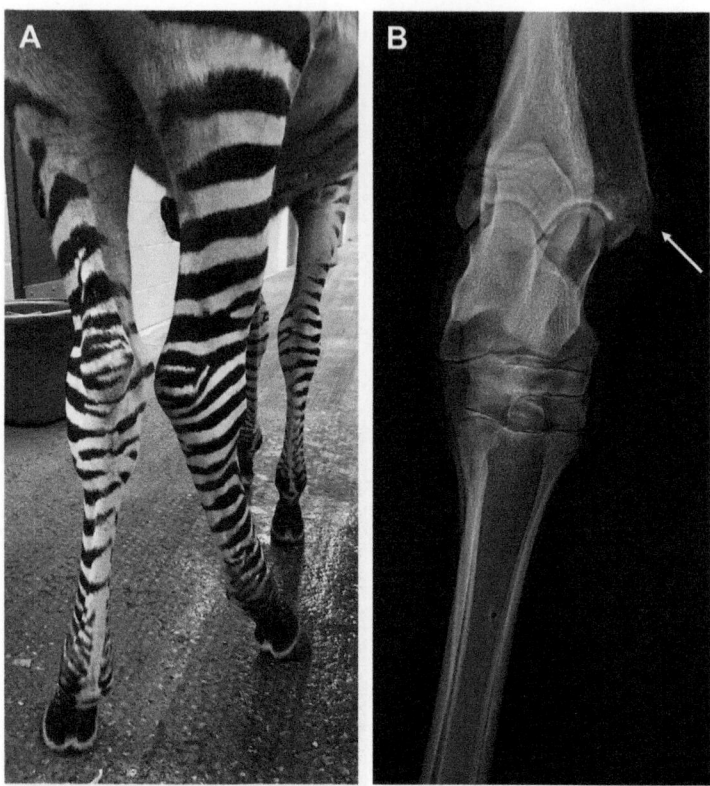

Fig. 3. (*A*) A 7-month-old zebra presented for severe left tarsal valgus. History of development was unknown. Based on clinical examination, a medial trasphyseal screw is an appropriate treatment. Further radiographic projections (not shown here) revealed evidence of a healed, misaligned physeal fracture. (*B*) The medial aspect of the distal tibial physis has a bony bridge and is closed (*arrow*); therefore, no benefit would be gained by performing a growth retardation procedure. This case emphasizes the importance of radiographic evaluation when determining treatment options.

Table 1
End of the rapid growth phase, age at transphyseal screw and screw and wire transphyseal bridge placement, and the numbers of days postoperatively that implants were removed for the distal metacarpus/metatarsus III, distal tibia, and distal radius with angular limb deformities. Data presented as range alone (ie. 2–3 months) or mean (min – max) (ie. 3 [0.7–3.7])

		Distal Metacarpus/ Metatarsus III	Distal Tibia	Distal Radius
Rapid growth ends (mo)		2–3[8,24]	4–6[8,24]	6,[8] 8–10[7,a]
Trasnphyseal screw	Age placed (mo)	3 (0.7–3.7)[20] 3.7 (3–4.8)[18]	7.3 (3.9–12)[19]	12.6[21] 13 (10.5–19)[22]
	Time to removal (d)	28–35[20] 31.1 (9–65)[18]	62 (39–89)[19]	38[21] 39.5 (14–125)[22]
Screw and wire	Age placed (mo)	3 (1–5.8)[18]	—	12[21]
	Time to removal (d)	42.8 (19–86)[18]	—	54[21]

[a] A second rapid growth phase occurs between 8 months to 10 months of age.

age with carpal valgus were included. Improvement in radiographic measurements at the time of removal revealed improvement in only 76% of horses. The investigators suggested that the older age of some cases may have contributed to the result. Only 55% of staples, however, were intact with no distortion at the time of removal. Complications included spreading of the legs of the staple (34%), broken staple, and staple migration out of the bone.[12] Other reported complications include difficulty placing the staple correctly, poorer incisional cosmesis, and difficulty removing the staple.[17,18] Based on the inferior results, the procedure has been largely abandoned in favor of the screw and wire or single transphyseal screw.[8,17]

Screw and Wire Transphyseal Bridge

The screw and wire technique was developed next and was advantageous because it was easier to place accurately, less prone to implant failure, could be placed through stab incisions, and was easier to remove. The transphyseal screw has replaced the screw and wire for many indications; however, for reasons discussed later, the screw and wire technique can still be of value for correction of angular limb deformities in foals. This technique is also used for physeal fracture repair in the distal physis of metacarpal/metatarsal III, distal radial physis, and proximal tibial physis.

Surgical procedure

Currently, the screw and wire transphyseal bridge is most commonly performed in the distal radius (**Fig. 4**). The horse is positioned in dorsal recumbency with the limb suspended. The hair is clipped and the skin prepared for aseptic surgery. The limb is draped to isolate the surgical field. A 20G needle is inserted in the distal radial physis. A needle may also be placed to mark the radiocarpal joint; however, this is readily palpable. Stab incisions are made full thickness through the skin, subcutaneous tissue, and periosteum in the center of the epiphysis and within the metaphysis of the distal radius ensuring the screws are in the center of the bone. A tunnel connecting the 2 stab incisions is created using a curved hemostatic forceps. A 3.2-mm drill bit is used to drill thread holes for 4.5-mm screws at the site of each stab incision and the holes are tapped. The thread holes should be drilled so that the distal screw is parallel to the radiocarpal joint and the screws are parallel to one another or slightly converging. A prebent 18G wire is fed into the tunnel so that the loop is positioned distally on the limb (the ends should exit the proximal incision). The top and bottom screw are placed but not tightened. The wire is then pulled proximally so it sits snug against the distal screw and the free ends are twisted (caution to avoid overtightening, which breaks the wire). The twisted end of the wire is held stable while the screws are tightened. Only 1 wire is required. The excess wire ends are cut and the twist is pressed into the bone to avoid soft tissue irritation. Intraoperative radiographs confirm correct placement. The subcutaneous tissue and skin are closed and the carpus is bandaged.

Perioperative and postoperative care

A single preoperative dose of broad spectrum systemic antimicrobials is sufficient. Anti-inflammatories are administered for 5 days to 7 days postoperatively. The horse is confined to a stall or small pen for 10 days until suture and bandage removal, after which it may be turned out in a small paddock for an additional 2 weeks. Normal turnout can resume if there have been no complications. Progress should be evaluated every 2 weeks and implants removed as soon as correction is achieved but no later. Implant removal can be performed standing or under general anesthesia. Complications are discussed in comparison with the transphyseal screw.

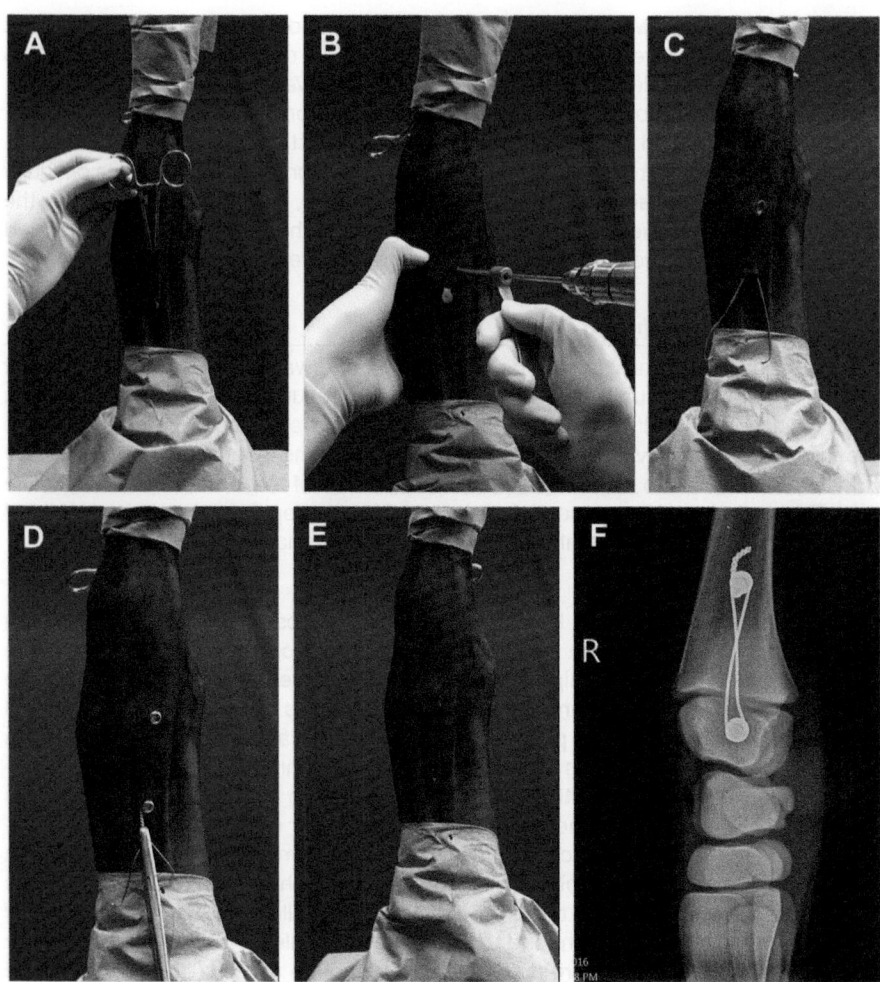

Fig. 4. Surgical procedure and intraoperative radiograph: placing a screw and wire construct in the distal radial physis. (*A*) Kelly forceps are passed subcutaneously to connect stab incisions. (*B*) Holes are drilled at each stab incision. (*C*) The wire is passed through the subcutaneous tunnel. (*D*) Screws are place through proximal and distal drill holes and the wire is twisted to tighten. (*E*) The screws are tightened and incisions are closed. (*F*) Post-operative radiograph.

Transphyseal Screw

The transphyseal screw differs from previous growth retardation techniques in that, rather than bridging the physis, the screw penetrates the physis. The technique for placing the transphyseal screw has been described for the distal physis of the tibia,[19] distal physis of metacarpal/metatarsal III,[18,20] and distal radial physis.[21,22] The procedure in the carpus is predominantly performed on yearlings; therefore, only the procedures for fetlock and tarsal angular limb deformity correction are described.

Surgical procedure

For both the fetlock and tarsus, the foal is anesthetized and positioned in dorsal recumbency. The limb is suspended, clipped, and aseptically prepared. The surgical site is isolated using sterile drapes. A 20G needle is placed to identify the physis of interest.

Fetlock A stab incision through the skin, subcutaneous tissue, and periosteum is made approximately 1 cm to 1.5 cm proximal to the physis in the center of the bone (**Fig. 5**). The skin should be manipulated so that the incision is not directly

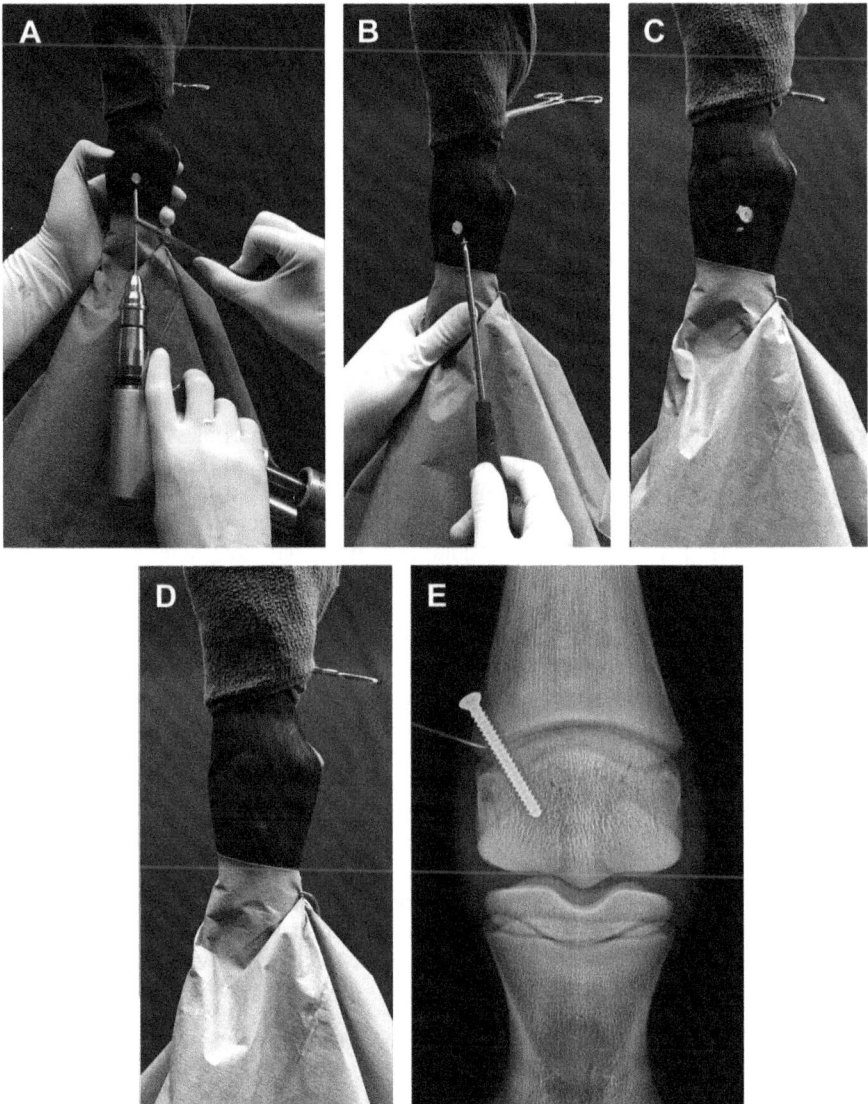

Fig. 5. Surgical procedure and intraoperative radiograph: placing a transphyseal screw in the distal metacarpal physis. (A) A needle is placed in the physis and a drill is used to prepare the screw hole. (B) Final tightening of the screw with a screw driver. (C) The screw is placed until the screw head just contacts the bone. (D) The needle is removed, notice the skin incision slides over the screw head so the incision does not lie directly over the screw. (E) Intraoperative radiograph after screw placement.

over the screw head at the end of surgery. A 2.5-mm drill bit (if placing a 3.5-mm self-tapping screw) or 3.2-mm drill bit (if placing a 4.5-mm cortical screw) is initially seated in to the cortex and then directed distally maintaining alignment with the dorsal cortex of metacarpal/metatarsal III. Penetration of the physis can be detected by an increase and then sudden decrease in bone density when drilling. The thread hole is tapped if needed and the screw placed. The screw should not be tightened but should be advanced only until the screw head contacts the bone to avoid bending the screw or breaking the screw head. Intraoperative radiographs confirm correct placement. The screw should engage 60% to 75% of the epiphysis, should be as vertical as possible, and should not cross midline.[23] The subcutaneous tissue and skin is closed and the limb is bandaged.

Tarsus A stab incision is made over the distal aspect of the medial malleolus. Radiographic guidance is used to confirm correct placement and angulation of a 3.2-mm drill bit prior to drilling the thread hole. The drill bit is advanced from distal to proximal to cross the physis and enter the metaphysis. The thread hole is tapped and a 4.5-mm cortical screw is placed. Again, the screw should not be tightened but advanced just until the screw head contacts bone. Intraoperative radiographs confirm correct placement, the incision is closed, and the limb bandaged.

Variations of the procedures have been described. The initial report in the distal tibial physis placed a 4.5-mm cortical screw in lag fashion; however, a later report stated that the technique had been modified to a position screw technique.[19,24] One report described drilling the cortex of the distal metacarpus with a 5.5-mm bit to create a shelf to seat the screw head, elevation of periosteum, and suturing of periosteum over the screw head.[18] As pointed out by another investigator, these steps are unnecessary and may create further trauma and complications.[20]

Wall and colleagues[25] described angular limb deformity correction in 6 foals with fetlock varus using a 4.5-mm absorbable transphyseal screw. Surgery was only performed when the investigators were confident overcorrection would not occur (mean age 137 days, range 106–156 days) since the implant is not removed. Although foals improved, only 2 foals achieved straight limb conformation. The principal advantage stated was that a second surgery was not needed for implant removal. Important questions need to be answered, however, prior to use in routine clinical practice. How long does the screw maintain sufficient mechanical strength to effect growth retardation? If the surgical site becomes infected, does the absorbable screw need to be removed to resolve the infection and can this be accomplished? How long does the screw persist in the bone? A clear radiolucent outline of the screw was still apparent on radiographs 9 months after surgery and the investigators stated that the material can last up to 3 years in people.[25] Will the persistent radiographic appearance of the screw effect the value of young horse going to sale? How might persistence of the material have an impact on bone remodeling in horses that are started into heavy training?

Perioperative and postoperative care
Management is similar to that of the screw and wire procedure except that foals are not confined to a stall but allowed turnout in a small pen.

Screw and Screw and Wire Removal

Removal can be performed in the standing sedated foal with a subcutaneous local block or under general anesthesia (**Fig. 6**). Removal under general anesthesia should be performed in all cases with bony overgrowth of the screw head that may require removal of excess bone. Local anesthetic should not be injected directly over the

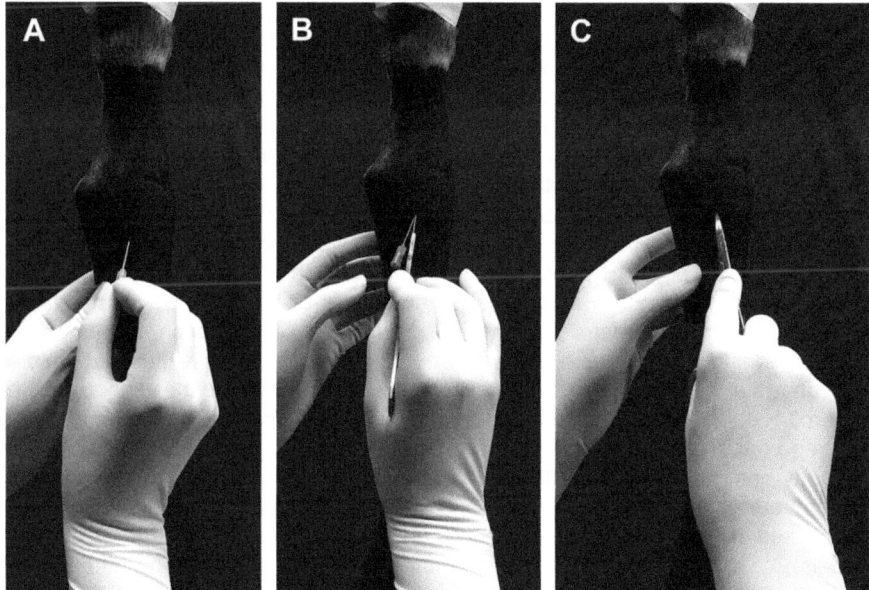

Fig. 6. Removal of a transphyseal screw from the distal metacarpal physis. (*A*) The screw head is identified using a needle. (*B*) A stab incision is made over the screw head. (*C*) A mosquito forcep is inserted to identify the depression in the screw head and to remove soft tissue if necessary, then a screwdriver is inserted along the same plane and the screw is removed.

screw head because it makes palpation to identify the screw head more difficult; rather, the local anesthetic should be injected in an inverted "V" shape around the screw head or screw and wire construct. A 20G needle is inserted in the skin and used to probe for the metal screw head. Once identified, a stab incision is made down to the screw head (this step is performed for each screw in the screw and wire; recording the distance between the screws placed at surgery can make finding the second screw easier at the time of removal). A curved hemostatic forceps is introduced through the stab incision and used to find the center of the screw head. The forceps can also be used to remove soft tissue that may be filling the driver site. The screw driver is then firmly seated into the screw head. It is of utmost importance that attempts to remove the screw are not made until the screw driver is convincingly seated well into the screw head, otherwise, the screw head can be stripped. The smaller 3.5-mm screws are subjectively more prone to this problem. The screw is removed. In the case of the screw and wire, the first screw is back out until it is visible outside of the skin, and then the second screw is removed followed by the first. The wire may need to be elevated from the bone using a forceps. It is then grasped and tugged sharply to pull it from the distal stab incision. The stab incisions may be sutured or closed with adhesive tape, a sterile bandage is placed, and the foal is maintained in a bandage until 10 days postoperatively.

SCREW AND WIRE VERSUS TRANSPHYSEAL SCREW: ADVANTAGES, DISADVANTAGES, AND COMPLICATIONS

Potential complications associated with all growth retardation surgeries include surgical site infection, overcorrection, bony overgrowth, and cosmetic defects.

Complications specific to the screw and wire include wound dehiscence (if a long incision is used rather than 2 stab incisions), wire breakage, soft tissue thickening, and seroma.[18] Surgical complications during transphyseal screw placement or removal include breaking the screw, stripping the screw, and difficulty locating the screw head.[20] Witte and colleagues[19] reported no surgical or postoperative complications for transphyseal screws placed in the distal tibial physis. Superficial surgical site infections after surgery to place a transphyseal screw were attributed by several investigators to postoperative bandaging problems.[18,20,24] This may be related to exposure of the incisions before wound healing was complete or bandaging too tightly, which can lead to pressure necrosis of the thin skin overlying the screw head. Advantages of the transphyseal screw in the distal metacarpus/metatarsus and distal tibia include faster surgery time, faster rate of correction, and improved cosmesis.[18–20] Concerns have been raised regarding the potential for spot welding of the physis at the site where the transphyseal screw penetrates the physis resulting in overcorrection after the screw is removed; however, specific examples have not been reported to date.[18]

A study comparing the complication rate after treatment of angular deformities of the carpus in yearlings with a screw and wire transphyseal bridge (n = 253) or a transphyseal screw (n = 315) was performed.[21] Although the focus of this article is on foals, the study highlights some important findings. There was no difference in any preoperative parameter including age, severity of deformity, gender, age at the time of surgery, and so forth. Correction of the deformity was significantly faster (16 days) in yearlings treated with a transphyseal screw compared with those treated with a screw and wire (see **Table 1**). There was no difference between groups for the incidence of incisional infections, seromas, or overcorrection. Significantly more yearlings treated with the transphyseal screw, however, developed physitis (17.1%) compared with the screw and wire (7.5%), and 4.4% of yearlings treated with a transphyseal screw developed a particular group of signs termed metaphyseal collapse, whereas no horses treated with a screw and wire developed this complication.[21] Metaphyseal collapse was defined by acute change in limb angulation associated with pain and lameness with no evidence of a bony bridge crossing the physis and occurring 2 months to 5 months after screw removal. Of the 14 affected horses, 4 required growth retardation on the opposite side of the limb to correct the acute deformity; 6 of 14 horses went on to race.[21] There are no large studies evaluating the use of the transphyseal screw in the distal radial physis when physitis is already present nor in foals with significant remaining growth potential. Growth retardation procedures are only performed in foals with severe angular deformities at the level of the distal radial physis that are not responsive to other therapies. The principal advantages of the transphyseal screw (faster correction and improved cosmesis) may be less critical in a foal with ample time for correction to occur and for swelling associated with the more bulky screw and wire construct to resolve. Therefore, until there is more evidence supporting the safe use of the transphyseal screw in foals and cases of physitis, it is advisable to continue to use the screw and wire transphyseal bridge.

SUMMARY

Growth retardation procedures are reserved for foals with angular limb deformities that are severe or not responsive to more conservative therapies or when insufficient time for physiologic correction remains for the degree of the deformity. Knowledge of normal growth patterns and appropriate timing for intervention is critical to successful treatment. The 2 principal surgical procedures used currently are the transphyseal screw and the screw and wire transphyseal bridge. The transphyseal screw is the preferred technique in the fetlock and tarsus because of the improved cosmesis and more rapid correction, which is of particular importance in the fetlock. The majority of distal radial growth plate manipulation is performed at 1 year of age; however, in young foals with severe deformity of the carpus necessitating growth retardation surgery, the screw and wire may be the preferred procedure.

REFERENCES

1. Santschi EM, Leibsle SR, Morehead JP, et al. Carpal and fetlock conformation of the juvenile thoroughbred from birth to yearling auction age. Equine Vet J 2006; 38(7):604–9.
2. Robert C, Valette JP, Denoix JM. Longitudinal development of equine forelimb conformation from birth to weaning in three different horse breeds. Vet J 2013; 198(Suppl 1):e75–80.
3. Ross MW. Conformation and lameness. In: Ross MW, Dyson SJ, editors. Diagnosis and management of lameness in the horse. St Louis (MO): W.B. Saunders; 2003. p. 15–31.
4. Anderson TM, McIlwraith CW, Douay P. The role of conformation in musculoskeletal problems in the racing thoroughbred. Equine Vet J 2004;36(7):571–5.
5. Weller R, Pfau T, Babbage D, et al. Reliability of conformational measurements in the horse using a three-dimensional motion analysis system. Equine Vet J 2006; 38(7):610–5.
6. Weller R, Pfau T, Verheyen K, et al. The effect of conformation on orthopaedic health and performance in a cohort of National Hunt racehorses: preliminary results. Equine Vet J 2006;38(7):622–7.
7. Bramlage LR, Embertson RM. Observations on the evaluation and selection of foal limb deformities for surgical treatment. AAEP 1990;36:273–9.
8. Auer JA. Angular limb deformities. In: Auer JA, Stick JA, editors. Equine surgery. 4th edition. St Louis (MO): Elsevier Saunders; 2012. p. 1201–21.
9. Barr AR. Management of angular limb deformities in the foal. Equine Vet Educ 1995;7(2):75–8.
10. Shamis LD, Auer J. Complete ulnas and fibulas in a pony foal. J Am Vet Med Assoc 1985;186(8):802–4.
11. Tyson R, Graham JP, Colahan PT, et al. Skeletal atavism in a miniature horse. Vet Radiol Ultrasound 2004;45(4):315–7.
12. Brauer TS, Booth TS, Riedesel E. Physeal growth retardation leads to correction of intracarpal angular deviations as well as physeal valgus deformity. Equine Vet J 1999;31(3):193–6.
13. Fretz PB, Cymbaluk NF, Pharr JW. Quantitative analysis of long-bone growth in the horse. Am J Vet Res 1984;45(8):1602–9.
14. Thompson KN. Skeletal growth rates of weanling and yearling thoroughbred horses. J Anim Sci 1995;73(9):2513–7.
15. Hintz HF, Hintz RL, Van Vleck LD. Growth rate of thoroughbreds, effect of age of dam, year and month of birth, and sex of foal. J Anim Sci 1979;48(3):480–7.
16. Campbell JR, Lee R. Radiological estimation of differential growth rates of the long bones of foals. Equine Vet J 1981;13(4):247–50.
17. Mitten LA, Bertone AL. Angular limb deformities in foals. J Am Vet Med Assoc 1994;204(5):717–20.

18. Roberts BL, Railton D, Adkins AR. A single screw technique compared to a two screw and wire technique as a temporary transphyseal bridge for correction of fetlock varus deformities. Equine Vet Educ 2009;21(12):666–70.
19. Witte S, Thorpe PE, Hunt RJ, et al. A lag-screw technique for bridging of the medial aspect of the distal tibial physis in horses. J Am Vet Med Assoc 2004; 225(10):1581–3.
20. Kay AT, Hunt RJ. Single screw transphyseal bridging of the distal metacarpus and metatarsus for correction of angular limb deformity in the foal. Equine Vet Education 2009;21(12):671–2.
21. Carlson ER, Bramlage LR, Stewart AA, et al. Complications after two transphyseal bridging techniques for treatment of angular limb deformities of the distal radius in 568 thoroughbred yearlings. Equine Vet J 2012;44(4):416–9.
22. Baker WT, Slone DE, Lynch TM, et al. Racing and sales performance after unilateral or bilateral single transphyseal screw insertion for varus angular limb deformities of the carpus in 53 thoroughbreds. Vet Surg 2011;40(1):124–8.
23. Aksahin E, Dogruyol D, Yuksel HY, et al. The comparison of the effect of corticosteroids and platelet-rich plasma (PRP) for the treatment of plantar fasciitis. Arch Orthop Trauma Surg 2012;132(6):781–5.
24. Witte S, Hunt R. A review of angular limb deformities. Equine Vet Educ 2009; 21(7):378–87.
25. Wall RA, Robinson P, Adkins AR. The use of an absorbable bone screw as a transphyseal bridge for the correction of fetlock varus deviations in six foals. Equine Vet Education 2010;22(11):571–5.

Osteochondritis Dissecans Development

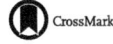

Stacy A. Semevolos, DVM, MS

KEYWORDS

- OCD • Cartilage • Osteochondrosis • Osteochondritis dissecans • Pathogenesis
- Development

KEY POINTS

- Blood supply to developing cartilage is very important because the articular-epiphyseal cartilage thickness far exceeds diffusion limits of synovial fluid.
- Anastomoses of cartilage canals and associated vessels along the ossification front are vulnerable to injury and may be an inciting factor in osteochondrosis (OC) development.
- Abnormal cartilage development and biomechanical trauma to cartilage canals or the osteochondral junction are etiologic factors for developing OC.
- Early OC lesions have the potential to heal intrinsically or develop into more advanced osteochondritis dissecans (OCD) lesions.
- Restricting exercise during the healing phase may help to prevent early OC lesions from becoming OCD flaps or fragments.

INTRODUCTION

Osteochondritis dissecans (OCD) and osteochondrosis (OC) are often interchangeably used to describe a defect in endochondral ossification leading to osteochondral fragmentation and/or cysts in joints of foals; however, they actually describe different stages of disease. OC represents the initial disease process, whereas OCD reflects secondary changes resulting in cartilage flap or osteochondral fragment formation (**Fig. 1**). This disease has been extensively studied in horses during the past 20 years, with more than 150 studies published during that time. The focus of this article is to provide a review of current knowledge of OCD development in horses, including normal cartilage development, early OC pathogenesis, and factors that result in healing or advancement to OCD fragments.

NORMAL CARTILAGE DEVELOPMENT

Articular cartilage covers the ends of long bones, creating a frictionless surface for normal movement of joints. In the postnatal period, dramatic changes occur in

Oregon State University, College of Veterinary Medicine, 200B Magruder Hall, Corvallis, OR 97322, USA
E-mail address: stacy.semevolos@oregonstate.edu

Vet Clin Equine 33 (2017) 367–378
http://dx.doi.org/10.1016/j.cveq.2017.03.009
0749-0739/17/© 2017 Elsevier Inc. All rights reserved.

vetequine.theclinics.com

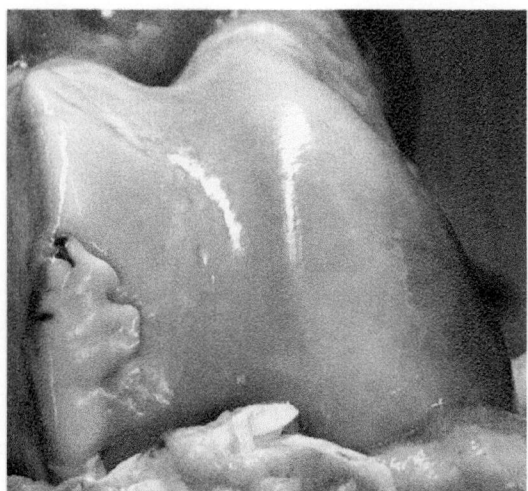

Fig. 1. OCD lesion on the lateral trochlear ridge of the distal femur in a yearling quarter horse filly.

articular cartilage and the underlying epiphyseal cartilage (so-called articular-epiphyseal [A-E] complex). The epiphyseal cartilage must be transformed into bone, whereas articular cartilage remains cartilage throughout the horse's life. Processes critical to normal cartilage development include endochondral ossification and cartilage canal formation and regression.

HOW DOES CARTILAGE TURN INTO BONE?
Endochondral Ossification Process

Endochondral ossification is an intricate process whereby a cartilage template is transformed into bone. This process occurs in physeal growth plates, A-E cartilage, and during fracture healing. Coordination of cell-to-cell signaling, cellular differentiation, and matrix modifications make this a highly orchestrated process.[1–3] Most of the literature describes the endochondral ossification process in growth plates but equally important is the transformation of A-E cartilage into subchondral bone.

In both the growth plate and A-E cartilage, several zones of cartilage cells (chondrocytes) are apparent, representing different stages of differentiation (**Fig. 2**). The resting zone contains round stem-like chondrocytes in a relatively quiescent state.[1] Resting chondrocytes produce parathyroid hormone-related protein (PTH-rP), which diffuses to nearby chondrocytes and helps to delay the differentiation of chondrocytes through its negative feedback on another protein called Indian hedgehog (Ihh).[3] Resting chondrocytes nearest the proliferative zone are recruited to enter the proliferative phase, where they develop a flattened appearance and line up in columns. As cells stop proliferation, they become rounder in appearance (prehypertrophic chondrocytes) and begin producing Ihh.[1] Ihh regulates cartilage differentiation and stimulates production of PTH-rP by resting chondrocytes. The classic feedback loop of Ihh and PTH-rP controls the pace of chondrocyte differentiation. Regulation of cartilage maturation is also coordinated by multiple signaling pathways including Wnts, bone morphogenetic proteins, retinoic acid, fibroblast growth factors, and many others.[2,4–6] Following the prehypertrophic phase, chondrocytes enter the hypertrophic phase, which is characterized by cytoplasmic enlargement and secretion

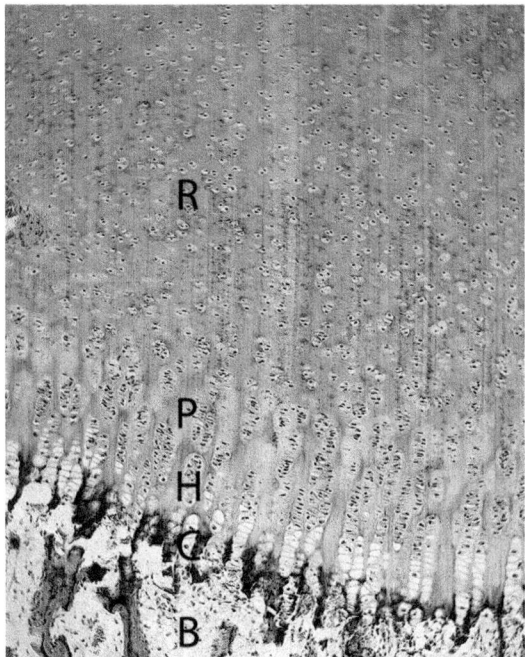

Fig. 2. Growth plate cartilage from a 3-day-old foal (hematoxylin). B, primary spongiosa; C, calcified cartilage zone; H, hypertrophic zone; P, proliferative zone; R, resting zone [H&E, original magnification x100].

of multiple paracrine factors, growth factors, and matrix molecules. Hypertrophic chondrocytes direct mineralization of surrounding matrix (calcified zone), secrete specialized collagen (type X), and produce vascular endothelial growth factor, which recruits blood vessels into the region. With the invasion of blood vessels into calcified cartilage, cartilage is removed by chondroclasts and new bone is laid down by osteoblasts (primary spongiosa). This bone is then remodeled into secondary spongiosa of trabecular bone in the epiphyseal (secondary center of ossification) or metaphyseal region (growth plate).

Nutrition of Postnatal Cartilage: Role of Cartilage Canals

Blood supply to developing cartilage is very important because the A-E cartilage thickness far exceeds the diffusion limits of synovial fluid. Cartilage canals provide the conduit for blood vessels to reach deeper layers of cartilage during the first 6 months of life (**Fig. 3**).[7,8] Each cartilage canal contains an arteriole and several venules. The cartilage canals run either transversely near the periphery (perichondrium) or perpendicularly along the ossification front (osteochondral junction).[9] As the ossification front moves toward the articular surface, cartilage canals fill in (chondrification) and are eventually converted to bone along with surrounding cartilage. In the hypertrophic zone of A-E cartilage, small rounded chondrocytes directly surrounding cartilage canals appear to be held in a resting phase compared with larger hypertrophic chondrocytes further away (**Fig. 4**).[2] Anastomoses of cartilage canals and associated vessels occur along the ossification front during the postnatal period, creating a vulnerable time period for injury, which may be an inciting factor for OC development.[10]

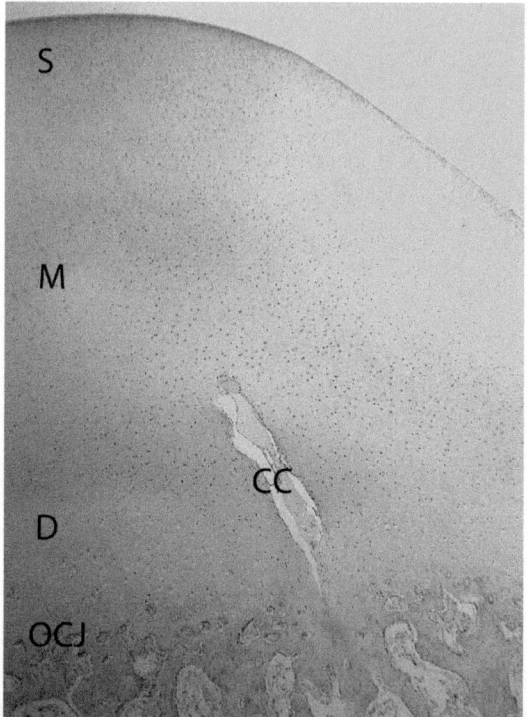

Fig. 3. Articular epiphyseal cartilage from 6-month-old quarter horse filly with cartilage canal (CC) in the deep layer (D) of cartilage near the osteochondral junction (OCJ) [H&E, original magnification x40]. M, middle layer; S, superficial layer.

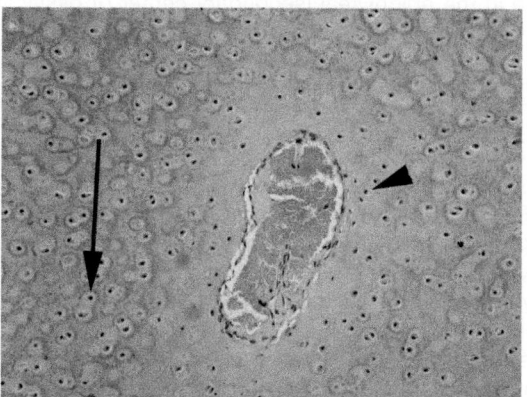

Fig. 4. Photomicrograph of cartilage canal in A-E cartilage of a 1-month-old foal. Smaller rounded chondrocytes (*arrowhead*) directly surround the cartilage canal, whereas larger hypertrophic chondrocytes (*arrow*) are further away in deep zone of cartilage [H&E, original magnification x100].

EARLY PATHOGENESIS OF OSTEOCHONDROSIS

OC has long been believed to be caused by a combination of factors, including genetic, nutritional, environmental, and biomechanical influences.[11–13] In recent years, the research focus has shifted to early OC pathogenesis in horses in an attempt to discover the origin of this disease.[14–20] From these studies, several theories of the causes of OC have emerged, including failure of cartilage canals, biomechanical shearing of the osteochondral junction, molecular alterations in endochondral ossification, and genetic basis.

Current Theories

Failure of cartilage canals

Failure of cartilage canals during the early postnatal period is believed to be a major factor in OC development and seems to be most susceptible along the ossification front.[7,8,10,16] As previously described, vessels form anastomoses between cartilage canals running parallel to and those running perpendicular to the ossification front. Failure of these anastomoses can lead to focal areas of chondronecrosis. A recent study has also illustrated a direct cause and effect in foals that have experimentally had the blood supply disrupted to the lateral trochlear ridge of the femur.[16] These foals developed areas of chondronecrosis and ultimately delayed endochondral ossification and OC lesions. Other studies have shown that young foals had evidence of chondronecrosis secondary to cartilage canal disruption and lack of blood supply.[10] Based on these studies and other research in pigs and horses, there is strong evidence that 1 cause of OC is directly related to failure of cartilage canals.

Shearing of osteochondral junction

Biomechanical forces also play an important role in the development and pathogenesis of OC.[21] Site predilections within joints often directly correlate to regions of high shear stress or impact. Shearing of bony trabeculae can occur as a primary event, with the cartilage-to-bone interface, providing a biomechanically weak region, particularly in 4-month-old foals (**Fig. 5**). Secondary shearing may also occur following cartilage canal failure and chondronecrosis or cartilage matrix weakening due to other factors, such as changes in collagen or glycosaminoglycans content or increased matrix metalloproteinases (MMPs).[17,22–25]

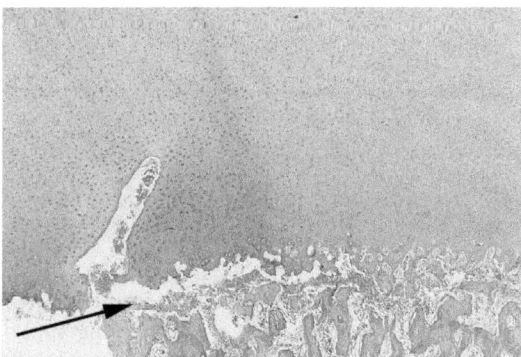

Fig. 5. Photomicrograph of articular epiphyseal cartilage in a 4-month-old foal having separation along the osteochondral junction (*arrow*) [H&E, original magnification x40].

Molecular alterations in endochondral ossification

Another theory for the cause of OC is that molecular alterations within the cartilage matrix and/or cell signaling pathways occur before OC development. Recent studies reveal molecular changes in early OC, providing evidence that an abnormal matrix is a significant factor in disease development.[15,17,22–25] Lecocq and colleagues[23] demonstrated that type II collagen synthesis is altered in OC cartilage and may be an initiating factor in weakening of cartilage matrix near cartilage canals and the osteochondral junction. Other studies in foals younger than 6 months of age reveal changes in gene expression of multiple growth factors and paracrine factors in chondrocytes surrounding cartilage canals and along the osteochondral junction in early OC.[17,18,20] Increased expression of MMP-13 and MMP-3 may also result in biomechanical weakening of matrix in these locations (**Fig. 6**).[17]

Growth factor and paracrine factor dysregulation may also cause a direct delay of endochondral ossification. In a recent study,[18] altered Wnt signaling in OC chondrocytes surrounding cartilage canals suggests that pathways associated with catabolism and inhibition of chondrocyte maturation are targeted in early OC pathogenesis. Other studies also support Wnt pathway dysregulation in OC development.[15,26,27] The Ihh/PTH-rP pathway is another signaling pathway altered in OC cartilage,[17,28,29] and increased expression of Ihh and PTH-rP may have a direct effect on chondrocytic differentiation and endochondral ossification in early OC cartilage. Mitochondrial dysfunction and endoplasmic reticulum (ER)-stress have also been linked to OC pathogenesis in the horse.[30]

Genetic factors

Heritability estimates of OC range from low to high (0.02–0.45) depending on the affected joint and breed of horse.[31] Numerous studies have elucidated genetic loci linked to OC.[32–37] Quantitative trait loci (QTL) are regions of the genome likely to have genes contributing to the trait of interest. More than 25 QTL have been discovered in equine OC through genome-wide studies using microsatellites or single nucleotide polymorphisms.[31–37] However, these loci are not consistent among breeds, and specific joints appear to have different QTL, making it a challenging process to uncover.

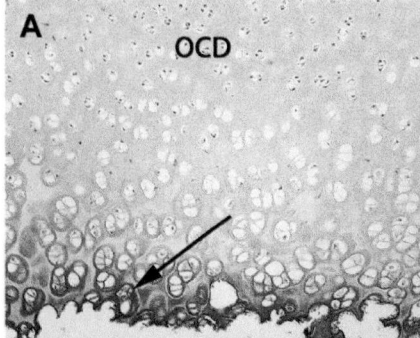 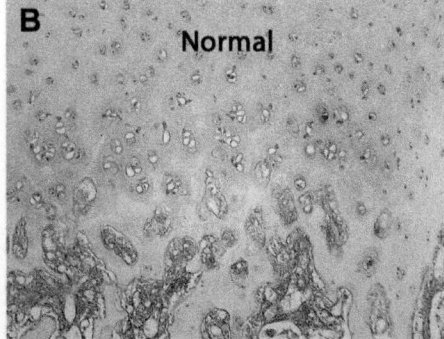

Fig. 6. Photomicrographs of the deep cartilage layer and osteochondral junction immunostained (brown) using MMP-13 primary antibody and DAB chromogen. (*A*) Deep cartilage layer showing strong MMP-13 immunostaining along the separated osteochondral junction in a foal having OCD (*arrow*). (*B*) Normal osteochondral junction showing mild expression of MMP-13 in the hypertrophic chondrocytes in a 4-month-old foal (H&E, Original magnification x100).

Studies of genome-wide gene expression in OC also reveal interesting results. One meta-analysis[38] of all known genome-wide studies reveals characteristic grouping of affected genes in OC. Genes tend to cluster into functional and biological processes, including pathways associated with protein secretion, extracellular matrix molecules, and growth plate maturation. Gene clusters of particular interest within these pathways include a collagen cluster, laminin cluster, cell signaling cluster, matrix turnover cluster, and posttranslational modification cluster.[38]

Early Detection

Biomarkers

Biomarkers are molecules that serve as early indicators of metabolic abnormalities in specific tissues of the body. Early detection of OC has been the focus of several studies, particularly as it relates to measurement of biomarkers in serum, synovial fluid, or blood.[19,39–43] The most promising early biomarker of OC is osteocalcin, which is increased in serum at 2 weeks of age in foals that develop OC at 5.5 months.[19] This biomarker also correlates with OC at 11 months of age when combined with radiographic assessment of the hock and stifle.[39] Products of collagen formation or degradation, and bone mineralization, in serum are also positively correlated with severity of OC, especially when combined with hock and stifle radiographs.[39] Strong correlations are present between radiographic appearance of OC at 5.5 months and serum CPII, a collagen type II formation marker.[19] The ratio of serum CPII to C2C, a cartilage degradation marker, is also significant at this time.

Synovial fluid biomarkers associated with OC in foals are mainly products of collagen (CPII:C2C) and aggrecan turnover (CS846).[24,40] Synovial fluid CPII:C2C ratios tend to be higher in OC joints at all ages but are significant at 5.5 months.[40] The aggrecan turnover marker, CS846, and insulin-like growth factor (IGF)-I are lower in OC-affected joints at 4.5 months of age.[40] In older foals (12–18 months of age), proteomic analysis of synovial fluid reveals dysregulation of pathways involving inflammation, coagulation, oxidative stress, and matrix damage, similar to those found in osteoarthritis.[41] Thus, secondary effects must be taken into account when sampling more mature animals because biomarkers are less likely to be specific to OC.

HEALING OR OSTEOCHONDRITIS DISSECANS DEVELOPMENT?

Early OC lesions have the potential to heal intrinsically or develop into more advanced OCD lesions, resulting in clinical disease. This balance between healing and OCD development hinges on several factors during the first year of life, including exercise level, nutrition, and growth rate, among others.[44–47] Healing requires endochondral ossification of retained cartilage and proper development of the articular cartilage-subchondral bone interface. Cartilage has some capacity to heal in younger foals. Once a foal reaches puberty (6–12 months), this capacity rapidly declines, corresponding to regression of cartilage canals and blood supply.[2,6,9] Therefore, OC lesions have a very limited window of time when healing can occur. By 1 year of age, remaining lesions are unlikely to heal further. Separation along the osteochondral junction results in fibrous tissue formation and development into OCD flaps or fragments.

Intrinsic Factors

Intrinsic factors associated with cartilage healing involve complex molecular interactions of cellular differentiation, matrix remodeling, energy production and metabolism, and endochondral ossification.[30,38,48,49] Increased MMP expression and production of markers of collagen formation indicate matrix remodeling in the deep articular cartilage layer and along the osteochondral junction in OC-affected foals.[17,24] Increased expression of growth factors such as IGF-I and transforming growth factor (TGF)-β1 likely reflect a healing response to damaged matrix, whereas increased expression of PTH-rP and Ihh in the deep layer of articular cartilage reveals modulation of cellular differentiation.[17,25,28,29] Blood supply to the affected area also plays an important role in determining whether OC lesions will heal or not. Invasion of new blood vessels into ischemic cartilage takes considerable time, during which abnormal cartilage may be subjected to biomechanical forces resulting in flap or fragment formation.[10]

Effect of Exercise

Exercise plays an important role in the development of normal articular cartilage and joint function.[50–52] In excess, however, exercise can cause progression of an early OC lesion by concentrating shear forces along the osteochondral junction, leading to fissures through abnormal OC matrix and, ultimately, OCD flaps. In a large field study of French performance horses (Thoroughbreds, Trotters, and Warmbloods), exercise history had a strong influence on manifestation and progression of OC.[13] Lack of exercise, irregular exercise or excessive exercise in the early developmental period (<6 months) has a negative effect on osteochondral status.[12,50,51] Irregular exercise, in particular, seems to result in the highest risk of poor osteochondral status in foals.[12] By 1 year of age, intrinsic trauma caused by excessive exercise is the most important factor in determining osteochondral status.[13] Therefore, foals having early clinical signs of OC should have a reduction of their exercise level to allow time for healing along the osteochondral junction.

THERAPEUTIC OPTIONS

Therapeutic options for early OC lesions mainly focus on decreased exercise level, decreased nutritional plane, and medical treatment of synovitis through joint injections of hyaluronic acid. Some younger foals with larger cartilage flaps with little subchondral bone attachment may also be amenable to reattachment to underlying subchondral bone via arthroscopically placed polydioxanone (PDS) pins.[53] Treatment with mesenchymal stem cells, platelet-rich plasma, or other biologics may be appropriate, depending on the type of OC lesion.[54] Arthroscopic removal of OCD flaps or fragments is generally recommended after foals have reached a year of age, when adequate cartilage-bone maturation has occurred. These and other treatment options will be discussed in greater detail in the next article.

SUMMARY

Several theories of the etiologic factors for OC have emerged over the past 20 years, including failure of cartilage canals, biomechanical shearing of the osteochondral junction, molecular alterations in endochondral ossification, and genetic contributors. From these theories, one can conclude the origin of OC in horses stems from 2 main sources: (1) factors contributing to abnormal cartilage matrix development around cartilage canals and the ossification front and (2) factors leading to biomechanical shearing or crushing of cartilage canals and/or the osteochondral junction. Regardless of the source, it is apparent that failure of cartilage canals near the ossification front during the early postnatal period is a major factor in OC development.

Early OC lesions have the potential to heal intrinsically or develop into more advanced OCD lesions, resulting in clinical disease. Healing of early OC lesions is most likely to occur in younger foals, when blood supply to developing cartilage is greatest. Healing requires endochondral ossification of retained cartilage and proper development of the articular cartilage to subchondral bone interface. Restricting exercise during the healing phase may help to prevent early OC lesions from becoming OCD flaps or fragments. Once horses have reached a year of age, the chance of intrinsic healing diminishes dramatically and surgical options may be better suited for treatment of OCD.

REFERENCES

1. Chagin AS, Kronenberg HM. G-proteins in differentiation of epiphyseal chondrocytes. J Mol Endocrinol 2014;53:R39–45.
2. Duesterdieck-Zellmer KF, Semevolos SA, Kinsley MA, et al. Age-related differential gene and protein expression in postnatal cartilage canal and osteochondral junction chondrocytes. Gene Expr Patterns 2015;17(1):1–10.
3. Kronenberg HM. Developmental regulation of the growth plate. Nature 2003;423: 332–6.
4. Andrade AC, Nilsson O, Barnes KM, et al. Wnt gene expression in the post-natal growth plate: regulation with chondrocyte differentiation. Bone 2007;40:1361–9.
5. Tamamura Y, Otani T, Kanatani N, et al. Developmental regulation of Wnt/beta-catenin signals is required for growth plate assembly, cartilage integrity, and endochondral ossification. J Biol Chem 2005;280:19185–95.
6. Semevolos SA, Nixon AJ, Fortier LA, et al. Age-related expression of molecular regulators of hypertrophy and maturation in articular cartilage. J Orthop Res 2006;24:1773–81.
7. Carlson CS, Cullins LD, Meuten DJ. Osteochondrosis of the articular-epiphyseal complex in young horses: evidence for a defect in cartilage canal blood supply. Vet Pathol 1995;32:641–7.
8. Shingleton WD, Mackie EJ, Cawston TE, et al. Cartilage canals in equine articular/epiphyseal growth cartilage and a possible association with dyschondroplasia. Equine Vet J 1997;29:360–4.
9. Olstad K, Ytrehus B, Ekman S, et al. Epiphyseal cartilage canal blood supply to the distal femur of foals. Equine Vet J 2008;40:433–9.
10. Olstad K, Ekman S, Carlson CS. An update on the pathogenesis of osteochondrosis. Vet Pathol 2015;52:785–802.
11. Semevolos SA, Nixon AJ. Equine osteochondrosis: etiologic factors. Compend Equine Ed 2007;2(3):158–64.
12. Lepeule J, Bareille N, Robert C, et al. Association of growth, feeding practices, and exercise conditions with the severity of the osteoarticular status of limbs in French foals. Vet J 2013;197:65–71.
13. van Weeren P, Denoix J-M. The Normandy field study on juvenile osteochondral conditions: Conclusions regarding the influence of genetics, environmental conditions, and management, and the effect on performance. Vet J 2013;197:90–5.
14. Mirams M, Avodele BA, Tatarczuch L, et al. Identification of novel osteochondrosis-associated genes. J Orthop Res 2016;34:404–11.
15. Mirams M, Tatarczuch L, Ahmed YA, et al. Altered gene expression in early osteochondrosis lesions. J Orthop Res 2009;27:452–7.
16. Olstad K, Hendrickson EHS, Carlson CS, et al. Transection of vessels in epiphyseal cartilage canals leads to osteochondrosis and osteochondritis dissecans in the femoro-patellar joint of foals; a potential model of juvenile osteochondritis dissecans. Osteoarthritis Cartilage 2013;21:730–8.

17. Riddick TL, Duesterdieck-Zellmer K, Semevolos SA. Gene and protein expression of cartilage canal and osteochondral junction chondrocytes and full-thickness cartilage in early equine osteochondrosis. Vet J 2012;194:319–25.

18. Kinsley M, Semevolos SA, Duesterdieck-Zellmer KF. Molecular characterization of Wnt/β-catenin signaling of cartilage canal and osteochondral junction chondrocytes in early equine osteochondrosis. J Orthop Res 2015;33:1433–8.

19. Donabedian M, van Weeren PR, Perona G, et al. Early changes in biomarkers of skeletal metabolism and their association to the occurrence of osteochondrosis (OC) in the horse. Equine Vet J 2008;40:253–9.

20. Semevolos SA, Duesterdieck-Zellmer K, Larson M. Role of Apoptosis in Development of Early Osteochondrosis. Proc Orthop Res Soc 2015;40:1273.

21. Pool R. Difficulties in definition of equine osteochondrosis; differentiation of developmental and acquired lesions. Equine Vet J 1993;(Suppl 16):5–12.

22. Laverty S, Girard C. Pathogenesis of epiphyseal osteochondrosis. Vet J 2013; 197:3–12.

23. Lecocq M, Girard CA, Fogarty U, et al. Cartilage matrix changes in the developing epiphysis: early events on the pathway to equine osteochondrosis? Equine Vet J 2008;40:442–54.

24. Laverty S, Okouneff S, Ionescu M, et al. Excessive degradation of type II collagen in articular cartilage in equine osteochondrosis. J Orthop Res 2002;20:1282–9.

25. Semevolos SA, Nixon AJ, Brower-Toland BD. Changes in molecular expression of articular cartilage collagen types I, II, and X, aggrecan, insulin-like growth factor-I, and transforming growth factor-beta1 in naturally acquired osteochondrosis. Am J Vet Res 2001;62:1088–94.

26. Power J, Hernandez P, Wardale J, et al. Alterations in sclerostin protein in lesions of equine osteochondrosis. Vet Rec 2014;1:e000005.

27. Serteyn D, Piquemal D, Vanderheyden L, et al. Gene expression profiling from leukocytes of horses affected by osteochondrosis. J Orthop Res 2010; 28:965–70.

28. Semevolos SA, Strassheim ML, Haupt JL, et al. Expression patterns of Hedgehog signaling peptides in naturally-acquired equine osteochondrosis. J Orthop Res 2005;23(5):1152–9.

29. Semevolos SA, Brower-Toland BD, Bent S, et al. Parathyroid hormone-related peptide and indian hedgehog expression patterns in naturally-acquired equine osteochondrosis. J Orthop Res 2002;20:1290–7.

30. Desjardin C, Chat S, Gilles M, et al. Involvement of mitochondrial dysfunction and ER-stress in the physiopathology of equine osteochondritis dissecans (OCD). Exp Mol Pathol 2014;96:328–38.

31. Distl O. The genetics of equine osteochondrosis. Vet J 2013;197:13–8.

32. McCoy AM, Beeson SK, Splan RK, et al. Identification and validation of risk loci for osteochondrosis in Standardbreds. BMC Genomics 2016;17:41.

33. Lampe V, Dierks C, Komm K, et al. Identification of a new quantitative trait locus in equine chromosome 18 responsible for osteochondrosis in Hanoverian warmblood horses. J Anim Sci 2009;87:3477–81.

34. Lampe V, Dierks C, Distl O. Refinement of a quantitative trait locus on equine chromosome 5 responsible for fetlock osteochondrosis in Hanoverian warmblood horses. Anim Genet 2009;40:553–5.

35. Lampe V, Dierks C, Distl O. Refinement of a quantitative locus on equine chromosome 16 responsible for osteochondrosis in Hanoverian warmblood horses. Animal 2009;3:1224–31.

36. Dierks C, Komm K, Lampe V, et al. Fine mapping of a quantitative trait locus for osteochondrosis on horse chromosome 2. Anim Genet 2010;41(Suppl 2):87–90.

37. Mittmann EH, Lampe V, Momke S, et al. Characterization of a minimal microsatellite set for whole genome scans informative in warmblood and coldblood horse breeds. J Hered 2010;10:246–50.

38. Bates JT, Jacobs JC, Shea KG, et al. Emerging genetic basis of osteochondritis dissecans. Clin Sports Med 2014;33:199–220.

39. Billinghurst RC, Brama PA, van Weeren PR, et al. Evaluation of serum concentrations of biomarkers of skeletal metabolism and results of radiography as indicators of severity of osteochondrosis in foals. Am J Vet Res 2004;65:143–50.

40. de Grauw JC, Donabedian M, van de Lest CHA, et al. Assessment of synovial fluid biomarkers in healthy foals and in foals with tarsocrural osteochondrosis. Vet J 2011;190:390–5.

41. Chiaradia E, Pepe M, Tartaglia M, et al. Gambling on putative biomarkers of osteoarthritis and osteochondrosis by equine synovial fluid proteomics. J Proteomics 2012;75:4478–93.

42. Verwilghen DR, Enzerink E, Martens A, et al. Relationship between arthroscopic joint evaluation and the levels of Coll2-1, Coll2-1NO$_2$, and myeloperoxidase in the blood and synovial fluid of horses affected with osteochondrosis of the tarsocrural joint. Osteoarthritis Cartilage 2011;19:1323–9.

43. Mendoza L, Piquemal D, Lejeune JP, et al. Age-dependent expression of osteochondrosis-related genes in equine leukocytes. Vet Rec Open 2015;2: e000058.

44. van Weeren PR, Sloet van Oldruitenborgh-Ooste, Barneveld A. The influence of birth weight, rate of weight gain, and final achieved height and sex on the development of osteochondrotic lesions in a population of genetically predisposed Warmblood foals. Equine Vet J Suppl 1999;31:26–30.

45. van Weeren PR, Barneveld A. The effect of exercise on the distribution and manifestation of osteochondrotic lesions in the Warmblood foal. Equine Vet J Suppl 1999;31:16–25.

46. Vander Heyden L, Lejeune J-P, Caudron I, et al. Association of breeding conditions with prevalence of osteochondrosis in foals. Vet Rec 2012;172:68.

47. McCoy AM, Toth F, Dolvik NI, et al. Articular osteochondrosis: a comparison of naturally-occurring human and animal disease. Osteoarthritis Cartilage 2013; 21(11):1638–47.

48. Desjardin C, Vaiman A, Mata X, et al. Next-generation sequencing identifies equine cartilage and subchondral bone miRNAs and suggests their involvement in osteochondrosis physiopathology. BMC Genomics 2014;15:798.

49. Desjardin C, Riviere J, Vaiman A, et al. Omics technologies provide new insights into the molecular physiopathology of equine osteochondrosis. BMC Genomics 2014;15:947.

50. van de Lest CH, Brama PA, van Weeren PR. The influence of exercise on the composition of developing equine joints. Biorheology 2002;39:183–91.

51. Brama PA, TeKoppele JM, Bank RA, et al. Development of biochemical heterogeneity of articular cartilage: influences of age and exercise. Equine Vet J 2002;34: 265–9.

52. Barneveld A, van Weeren PR. Conclusions regarding the influence of exercise on the development of the equine musculoskeletal system with special reference to osteochondrosis. Equine Vet J 1999;31:112–9.

53. Sparks HD, Nixon AJ, Fortier LA, et al. Arthroscopic reattachment of osteochondritis dissecans cartilage flaps of the femoropatellar joint: long-term results. Equine Vet J 2011;43:650–9.

54. Seo JP, Tanabe T, Tsuzuki N, et al. Effects of bilayer gelatin/β-tricalcium phosphate sponges loaded with mesenchymal stem cells, chondrocytes, bone morphogenetic protein-2, and platelet rich plasma on osteochondral defects of the talus in horses. Res Vet Sci 2013;95:1210–6.

Surgical Management of Osteochondrosis in Foals

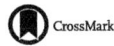

Kyla F. Ortved, DVM, PhD

KEYWORDS

- Osteochondrosis • Osteochondritis dessicans • Arthroscopy • Femoropatellar joint
- Tarsocrural joint • Fetlock joint

KEY POINTS

- Osteochondrosis is a common developmental disease in young horses.
- Osteochondrosis is caused by failure of normal endochondral ossification and most commonly affects the articular–epiphyseal cartilage.
- Osteochondrosis is a multifactorial disease with trauma, biomechanical forces, nutrition, exercise, cartilage vascularization, and genetics playing contributory roles.
- Horses with osteochondrosis often show lameness and joint effusion. Radiographs are usually diagnostic, although some lesions are only apparent arthroscopically.
- Arthroscopic debridement of abnormal cartilage and subchondral bone is the most common treatment and is indicated in horses with clinical signs.

INTRODUCTION

Osteochondrosis is a common developmental orthopedic disease and frequent cause of lameness in young, athletic horses.[1] It is a complex disorder, but can be primarily defined as focal failure of endochondral ossification leading to an area of growth cartilage that fails to undergo matrix calcification and vascular invasion and, therefore, is not converted to bone (**Fig. 1**).[2]

Osteochondrosis lesions are generally first seen as fissures in articular cartilage with cartilaginous or osteochondral fragments detaching from the parent bone, possibly forming free intraarticular fragments.[3] The term osteochondritis dessicans is used to describe lesions with loose or separated flaps of cartilage. Although the clinical manifestations of osteochondrosis are well-described, the definitive cause remains unknown and likely involves several factors, including biomechanical forces, nutrition, and genetics. In the horse, osteochondrosis most commonly affects the femoropatellar, tarsocrural, and metatarsophalangeal/metacarpophalangeal joints, although it can also be diagnosed in other joints.

Clinical Studies, New Bolton Center, University of Pennsylvania, 382 West Street Road, Kennett Square, PA 19348, USA
E-mail address: kortved@vet.upenn.edu

Vet Clin Equine 33 (2017) 379–396
http://dx.doi.org/10.1016/j.cveq.2017.03.010   **vetequine.theclinics.com**

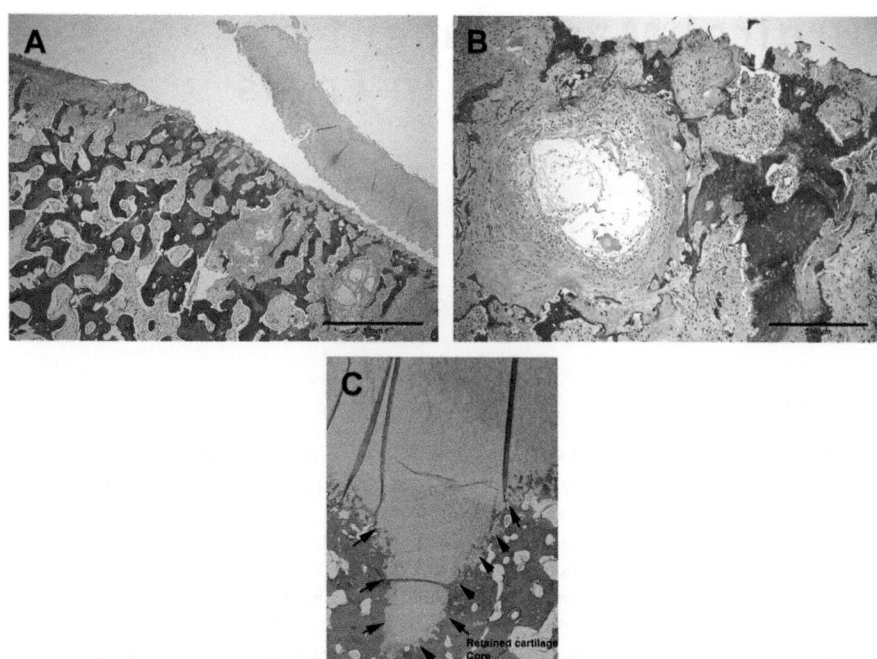

Fig. 1. (*A*) Hematoxylin and eosin (H&E)–stained osteochondral section from a humeral head of a Thoroughbred yearling with osteochondrosis. A cartilage flap is seen dissecting away from the subchondral bone. (*B*) H&E–stained section from the glenoid of the same yearling showing a subchondral cystic lesion and secondary osteoarthritis. (*C*) H&E–stained osteochondral section from the lateral trochlear ridge of the femur of a Standardbred yearling showing a retained cartilage core consistent with osteochondrosis. (*From* Engiles JB. Diseases of the skeletal system. In: Buergelt CD, Del Piero F, editors. Color atlas of equine pathology. Ames(IO):John Wiley & Sons, Inc.; 2013:301–43; with permission.)

This review discusses the etiology, causative factors, and clinical signs associated with osteochondrosis in the young horse with a focus on surgical treatment options for specific joints affected.

ETIOLOGY

The cartilaginous primordial skeleton begins the process of endochondral ossification during early fetal development with longitudinal growth of long bones extending from physes after birth.[4] During endochondral ossification, chondrocytes proliferate, hypertrophy, and then undergo apoptosis followed by calcification. Osteoblasts are responsible for deposition of primary bone after calcification, which is then successively remodeled into bony trabeculae. This remodeling process continues into adulthood. In long bones, the articular–epiphyseal cartilage undergoes a similar ossification process to the physis. Although osteochondrosis can develop at either location, the articular–epiphyseal cartilage is the more common site of clinical osteochondrosis in horses.[5]

CAUSATIVE FACTORS

Many causative factors have been proposed, including trauma and biomechanical forces, exercise, nutrition and hormonal factors, failure of vascularization, and genetics. The influence of trauma and biomechanical forces is supported by the consistency of predilection sites in specific joints.[6] It is hypothesized that excessive forces on normal tissues or normal forces on abnormal tissues may lead to disruption of vascular supply in cartilage undergoing endochondral ossification or cause shearing of cartilage flaps.[7,8] Other factors, including body size, conformation, and exercise, obviously influence biomechanical forces within the joint. Sandgren and colleagues (1993) found a relationship between conformation and osteochondrosis in Standardbred foals. The authors found that foals with externally rotated tarsi had a significantly higher incidence of tarsocrural osteochondrosis than foals with normal conformation. There is conflicting evidence regarding the role of exercise in development of osteochondrosis; however, most researchers agree that moderate exercise is necessary for normal functional adaptation of cartilage during early development, and that too little or excessive exercise can contribute to the development of osteochondrosis.[9]

The role of nutrition, including digestible energy and mineral concentration, has been implicated in the pathogenesis of osteochondrosis for many years. Originally, copper deficiency was proposed to cause osteochondrosis owing to the requirement for copper as a cofactor in lysyl oxidase, which is needed for collagen cross-linking.[10–12] More recently, adequate copper has been shown to have a beneficial effect on repair of lesions but no direct relationship with pathogenesis.[13] There are differing opinions on whether fast growth rate or high-energy feeding leads to osteochondrosis. Donabedian and colleagues[14] (2006) showed that osteochondrosis lesions increased with fast growth rate regardless of diet, whereas Savage and colleagues[15] (1993) found increased osteochondrosis in foals fed high-energy diets. It has been proposed that high-energy diets cause postprandial hyperinsulinemia and upregulation of insulin-like growth factor-I, which has mitogenic and antiapoptotic effects in chondrocytes.[16] Insulin also stimulates removal of thyroxine (T3 and T4) from circulation, both of which are required for normal chondrocyte differentiation and vascularization of growth cartilage.[17] Interruption of chondrocyte differentiation associated with hyperinsulinemia could, therefore, lead to the development of osteochondrosis.

Failure of vascularization has also been implicated in osteochondrosis. In early skeletal development, cartilage canals are needed to supply nutrition to deep cartilage that cannot be nourished by synovial fluid alone. However, these canals are obliterated during endochondral ossification.[18] Areas of chondronecrosis associated with obliterated cartilage canals have been seen in pigs with naturally occurring osteochondrosis. Additionally, the presence of cartilage plugs have been observed after experimental devascularization of deep cartilage in pigs.[19] These findings suggest that premature interruption of the vascular supply may lead to ischemic necrosis of cartilage and development of osteochondrosis lesions.[20]

Several studies have also shown that osteochondrosis is a polygenic trait with complex inheritance.[21–24] Progeny from stallions affected with osteochondrosis have a higher incidence of osteochondrosis[25] and osteochondrosis is uncommon in ponies and feral horses.[26,27] Although it is clear that heritability contributes to the disease, there is significant phenotypic variance.

CLINICAL SIGNS

Any breed of horse can develop osteochondrosis; however, the reported incidence is greatest in Standardbreds (10.5%–35%),[28–30] Thoroughbreds (20%), and Warmbloods (20%).[31,32] Clinical signs associated with osteochondrosis can range from minimal to severe, with the majority being mild to moderate. Most osteochondrosis lesions develop before 7 months of age,[33] but may not be diagnosed until later in life when the horse commences training and the joint is biomechanically stressed. Clinical signs include effusion of the affected joint(s) and variable, but generally mild, lameness. The majority of osteochondrosis lesions can be definitively diagnosed with radiography, although some lesions are radiographically occult yet present on arthroscopic examination. McIlwraith (2013)[34] described 3 main clinical categories of osteochondrosis:

1. Both clinical signs and radiographic signs are present.
2. Clinical signs without radiographic signs but arthroscopic signs are present.
3. Radiographic signs are present but no clinical signs are present.

A study following the radiographic progression of osteochondrosis lesions in Warmblood foals revealed that some radiographic lesions heal or stabilize.[33] In this study, lesions at the cranial intermediate ridge of the distal tibia (C1RDT) and lateral trochlear ridge (LTR) of the talus showed healing in horses less than 5 months of age. Lesions in these locations present past 5 months were unlikely to heal. Similarly, lesions on the LTR of the femur present past 8 months were unlikely to heal (**Fig. 2**). In addition, caution must be taken when interpreting radiographs in very young foals, because delayed endochondral ossification is normal in the trochlear ridges of the femur and talus.

DISTRIBUTION OF LESIONS

In the horse, the most commonly affected joints are the tarsocrural joint, femoropatellar joint, and metacarpophalangeal and metatarsophalangeal (fetlock) joints followed by the carpal joint, elbow joint, shoulder joint, and cervical articular facet joints.[35] The LTR of the femur is most commonly affected in the femoropatellar joint. Within the tarsocrural joint, the cranial intermediate ridge of the distal tibia, LTR of the talus, and medial malleolus are affected in descending order.[36] Within the metacarpophalangeal and metatarsophalangeal joints, the sagittal ridge is the most commonly affected. Osteochondrosis lesions are commonly found bilaterally, therefore, radiography of the contralateral joint or all 4 fetlock joints should be strongly considered.[28]

TREATMENT
Conservative Management

Conservative management generally consists of stall or small paddock confinement, and appropriate nutritional management. Systemic nonsteroidal antiinflammatory drug and/or intraarticular medication with corticosteroids and/or hyaluronic acid may be administered; however, they do not seem to be very effective.[37] Affected horses should be monitored for increased joint effusion, changes in gait, and/or increased lameness. They should also be followed radiographically to assess temporal changes in the lesion. Horses less than 5 months of age with osteochondrosis lesions in the tarsus or fetlock can be treated conservatively and monitored radiographically; many of these lesions will heal spontaneously. Horses less than 8 months of age with osteochondrosis lesions in the stifle can also be treated conservatively and monitored radiographically. Spontaneous healing of osteochondrosis lesions is almost always superior to healing after surgical debridement, therefore, allowing time for spontaneous resolution is recommended if possible.

Surgical Management

Surgical management of osteochondrosis lesions is common, because it generally leads to resolution of clinical signs, including joint effusion and lameness, and decreases the potential for future joint damage caused by loose flaps or free fragments. Additionally, surgical intervention improves radiographic signs, which is an important consideration in the presale horse.

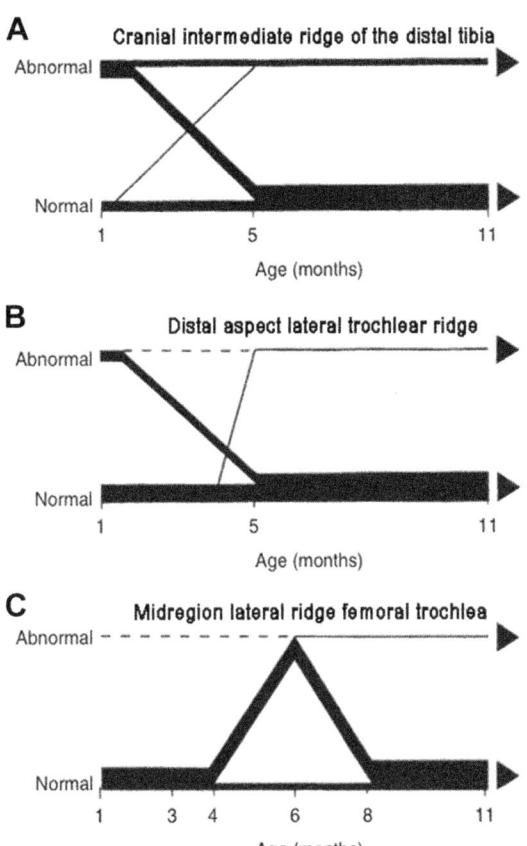

Fig. 2. Radiologic development of osteochondrosis in young horses. (*A*) The majority of osteochondrosis lesions in the cranial intermediate ridge of the distal tibia are present at 1 month of age, with few appearing after 1 month. The majority of these lesions resolve over the next 4 months. After 5 months, the radiographic appearance of lesions is stable. (*B*) A similar pattern is noted for osteochondrosis lesions of the lateral trochlear ridge of the talus. (*C*) Early development of osteochondrosis lesions of the lateral trochlear ridge of the femur seems to be different with most lesions becoming radiographically apparent after 3 months with a peak at 6 months. Many lesions will resolve by 8 months with remaining lesions being stable after 8 months. (*From* Dik KJ, Enzerink EE, van Weeren PR. Radiographic development of osteochondral abnormalities, in the hock and stifle of Dutch Warmblood foals, from age 1 to 11 months. Equine Vet Suppl 1999;31:9; with permission.)

In the past, many osteochondrosis lesions were approached and debrided through an arthrotomy; however, with the advancement of minimally invasive surgery, the vast majority of osteochondrosis lesions are now treated arthroscopically. Arthroscopic debridement of abnormal cartilage and subchondral bone is used most commonly; however, surgical management for specific joints and different manifestations of osteochondrosis is discussed elsewhere in this article.

Femoropatellar Joint

The femoropatellar joint is a common site of osteochondrosis with most lesions occurring on the LTR (**Fig. 3**). Lesions can also occur on the medial trochlear ridge, trochlear

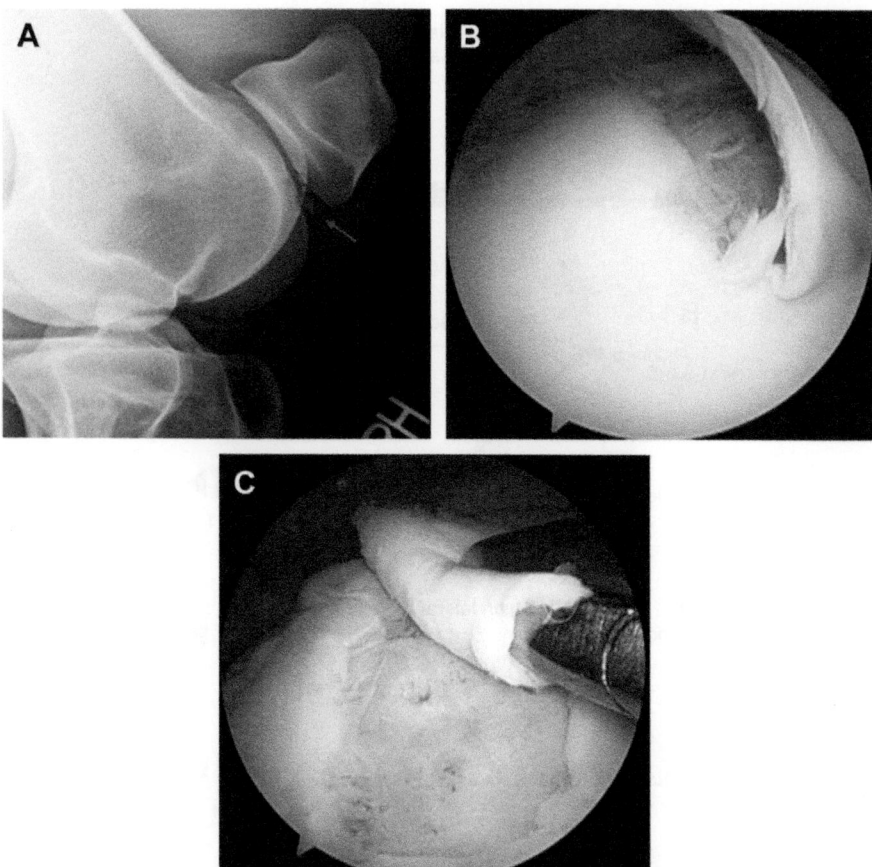

Fig. 3. (*A*) Lateromedial radiographic view of the stifle of a horse showing an osteochondrosis lesion on the lateral trochlear ridge (*red arrow*). (*B*) Arthroscopic image of the osteochondrosis lesion seen in A before debridement. (*C*) Arthroscopic image of the same osteochondrosis lesion during debridement.

groove, and, less commonly, the articular surface of the patella.[38] Joint effusion with variable lameness including stiffness and/or uneven gait, is generally present, with most horses showing clinical signs at less than 1 year of age.[39] Small lesions (<2 cm long, <5 mm deep) without radiographic fragmentation in younger horse may respond to conservative management. It should be noted that healing in the femoropatellar joint is generally complete by 8 months of age.[33] Radiographic signs can be variable, including no radiographic abnormalities, flattening of the trochlear ridge, irregular defects and areas of mineralization associated with the trochlear ridge, and free osteochondral fragments within the joint space.[40] Lesions are often more severe arthroscopically than radiographically.

Arthroscopic debridement of lesions is indicated in horses with lameness and joint effusion and in horses greater than 11 months of age. It is also indicated to debride lesions in horses that are intended for sale to improve the radiographic appearance of the joint. Routine femoropatellar joint arthroscopy with the horse positioned in dorsal recumbency allows access to most lesions. Removal of loose cartilaginous and osteochondral flaps followed by conservative debridement down to healthy subchondral bone is recommended (see **Fig. 3**B, C). Free osteochondral fragments may accumulate in the suprapatellar pouch necessitating long arthroscopic instruments or a suprapatellar instrument portal.

Reattachment of cartilage flaps using polydioxanone (PDS) pins (Orthosorb Pins, DePuy Synthes, Warsaw, IN) has been described.[41,42] Polydioxanone pinning has resulted in reattachment of flaps and improved radiographic outcomes; however, the technique should be reserved for lesions with persisting perimeter continuity, surfaces that are not deeply fissured or irregular, and cartilage flaps that are not extensively mineralized. The pins are arthroscopically placed into small drill holes 10 to 15 mm apart with 1 to 2 mm of pin left protruding from the surface to allow for flattening of the head and stabilization (**Fig. 4**). Sparks and colleagues[42] (2011) reviewed polydioxanone pinning of 40 LTR lesions in 27 horses. Radiographic resolution was observed by 6 months in all joints. Twenty horses had long-term follow-up with 19 being sound and athletic. The overall success rate was reported to be 95%.

Postoperative management includes 2 weeks of box stall rest, at which point the sutures are removed and hand walking commences. Controlled, gradually increasing periods of hand walking are recommended for 6 to 10 weeks after suture removal. Small paddock turnout is recommended in the fourth postoperative month with return to training 5 to 6 months postoperatively.

Overall, the prognosis for arthroscopic debridement of femoropatellar osteochondrosis is fair to good, depending on severity. Several studies have reported approximately 65% of horses performed at their intended level after arthroscopic debridement of LTR lesions.[39,43] Horses with trochlear ridge osteochondrosis seem to have fewer starts, fewer placed finishes, and earn less money than their age matched controls.[44] Foland and colleagues[39] (1992) further categorized lesions and found that grade I lesions (<2 cm) had a significantly better prognosis (78%) than grade II (2-4 cm; 63%) or grade III lesions (>4 cm; 54%). A more recent study in sport horses found that involvement of structures other than the LTR, including the patella and medial trochlear ridge, resulted in a worse prognosis.[43]

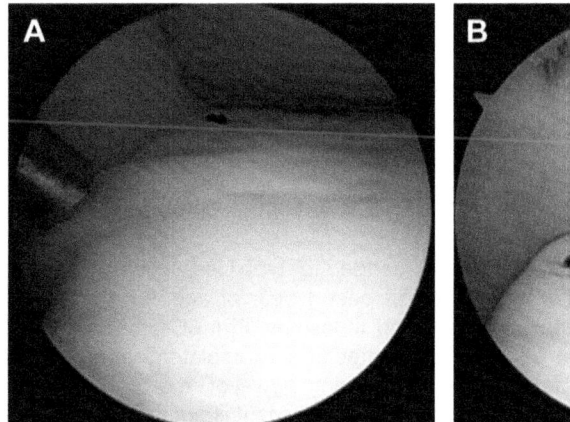
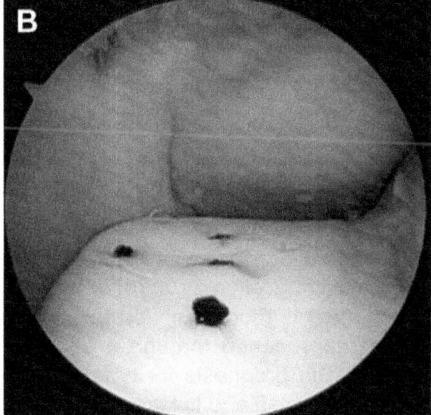

Fig. 4. (*A*) An arthroscopic image of a large osteochondrosis lesion of the lateral trochlear ridge of the femur being reattached with polydioxanone (PDS) pins. The cannula for pin insertion is seen on the left of the image. (*B*) An arthroscopic image of the lateral trochlear ridge after insertion of all PDS pins. The cartilage flap has been stabilized by the pins.

Tarsocrural Joint

Joint effusion (bog spavin) is the most common clinical sign of tarsocrural osteo-chondrosis and effusion can be marked. Lameness is variable and not necessarily correlated with the degree of effusion.[45] Lameness tends to become more prevalent in horses with osteochondrosis once they begin training or racing.[36] The cranial inter-mediate ridge of the distal tibia is the most common location for osteochondrosis in the tarsocrural joint, followed by the LTR and the medial malleolus.[46]

Four view radiographs of the tarsus are used to evaluate all aspects of the joint. Medial malleolar lesions can be difficult to see necessitating several slightly off-angled dorsoplantar views to highlight the lesion. Radiographically silent lesions are not uncommon in this joint; therefore, persistent effusion can be an indication for surgery.

Arthroscopic debridement of osteochondrosis lesions in the tarsocrural joint is commonplace. Although the clinical relevance of cranial intermediate ridge of the distal tibia lesions has been questioned in the past, most surgeons recommend arthro-scopic debridement in all cases with clinical signs and an athletic career planned.[34] A routine dorsomedial arthroscopic portal with the animal placed in dorsal recumbency is suitable to visualize lesions (**Fig. 5**C). Lesions on the cranial intermediate ridge of the distal tibia and LTR can be accessed via a dorsolateral instrument portal, whereas medial malleolar lesions require a dorsomedial instrument portal.

The prognosis for arthroscopic debridement of cranial intermediate ridge of the distal tibia and LTR lesions has been reported to be good.[47,48] McIlwraith and associates (1991) found that 76.5% of horses raced or performed their intended use after surgery. Additionally, Standardbreds with arthroscopically treated cranial intermediate ridge of the distal tibia lesions were found to perform as well as matched controls.[45]

Fetlock Joint

In the metacarpophalangeal and metatarsophalangeal joints, fragmentation and irreg-ularity of the dorsal sagittal ridges and condyles are most common. Joint effusion is the most common clinical sign. Lameness generally only occurs in horses with large or unstable lesions, with a flexion test of the joint being positive. Lesions can occur bilaterally or quadrilaterally; therefore, all fetlock joints should be evaluated radio-graphically if a lesion is recognized in one joint. Lesions are best diagnosed using a flexed lateral–medial radiograph, which highlights the dorsal sagittal ridge (**Fig. 6**A, B). Three types of sagittal ridge osteochondrosis have been described[49]:

1. Type I: Flattening of the sagittal ridge.
2. Type II: Discrete fragment located within area of flattening.
3. Type III: Flattening with or without a discrete fragment and loose fragments within the joint.

Conservative management has been recommended for type I lesions unless clinical signs, including effusion and lameness, persist past 1 year of age.[50] Arthroscopic debridement is recommended for all type II and III lesions (**Fig. 6**C–F). The sagittal ridge is approached through a standard dorsomedial or dorsolateral approach to the joint. The prognosis for type I lesions is excellent; however, the prognosis de-creases for type II and III lesions if timely surgical management is not instituted. Addi-tionally, prognosis is decreased if cartilage erosion or wear lines are noted in the condyles during arthroscopic examination.[50]

Osteochondral fragments at the plantar/palmar aspect of proximal P1 are consid-ered by some to be a manifestation of osteochondrosis[51] owing to their presence in

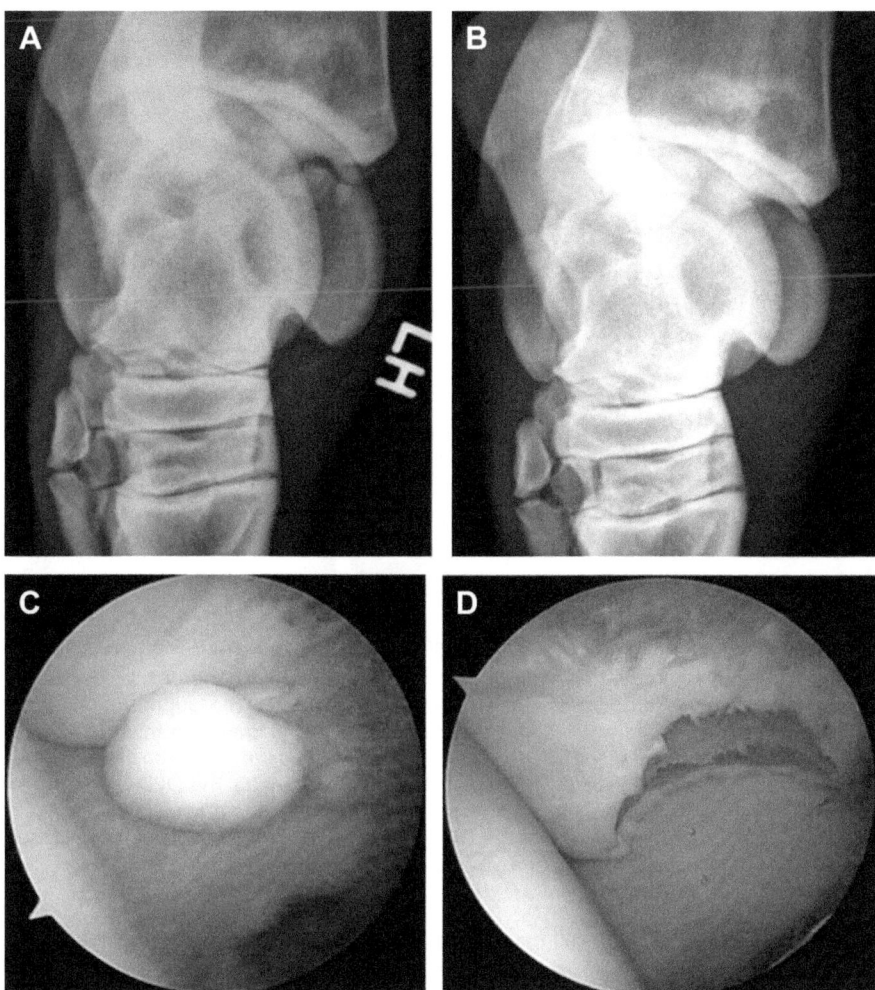

Fig. 5. (*A*) A dorsomedial-plantarolateral oblique (DMPLO) radiographic view of the tarsus highlighting an osteochondrosis lesion at the cranial intermediate ridge of the tibia. (*B*) A DMPLO radiographic view of the tarsus after complete debridement of a cranial intermediate ridge of the distal tibia (CIRDT) lesion. (*C*) Arthroscopic image of a CIRDT lesion. (*D*) An arthroscopic image of the lesion after fragment removal. (*Courtesy of* Dr Michael Ross, New Bolton Center, University of Pennsylvania, Kennett Square, PA.)

young, untrained horses and their predictable location. Several others have argued that these lesions are traumatic in origin,[52,53] because the histologic appearance of these fragments is not consistent with osteochondrosis and the location of the fragments is consistent with an avulsion fracture of the short sesamoidean ligaments. These fragments are much more common in the hindlimbs than the forelimbs, and are most common in Standardbreds. Lameness can be present; however, these osteochondral fragments are often identified on survey radiographs without any clinical signs. Arthroscopic removal of these fragments is often elected either prophylactically or to alleviate associated lameness. Arthroscopy of the palmar/plantar fetlock joint is undertaken to identify the fragment, which is generally embedded in the short

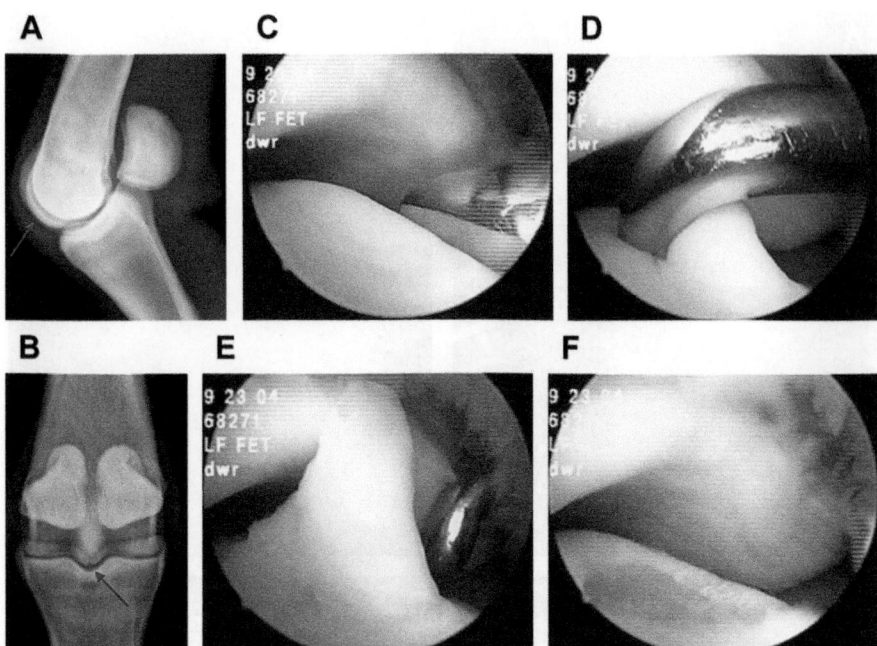

Fig. 6. (A) Flexed lateromedial radiographic view of an osteochondrosis lesion on the sagittal ridge of the third metacarpus (*Red arrow*) of a 2-year-old Thoroughbred racehorse. (*B*) Dorsopalmar radiographic view of the same lesion (*Red arrow*) seen in A. (*C*) Arthroscopic image of the lesion seen in A. (*D*) An arthroscopic image of the osteochondritis dessicans (OCD) lesion being elevated with an arthroscopic probe. (*E*) The OCD lesion once it has been loosened. The fragment is now ready for removal using a Ferris-Smith rongeur. (*F*) The sagittal ridge after removal of the OCD fragment. (*Courtesy of* Dr Dean Richardson, New Bolton Center, University of Pennsylvania, Kennett Square, PA.)

sesamoidean ligament just proximal to palmar/plantar eminence of proximal P1. Fragments are cut free from their ligamentous attachments and removed. Prognosis is excellent after arthroscopic removal.[54]

Elbow Joint

Osteochondrosis of the elbow joint is uncommon in the horse. Osteochondrosis of the distal humerus and/or proximal radius can be a cause of lameness and is generally diagnosed after intraarticular analgesia and radiographs. Osteochondral flaps on the humeral condyles or osseous cystlike lesions in the proximal radius are most common.[55] Radiography is used to identify osseous cystlike lesions or areas of lysis consistent with osteochondral flap lesions. Osteochondral flaps on the caudal humerus can be accessed via a caudomedial or caudolateral arthroscopic approach and are amenable to debridement. Owing to the complex anatomy of the elbow joint and the substantial collateral ligaments limiting joint distraction, arthroscopy of the proximal radius is extremely limited.[55] Extraarticular curettage of osseous cystlike lesions in the proximal radius has some success,[56] although conservative management of these cysts has been advocated by others.[57] Overall, the results of conservative and surgical management of elbow osteochondrosis have been disappointing, with secondary osteoarthritis being a common sequela.

Shoulder Joint

Fortunately, osteochondrosis of the shoulder is not common as it is the most debilitating form of osteochondrosis in the horse. Large areas of the articular surface of the humeral head and glenoid are often involved and secondary osteoarthritis is common. Young horses (usually less 1 year of age) tend to present with forelimb lameness of variable severity.[55]

Diagnosis of shoulder osteochondrosis is generally made after intraarticular analgesia and radiography. Flattening, indentation, or osseous cystlike lesions of the humeral head and/or glenoid are commonly seen. Some horses have secondary degenerative changes, including osteophytosis of the caudal glenoid cavity.[58]

Arthroscopic surgery is recommended in moderate to severe cases, before the development of secondary osteoarthritis.[55,58] The shoulder joint can be accessed via a craniolateral or lateral approach for debridement of the humeral head and/or glenoid lesions. The arthroscopic approach largely depends on lesion location and surgeon preference.

The overall prognosis for shoulder osteochondrosis seems to be significantly worse than other joints with prognoses ranging from poor (30%)[59] to good (80%)[58] for return to soundness. The prognosis decreases further if secondary osteoarthritis is identified and if lesions are present on both the humeral head and glenoid. It should be noted that conservative treatment of shoulder osteochondrosis has minimal reported success.[55] Early surgical intervention, before the onset of osteoarthritis, is recommended to achieve the best chance of a successful outcome.

Subchondral Cystic Lesions

Subchondral cystic lesions (SCLs) are considered by some to be part of the osteochondrosis complex[60,61]; however, many aspects of SCLs are pointedly different. Whereas most osteochondrosis lesions occur at the junction of non–weight-bearing and weight-bearing surfaces, SCLs primarily occur at weight-bearing surfaces. Additionally, SCLs have been found to have increased prostaglandin E2, matrix metalloproteinase, nitric oxide, and osteoclast activity within their fibrous lining.[62] SCLs have also been produced after experimentally created chondral or osteochondral lesions in horses, which supports a traumatic etiology.[63,64] Overall, several theories for the development of SCLs beyond osteochondrosis have been proposed, including the following.

1. Hydraulic theory: Synovial fluid is pulled through the subchondral bone into the cancellous bone via a slitlike lesion in the cartilage.[65]
2. Inflammatory theory: SCLs become lined with fibrous tissue that secretes inflammatory mediators including prostaglandin E2 and interleukin-6.[62]
3. Trauma: SCLs develop after primary damage of the subchondral bone with collapse of the articular surface.[63,65]

Although this author is under the impression that SCLs are a sequela of chondral or osteochondral trauma, a brief discussion of the surgical management of SCLs is included in this review.

A review of SCLs in the horse found that the medial femoral condyle is the most common location (45%), followed by phalanges and navicular bone (26.2%), carpal bones (7.1%), and MC3 and MT3 (6%). Less than 5% of lesions were identified in the proximal tibia, radius, proximal sesamoid bones, patella, scapula, and distal tarsal bones combined.[66] In this study, Thoroughbreds were the most commonly affected (39.5%), followed by Quarter Horses (14.1%), Standardbreds (9.9%), Arabs (8.5), and Warmbloods (7.3%).

Horses show variable lameness and variable joint effusion. Pain is thought to be associated with increased intraosseous or intracystic pressure.[65] Clinical signs are most common when affected horses begin athletic training, although many SCLs are found on survey films before sales or during prepurchase examinations. Diagnosis is generally confirmed by radiography; however, computed tomography can be helpful in determining the exact location and presence of articular communication. A radiolucent area outlined by a sclerotic rim characterizes radiographic changes (**Fig. 7**A). SCLs are most often in the subchondral bone underlying the articular surface, with or without articular communication. Less commonly, SCLs are found in the metaphysis. Contralateral joints should be radiographed because bilateral lesions are common.

Conservative management of SCLs includes nonsteroidal antiinflammatory drugs, rest, intraarticular corticosteroids, and direct injection of the cyst with corticosteroids. Generally disappointing results with conservative treatment (33%–65%)[66,67] have encouraged many equine veterinarians to treat these surgically. Surgical management has been strongly advocated in horses showing lameness attributable to the lesion and older horses with secondary changes owing to their poor response to medical therapy.

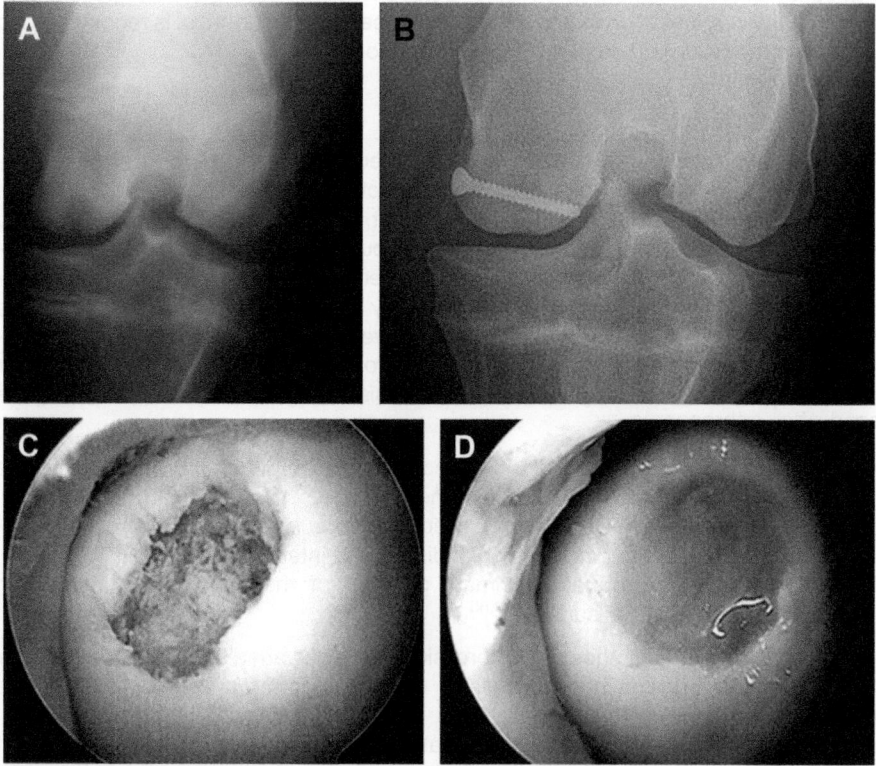

Fig. 7. (*A*) A caudal–cranial radiographic view showing a subchondral cystic in the medial femoral condyle. (*B*) A caudal–cranial radiograph demonstrating placement of a cortical bone screw placed across the medial femoral condyle to treat a subchondral cystic lesion (SCL). (*C*) An arthroscopic image of a debrided SCL. (*D*) An arthroscopic image of a SCL grafted with allogeneic chondrocytes in fibrin. (*Courtesy of* [*A, B*] Dr Elizabeth Santschi, Kansas State University, Manhattan, Kansas.)

Surgical debridement of SCLs through an arthrotomy has largely been replaced with arthroscopic debridement. Regardless of location, arthroscopy allows visualization of the articular component of the cyst and facilitates debridement of abnormal articular cartilage, cyst lining, and subchondral bone (**Fig. 7**C). After debridement, the joint should be flushed thoroughly to remove debris. To promote filling of the cyst postoperatively and to improve the articular surface after debridement, some advanced techniques have been evaluated. Cancellous bone grafting to improve cyst filling was investigated; however, studies found that grafting led to poorer outcomes than debridement alone, with some horses actually showing an increase in cyst size.[68,69] Mosaic arthroplasty has been described in SCLs of the medial femoral condyle, lateral femoral condyle, distal metacarpus, and distal metatarsus.[70,71] Allogeneic chondrocyte implantation has been shown to improve outcomes in older and arthritic horses (**Fig. 7**D).[72]

Some SCLs cannot be accessed through an articular approach, thereby necessitating transosseous debridement and treatment. Radiographic or fluoroscopic guidance is extremely useful to guide careful entry into the cyst. Recently, transcondylar screw placement has been evaluated for treatment of SCLs of the medial femoral condyle (**Fig. 7**B).[73] Santschi and colleagues (2015) found that screws decreased cyst area and eliminated lameness in ~75% of horses by 120 days. The authors hypothesized that transcondylar screws returned trabecular bone strain to the interior of the SCL thereby promoting formation of new woven bone and filling of the defect.

Intralesional corticosteroid injection has been successfully used to treat SCLs, especially when performed under arthroscopic guidance.[74] Injections can also be performed under ultrasonographic guidance although this technique is less precise and evaluation of cartilage lesions is not possible. Multiple injections into the cyst lining during the procedure are recommended. Return to soundness was reported in 67% of horses undergoing arthroscopic guided corticosteroid injection of medial femoral condyle cysts.[74]

The majority of studies evaluating surgical outcomes are in reference to SCLs of the medial femoral condyle because this is the most common location. Smith and colleagues[75] found that 64% of horses less than 3 years of age with SCLs of the medial femoral condyle were successful after debridement, whereas only 35% of horses greater than 3 years of age were successful. In another study, 64% of Thoroughbreds raced after arthroscopic debridement, with horses having smaller articular surface areas debrided (<15 mm) having significantly better prognoses than horses with larger areas.[76] Hogan and colleagues[77] (1997) reported good outcome (80% return to soundness) in horses undergoing debridement of third metacarpal bone SCLs. Arthroscopic debridement of SCLs of the distal phalanx has also been successful with 00% of horses returning to athletic soundness.[78]

SUMMARY

Osteochondrosis is a commonly encountered disease in young and athletic horses. Some lesions respond well to conservative therapy, depending on age, location, and severity. However, for the majority of osteochondrosis lesions, surgical management is the mainstay of treatment. Arthroscopic debridement is most useful in the femoropatellar joint, tarsocrural joint, fetlock joint, and shoulder joint. Debridement is generally associated with good outcomes, except in the shoulder joint, where results have been less promising. Osteochondrosis lesions in the elbow may be difficult to access arthroscopically, necessitating transosseous debridement. Surgical management of SCLs of the medial femoral condyle consists of a variety of different techniques including debridement, debridement with grafting, transcondylar screws, and intralesional corticosteroid injection. Overall, surgical management of osteochondrosis is indicated in horses with clinical signs, including lameness and persistent effusion, and in many horses intended for athletic use.

REFERENCES

1. McIlwraith CW. lameness in the young horse: osteochondrosis. In: Baxter GM, editor. Adams and Stashak's lameness in horses. 6th edition. Blackwell Publishing Ltd; 2011. p. 1155–64.
2. Ekman S, Carlson CS. The pathophysiology of osteochondrosis. Vet Clin North Am Small Anim Pract 1998;28(1):17–32.
3. Olsson SE, Reiland S. The nature of osteochondrosis in animals. Summary and conclusions with comparative aspects on osteochondritis dissecans in man. Acta Radiol Suppl 1978;358:299–306.
4. Ytrehus B, Carlson CS, Ekman S. Etiology and pathogenesis of osteochondrosis. Vet Pathol 2007;44(4):429–48.
5. Hurtig MB, Pool RR. Pathogenesis of equine osteochondrosis. In: McIlwraith CW, Trotter GW, editors. Joint disease in the horse. 2nd edition. Saunders; 1996. p. 335.
6. McIlwraith CW. Inferences from referred clinical cases of osteochondritis dissecans. Equine Vet J 1993;25(S16):27–30.
7. Whitton RC. Equine developmental osteochondral lesions: the role of biomechanics. Vet J 1998;156(3):167–8.
8. Pool RR. Difficulties in definition of equine osteochondrosis: differentiation of developmental and acquired lesions. Equine Vet J Suppl 1993;16:5.
9. Brommer H, Brama PA, Barneveld A, et al. Differences in the topographical distribution of articular cartilage degeneration between equine metacarpo- and metatarsophalangeal joints. Equine Vet J 2004;36(6):506–10.
10. Bridges CH, Womack JE, Harris ED, et al. Considerations of copper metabolism in osteochondrosis of suckling foals. J Am Vet Med Assoc 1984;185:173–8.
11. Bridges CH, Harris ED. Experimentally induced cartilaginous fractures (osteochondritis dissecans) in foals fed low-copper diets. J Am Vet Med Assoc 1988; 193:215–21.
12. Knight D, Gabel A, Reed S, et al. Correlation of dietary mineral to incidence and severity of metabolic bone disease in Ohio and Kentucky. Proc Am Assoc Eq Prac 1985;445.
13. van Weeren PR, Knaap J, Firth EC. Influence of liver copper status of mare and newborn foal on the development of osteochondrotic lesions. Equine Vet J 2003; 35(1):67–71.
14. Donabedian M, Fleurance G, Perona G, et al. Effect of fast vs. moderate growth rate related to nutrient intake on developmental orthopaedic disease in the horse. Anim Res 2006;(55):471–86.
15. Savage C, McCarthy R, Jeffcott L. Effects of dietary energy and protein induction on dyschondroplasia in foals. Equine Vet J Suppl 1993;16:74.
16. Henson FM, Davenport C, Butler L, et al. Effects of insulin and insulin-like growth factors I and II on the growth of equine fetal and neonatal chondrocytes. Equine Vet J 1997;29(6):441–7.
17. Jeffcott LB, Henson FM. Studies on growth cartilage in the horse and their application to aetiopathogenesis of dyschondroplasia (osteochondrosis). Vet J 1998; 156(3):177–92.

18. Ekman S, Rodriguez-Martinez H, Plöen L. Morphology of normal and osteochon-drotic porcine articular-epiphyseal cartilage. A study in the domestic pig and min-ipig of wild hog ancestry. Acta Anat (Basel) 1990;139(3):239–53.

19. Carlson CS, Meuten DJ, Richardson DC. Ischemic necrosis of cartilage in spon-taneous and experimental lesions of osteochondrosis. J Orthop Res 1991;9(3):317–29.

20. Carlson CS, Cullins LD, Meuten DJ. Osteochondrosis of the articular-epiphyseal cartilage complex in young horses: evidence for a defect in cartilage canal blood supply. Vet Pathol 1995;32:641–7.

21. Grøndahl AM, Dolvik NI. Heritability estimations of osteochondrosis in the tibiotar-sal joint and of bony fragments in the palmar/plantar portion of the metacarpo-and metatarsophalangeal joints of horses. J Am Vet Med Assoc 1993;203(1):101–4.

22. Lykkjen S, Olsen HF, Dolvik NI, et al. Heritability estimates of tarsocrural osteo-chondrosis and palmar/plantar first phalanx osteochondral fragments in Stan-dardbred trotters. Equine Vet J 2014;46(1):32–7.

23. Hilla D, Distl O. Heritabilities and genetic correlations between fetlock, hock and stifle osteochondrosis and fetlock osteochondral fragments in Hanoverian Warm-blood horses. J Anim Breed Genet 2014;131(1):71–81.

24. Distl O. The genetics of equine osteochondrosis. Vet J 2013;197(1):13–8.

25. Strömberg B, Rejnö S. Osteochondrosis in the horse. I. A clinical and radiologic investigation of osteochondritis dissecans of the knee and hock joint. Acta Radiol Suppl 1978;358:139–52.

26. Valentino L, Lillich JD, Gaughan EM, et al. Radiographic prevalence of osteo-chondrosis in yearling feral horses. Vet Comp Orthop Traumatol 1999;12(3):56–60.

27. Voute LC, Henson FMD, Platt D, et al. Osteochondrosis lesions of the lateral trochlear ridge of the distal femur in four ponies. Vet Rec 2011;168(10):265.

28. Sandgren B, Dalin G, Carlsten J. Osteochondrosis in the tarsocrural joint and os-teochondral fragments in the fetlock joints in Standardbred trotters. Equine Vet J Suppl 1993;16:31.

29. Hoppe F, Phillipson J. A genetic study of osteochondrosis dissecans in Swedish horses. Equine Pract 1985;7:7.

30. Alvarado AF, Marcoux M, Breton L. The incidence of osteochondrosis in a Stan-dardbred breeding farm in Quebec. Proc Am Assoc Eq Prac 1989;295.

31. O'Donohue D, Smith F, Strickland K. The incidence of abnormal limb develop-ment in the Irish Thoroughbred from birth to 18 months. Equine Vet J 1992;24:305.

32. Lepeule J, Bareille N, Robert C, et al. Association of growth, feeding practices and exercise conditions with the prevalence of Developmental Orthopaedic Dis-ease in limbs of French foals at weaning. Prev Vet Med 2009;89(3–4):167–77.

33. Dik KJ, Enzerink E, van Weeren PR. Radiographic development of osteochondral abnormalities, in the hock and stifle of Dutch Warmblood foals, from age 1 to 11 months. Equine Vet J Suppl 1999;31:9–15.

34. McIlwraith CW. Surgical versus conservative management of osteochondrosis. Vet J 2013;197(1):19–28.

35. van Weeren PR, Barneveld A. The effect of exercise on the distribution and mani-festation of osteochondrotic lesions in the Warmblood foal. Equine Vet J Suppl 1999;31:16–25.

36. McIlwraith CW, Foerner JJ, Davis DM. Osteochondritis dissecans of the tarsocrural joint: results of treatment with arthroscopic surgery. Equine Vet J 1991;23(3): 155–62.

37. Carmona J, Arguelles D, Deulofeu R, et al. Effect of the administration of an oral hyaluronan formulation on clinical and biochemical parameters in young horses with osteochondrosis. Vet Comp Orthop Traumatol 2009;22(6):455–9.

38. Bourzac C, Alexander K, Rossier Y, et al. Comparison of radiography and ultrasonography for the diagnosis of osteochondritis dissecans in the equine femoropatellar joint. Equine Vet J 2009;41(7):685–92.

39. Foland JW, McIlwraith CW, Trotter GW. Arthroscopic surgery for osteochondritis dissecans of the femoropatellar joint of the horse. Equine Vet J 1992;24(6): 419–23.

40. Butler JA, Colles CM, Dyson SJ. The stifle and tibia. In: Clinical Radiology of the Horse. 4th edition. Somerset (NJ): Wiley-Blackwell; 2016.

41. Nixon AJ, Fortier LA, Goodrich LR, et al. Arthroscopic reattachment of osteochondritis dissecans lesions using resorbable polydioxanone pins. Equine Vet J 2004; 36(5):376–83.

42. Sparks HD, Nixon AJ, Fortier LA, et al. Arthroscopic reattachment of osteochondritis dissecans cartilage flaps of the femoropatellar joint: long-term results. Equine Vet J 2011;43(6):650–9.

43. UpRichard K, Elce YA, Piat P, et al. Outcome after arthroscopic treatment of lateral femoral trochlear ridge osteochondrosis in sport horses. A retrospective study of 37 horses. Vet Comp Orthop Traumatol 2013;26(2):105–9.

44. Clarke KL, Reardon R, Russell T. Treatment of osteochondrosis dissecans in the stifle and tarsus of juvenile thoroughbred horses. Vet Surg 2015;44(3):297–303.

45. Laws EG, Richardson DW, Ross MW, et al. Racing performance of Standardbreds after conservative and surgical treatment for tarsocrural osteochondrosis. Equine Vet J 1993;25(3):199–202.

46. Richardson DW. Diagnosis and management of osteochondrosis and osseous cyst-like lesions. In: Ross MW, Dyson SJ, editors. Diagnosis and management of lameness in the horse. 1st edition. Saunders Elsevier; 2003. p. 549–56.

47. Beard WL, Bramlage LR, Schneider RK, et al. Postoperative racing performance in Standardbreds and thoroughbreds with osteochondrosis of the tarsocrural joint: 109 cases (1984-1990). J Am Vet Med Assoc 1994;204:1655–9.

48. Brink P, Dolvik NI, Tverdal A. Lameness and effusion of the tarsocrural joints after arthroscopy of osteochondritis dissecans in horses. Vet Rec 2009;165(24): 709–12.

49. Yovich JV, Stashak TS, Bertone AL. Incarceration of small intestine through rents in the gastrosplenic ligament in the horse. Vet Surg 1985;14(4):303–6.

50. McIlwraith CW, Vorhees M. Management of osteochondritis dissecans of the dorsal aspect of the distal metacarpus and metatarsus. Proc Am Assoc Eq Prac 1990;547.

51. Foerner JJ, Barclay WP, Phillips TN, et al. Osteochondral fragments of the palmar/plantar aspect of the fetlock joint. 33rd Proc Am Assoc Eq Pr 1987;739–44.

52. Dalin G, Sandgren B, Carlsten J. Plantar osteochondral fragments in the metatarsophalangeal joints in Standardbred trotters: results of osteochondrosis or trauma? Equine Vet J 1993;25:62–5.

53. Nixon AJ, Pool RR. Histologic appearance of axial osteochondral fragments from the proximoplantar/proximopalmar aspect of the proximal phalanx in horses. J Am Vet Med Assoc 1995;207(8):1076–80.

54. Fortier LA, Foerner JJ, Nixon AJ. Arthroscopic removal of axial osteochondral fragments of the plantar/palmar proximal aspect of the proximal phalanx in horses: 119 cases (1988-1992). J Am Vet Med Assoc 1995;206:71–4.

55. McIlwraith CW, Wright I, Nixon AJ. Diagnostic and surgical arthroscopy in the horse. Edinburgh (United Kingdom); New York: Mosby Elsevier; 2005.

56. Bertone AL, McIlwraith CW, Powers BE, et al. Subchondral osseous cystic lesions of the elbow of horses: conservative versus surgical treatment. J Am Vet Med Assoc 1986;189(5):540–6.

57. Hopen LA, Colahan PT, Turner TA, et al. Nonsurgical treatment of cubital subchondral cyst-like lesions in horses: seven cases (1983 1007). J Am Vet Med Assoc 1992;200(4):527–30.

58. Bertone AL, McIlwraith CW. Arthroscopic surgery for the treatment of osteochondrosis in the equine shoulder joint. Vet Surg 1987;16(4):303–11.

59. Jenner F, Ross MW, Martin BB, et al. Scapulohumeral osteochondrosis. A retrospective study of 32 horses. Vet Comp Orthop Traumatol 2008;21(5):406–12.

60. Baxter GM. Subchondral cystic lesions in horses. In: McIlwraith CW, Trotter GW, editors. Joint disease in the horse, vol. 1. Philadelphia: W.B. Saunders Co.; 1996. p. 384–97.

61. Rejnö S, Strömberg B. Osteochondrosis in the horse. II. Pathology. Acta Radiol Suppl 1978;358:153–78.

62. von Rechenberg B, Guenther H, McIlwraith CW, et al. Fibrous tissue of subchondral cystic lesions in horses produce local mediators and neutral metalloproteinases and cause bone resorption in vitro. Vet Surg 2000;29(5):420–9.

63. Ray CS, Baxter GM, McIlwraith CW, et al. Development of subchondral cystic lesions after articular cartilage and subchondral bone damage in young horses. Equine Vet J 1996;28(3):225–32.

64. Kold SE, Hickman J. Results of treatment of subchondral bone cysts in the medial condyle of the equine femur with an autogenous cancellous bone graft. Equine Vet J 1984;16(5):414–8.

65. Kold SE, Hickman J, Melsen F. An experimental study of the healing process of equine chondral and osteochondral defects. Equine Vet J 1986;18(1):18–24.

66. Rechenberg B, McIlwraith CW, Auer JA. Cystic bone lesions in horses and humans: a comparative review. Vet Comp Orthop Traumatol 1998;11:8.

67. Textor JA, Nixon AJ, Lumsden J, et al. Subchondral cystic lesions of the proximal extremity of the tibia in horses: 12 cases (1983-2000). J Am Vet Med Assoc 2001; 218(3):408–13.

68. Kold SE, Hickman J. Use of an autogenous cancellous bone graft in the treatment of subchondral bone cysts in the medial femoral condyle of the horse. Equine Vet J 1983;15(4):312–6.

69. Jackson WA, Stick JA, Arnoczky SP, et al. The effect of compacted cancellous bone grafting on the healing of subchondral bone defects of the medial femoral condyle in horses. Vet Surg 2000;29(1):8–16.

70. Bodo G, Hangody L, Szabo Z, et al. Arthroscopic autologous osteochondral mosaicplasty for the treatment of subchondral cystic lesion in the medial femoral condyle in a horse. Acta Vet Hung 2000;48(3):343–54.

71. Bodo G, Vasarhelyi G, Hangody L, et al. Mosaic arthroplasty of the medial femoral condyle in horses - an experimental study. Acta Vet Hung 2014;62(2): 155–68.

72. Ortved KF, Nixon AJ, Mohammed HO, et al. Treatment of subchondral cystic lesions of the medial femoral condyle of mature horses with growth factor

enhanced chondrocyte grafts: a retrospective study of 49 cases. Equine Vet J 2012;44(5):606–13.

73. Santschi EM, Williams JM, Morgan JW, et al. Preliminary investigation of the treatment of equine medial femoral condylar subchondral cystic lesions with a transcondylar screw. Vet Surg 2015;44(3):281–8.

74. Wallis TW, Goodrich LR, McIlwraith CW, et al. Arthroscopic injection of corticosteroids into the fibrous tissue of subchondral cystic lesions of the medial femoral condyle in horses: a retrospective study of 52 cases (2001-2006). Equine Vet J 2008;40(5):461–7.

75. Smith MA, Walmsley JP, Phillips TJ, et al. Effect of age at presentation on outcome following arthroscopic debridement of subchondral cystic lesions of the medial femoral condyle: 85 horses (1993–2003). Equine Vet J 2005;37(2):175–80.

76. Sandler EA, Bramlage LR, Embertson RM, et al. Correlation of lesion size with racing performance in thoroughbreds after arthroscopic surgical treatment of subchondral cystic lesions of the medial femoral condyle: 150 cases (1989-2000). Proc Annu Conv AAEP 2002;48:255–6.

77. Hogan PM, McIlwraith CW, Honnas CM, et al. Surgical treatment of subchondral cystic lesions of the third metacarpal bone: results in 15 horses (1986-1994). Equine Vet J 1997;29(6):477–82.

78. Story MR, Bramlage LR. Arthroscopic debridement of subchondral bone cysts in the distal phalanx of 11 horses (1994-2000). Equine Vet J 2004;36(4):356–60.

Foal Fractures

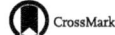

Osteochondral Fragmentation, Proximal Sesamoid Bone Fractures/Sesamoiditis, and Distal Phalanx Fractures

Heidi L. Reesink, VMD, PhD

KEYWORDS

- Fracture • Foal • Musculoskeletal • Sesamoid • Sesamoiditis • Coffin bone
- Distal phalanx

KEY POINTS

- Osteochondral fragmentation of the fetlocks is common in foals. Foals are also susceptible to fractures of the proximal sesamoid bones and distal phalanx.
- Non–long bone fractures, including proximal sesamoid bone and distal phalanx fractures, are more likely to heal via bony union and carry a better prognosis in foals compared with adults.
- Surgery is rarely indicated for the treatment of proximal sesamoid bone and distal phalanx fractures in foals. Arthroscopy may be appropriate for certain types of osteochondral fragmentation of the fetlocks.
- Although the prognosis for fracture healing is better for foals than adults, an early, accurate diagnosis and appropriate management are likely to improve the cosmetic appearance and functional outcome in foals.

FOAL FRACTURES

Foals are susceptible to many of the same types of fractures as adult horses, often secondary to external sources of trauma. In addition, some types of fractures are specific to foals and occur routinely in young horses under 1 year of age. These foal-specific fractures may present with distinct clinical signs, and treatment plans and prognoses are tailored specifically to young animals. Common fractures not affecting the long bones in foals are discussed in this article, including osteochondral fragmentation, proximal sesamoid bone fractures/sesamoiditis, and distal phalanx fractures.

Disclosure Statement: The authors have nothing to disclose.
Department of Clinical Sciences, College of Veterinary Medicine, Cornell University, C3-101 Vet Med Center, Ithaca, NY 14853, USA
E-mail address: hlr42@cornell.edu

OSTEOCHONDRAL FRAGMENTATION
Introduction

Osteochondral fragmentation may be due to either developmental orthopedic disease or trauma. Fragmentation occurring secondary to osteochondrosis of the stifle (trochlear ridges of the femur) and tarsus (distal intermediate ridge and malleoli of the tibia, trochlea of the talus) is discussed separately, and fragmentation of the proximal sesamoid bones is discussed later in this article. The proximal plantar and palmar tuberosities of the proximal phalanx (P1) are a predilection site for osteochondral fragmentation in young horses. Although developmental bone disease (osteochondrosis) has been proposed as a cause,[1,2] recent histopathologic evidence suggests a fracture etiology.[3,4] The proximal sesamoid bones, the dorsal proximal margins of the P1 and the sagittal ridges of the third metacarpal (MC3)/ third metatarsal (MT3) bones are also affected.[3,5] Occasionally, large fragments of the abaxial borders of the proximal plantar/palmar tuberosities of the P1 are observed in foals.[6]

Patient Evaluation Overview

Conformation may predispose to abnormal forces, leading to certain predilection sites for osteochondral fragmentation. Osteochondral fragmentation of the fetlock joints is often diagnosed on survey or prepurchase radiographs in foals and yearling horses because many of these fragments are clinically silent until high-speed exercise is introduced.[7] Occasionally, foals with larger, abaxial fragments of the proximal plantar/ palmar tuberosities of P1 present with lameness, heat, and swelling of the fetlock (**Fig. 1**). Synovial effusion may be present, and mild to moderate pain may be elicited by fetlock flexion.

Plantar/palmar osteochondral fragmentation of the fetlocks

The proximoplantaromedial aspect of the P1 is a common anatomic location for osteochondral fragmentation in the young horse, with the highest prevalence in Standardbreds.[5,8] Osteochondral fragments in this location are categorized as type I and type II fractures (**Fig. 2**). Type I fractures occur on the axial, proximal plantar/palmar rim of the P1 and are predominantly articular, whereas type II fractures are larger, are abaxially located, and involve minimal articular cartilage.[9] Routine oblique radiographic projections detect type II fractures but are not ideal for type I fractures, which are best delineated by elevating the radiographic beam 20° above horizontal and 15° to 20° dorsal to a standard lateromedial projection (see **Fig. 2**; **Fig. 3**).[9]

- Type I fragments: axial, articular, best viewed with an elevated oblique radiographic projection
- Type II fragments: abaxial, minimally articular or nonarticular, viewed with routine oblique radiographic projection

Dorsal osteochondral fragmentation of the fetlocks

Sites of osteochondral fragmentation in the dorsal aspect of the fetlock include the dorsal proximal margins of P1 (**Fig. 4**), the sagittal ridges of MC3/MT3, and synovial pad fragments, with a higher prevalence of dorsal fetlock fragmentation observed in Warmbloods compared with Thoroughbreds or Standardbreds.[5] Joint effusion may or may not be present, and lameness is variable. Flattening or defects in the dorsal aspect of the sagittal ridges of MC3/MT3 are typically considered osteochondrosis lesions; however, histologic studies do not support a developmental etiology for fragments of the proximodorsal aspects of P1[3] or

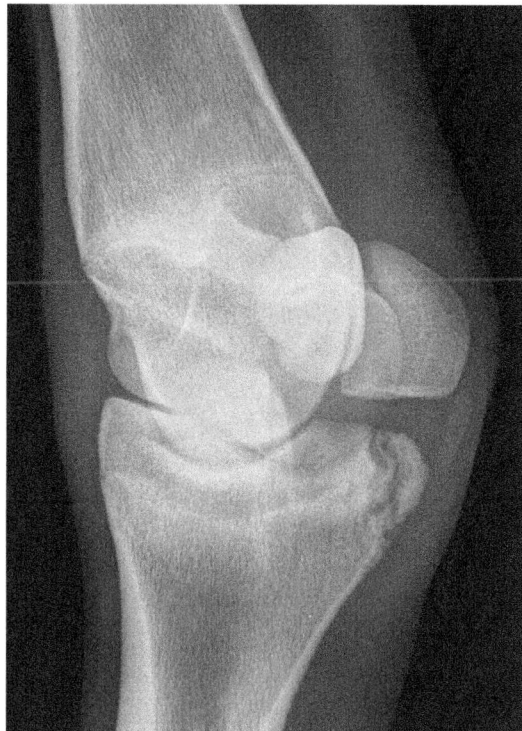

Fig. 1. Elevated oblique radiographic projection (D15Pr20L-PlDiMO) of the right hind fetlock of a 7-month-old Warmblood filly with a large, abaxial osteochondral fragment of the proximal plantarolateral tuberosity of the P1. Conservative treatment was recommended. (*Courtesy of* Dr Norm Ducharme, Ithaca, NY; with permission.)

synovial pad fragments.[10] Sagittal ridge defects are often best observed using flexed lateromedial radiographic projections (**Fig. 5**). It is not uncommon for sagittal ridge defects to be found bilaterally or for all 4 fetlocks to be involved. Fetlock flexion typically induces or exacerbates lameness. Dorsal P1 fragments are more common in the forelimbs than hindlimbs, and are more common medially than laterally.

Classification of dorsal sagittal ridge lesions[11]
- Type I: a defect or flattening as the only visible radiographic lesion
- Type II: a defect or flattening with fragmentation associated with the defect
- Type III: a defect or flattening with or without fragmentation plus one or more loose bodies

Pharmacologic Treatment Options

Anti-inflammatories/analgesics, including phenylbutazone, firocoxib, and meloxicam, may be administered in foals with traumatic osteochondral fragmentation, resulting in joint effusion or lameness. Nonsteroidal anti-inflammatory medications are administered postoperatively in horses undergoing arthroscopic fragment removal. Firocoxib and meloxicam may be associated with fewer adverse side effects in foals compared with phenylbutazone.[12,13]

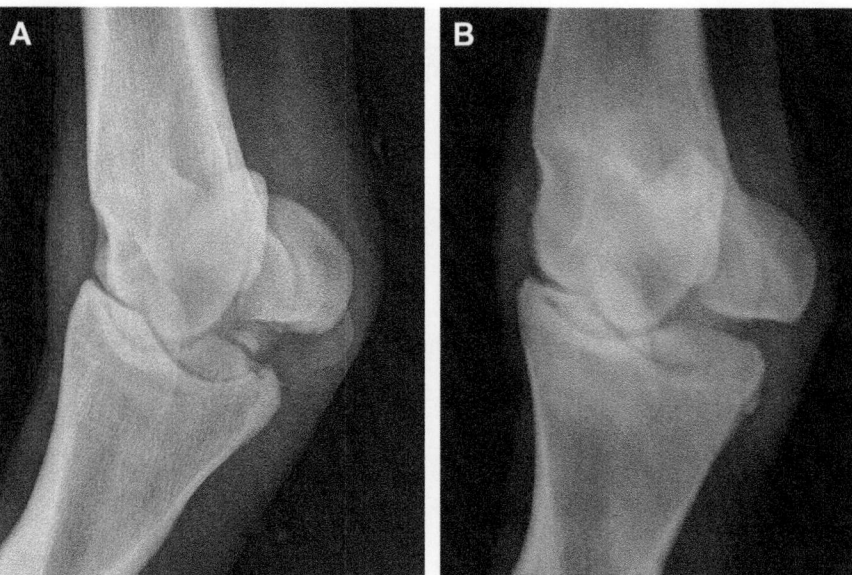

Fig. 2. (*A*) Elevated oblique radiographic projection (D15Pr20M-PlDiLO) of the left hind fetlock of a yearling Warmblood filly, demonstrating a type I (axial) osteochondral fragment of the proximoplantaromedial aspect of the proximal phalanx. This fragment was removed arthroscopically. (*B*) Elevated oblique radiographic projection (D15Pr20M-PlDiLO) of the right hind fetlock of a yearling Thoroughbred colt, demonstrating a type II (abaxial) osteochondral fragment of the P1.

Nonpharmacologic Treatment Options

Conservative treatment, consisting of box stall rest or exercise restriction, is appropriate for the majority of nonarticular osteochondral fragments. Foals should always be gradually reintroduced to exercise after a period of stall rest to prevent the risk of injury, especially biaxial proximal sesamoid bone fracture. In cases of fragments that are nonarticular and are no clinical signs, treatment is unnecessary. Abnormal radiographic findings can be evaluated with follow-up clinical and radiographic examination. The presence or absence of clinical signs, including lameness and joint effusion, should dictate appropriate therapy.

Fetlock osteochondral fragments amenable to conservative therapy
- Type II (abaxial) plantar/palmar P1 fragments
- Type I sagittal ridge MC3/MT3 lesions
- Small synovial pad fragments
- Small, apical proximal sesamoid bone fragments

Surgical Treatment Options

Arthroscopic surgical removal is recommended for osteochondral fragments causing persistent clinical signs, including joint effusion, synovitis, and lameness. Lameness is rare in young horses; however, type I plantar/palmar P1 fragments are typically removed in yearlings to prevent lameness during training. Type II fragments rarely warrant surgical removal. Surgical removal of dorsoproximal P1 fragments, synovial pad fragments, and type II–III sagittal ridge lesions is commonly performed to improve the appearance of prepurchase radiographs and to prevent the future development of lameness. As such, it is difficult to predict what proportion of horses with these lesions

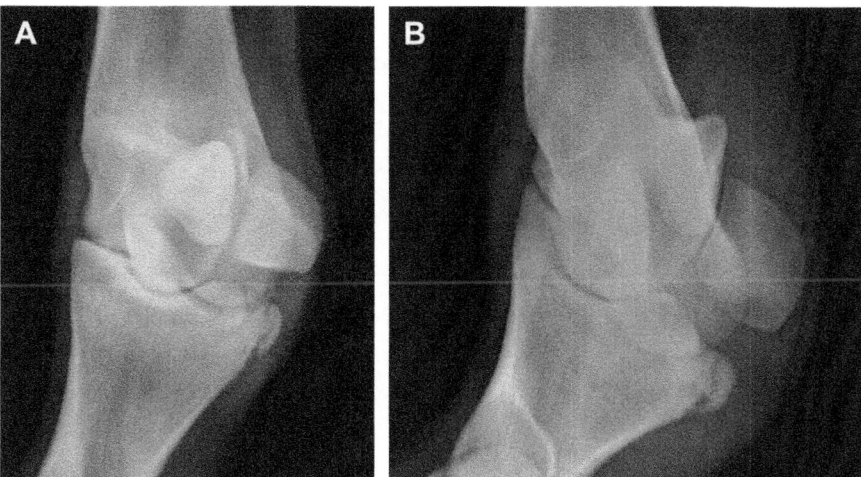

Fig. 3. (*A*) Elevated oblique radiographic projections of the right hind fetlock of a yearling Thoroughbred colt with a wedge-shaped axial osteochondral fragment, in addition to an abaxial (type II) fragment of the proximoplantarolateral tuberosity of the P1. (*B*) The axial fragment was removed arthroscopically, revealing a 1-cm fracture plane within the proximal margin of the fracture bed. Postoperative radiographs show removal of the axial but not the abaxial fragment. (*Courtesy of* Dr Alan Nixon, Ithaca, NY; with permission.)

would become symptomatic if not treated arthroscopically. In 1 report of 8 cases of type II sagittal ridge lesions treated conservatively, surgery was eventually performed in 2 due to persistent clinical signs, and clinical signs persisted in 5 others.[14]

Treatment Resistance/Complications

Horses that do not respond to conservative management or that develop clinical symptoms during training should have osteochondral fragments removed

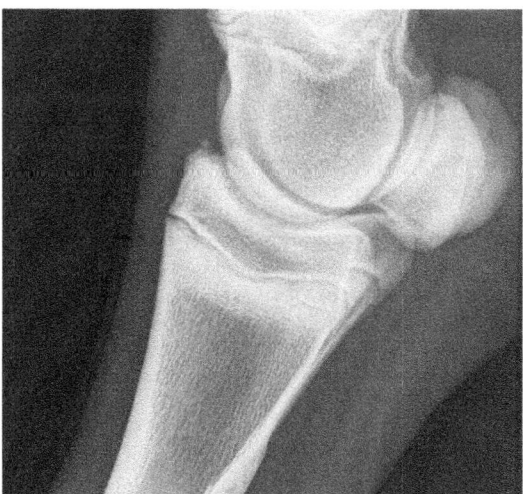

Fig. 4. Lateromedial radiograph of the fetlock of a 6-month-old Warmblood colt, revealing a small osteochondral fragment of the dorsal border of the P1.

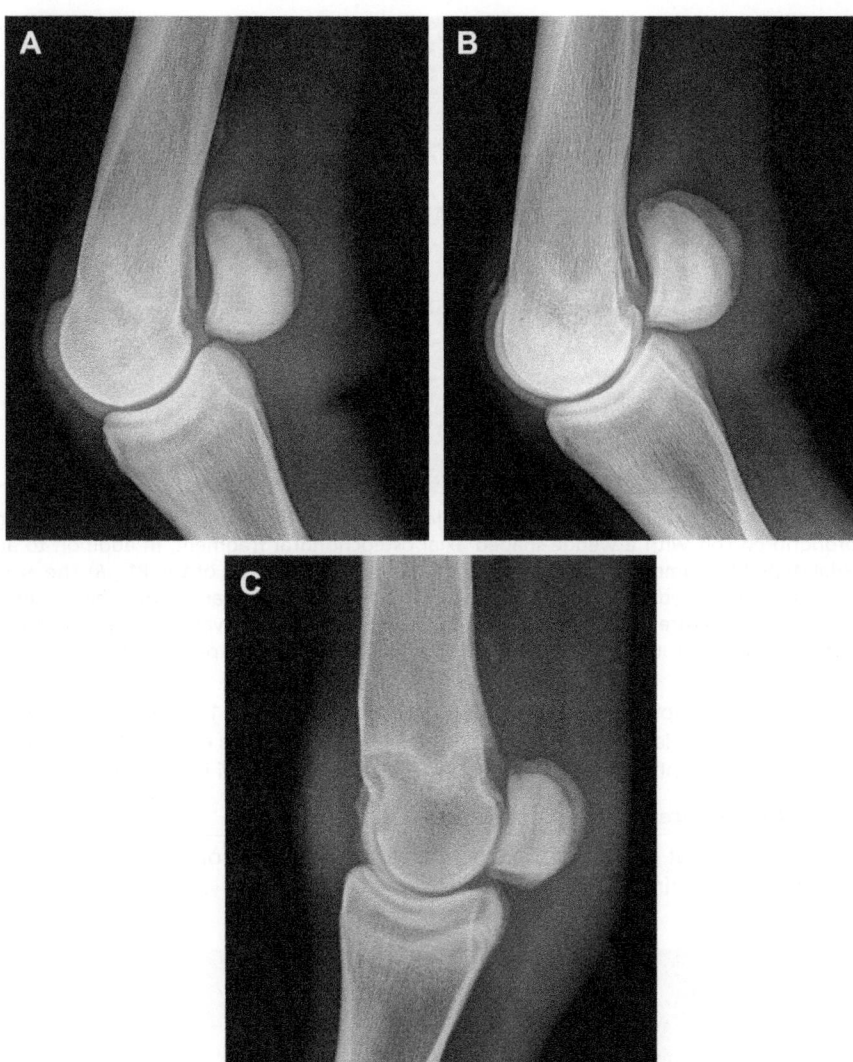

Fig. 5. Dorsal sagittal ridge osteochondrosis lesions. (*A*) Flexed lateromedial radiographic projection of the left front fetlock of a yearling Thoroughbred colt, revealing flattening of the distal aspect of the sagittal ridge of the MC3 bone (type I lesion). (*B*) Flexed lateromedial projection of the right front fetlock of a yearling Thoroughbred colt with a small defect and associated fragmentation of the proximal aspect of the sagittal ridge of MC3 (type II lesion). (*C*) Lateromedial projection of the right hind fetlock of a weanling Thoroughbred colt with a lucency of the proximal sagittal ridge of the MT3 bone with a loose fragment in the proximal plantar pouch of the joint (type III lesion). (*Courtesy of* Dr Alanna Zantingh, Cambridge, Waikato, New Zealand; with permission.)

arthroscopically. Large, articular and displaced fragments should be removed in young horses to prevent synovitis and articular damage secondary to impingement of osteochondral fragments between the metacarpal/metatarsal condyles and the P1.

Evaluation of Outcome and Long-term Recommendations

The prognosis for horses with plantar/palmar osteochondral fragments is good, with 55 of 87 (63%) of horses returning to racing at an equal or better level of performance.[7] In a study of 42 horses with dorsal sagittal ridge lesions of MC3/MT3, the success rate was approximately 60%, and evidence of cartilage erosion, wear lines, or extension of the lesion onto the condyles was associated with a poorer prognosis.[11] A recent retrospective evaluating postsurgical outcome of horses with distal sagittal ridge lesions of MC3 reported a good prognosis, with 13 of 14 (93%) horses performing athletically, including 11/12 (92%) Thoroughbreds that raced.[15]

Summary/Discussion

Osteochondral fragmentation is common in young horses. Whereas fragments in the stifle and tarsus are typically the result of osteochondrosis, osteochondral fragmentation in the fetlock seems to have multiple etiologies. Fetlock osteochondral fragments are often clinically silent in foals, weanlings, and yearlings; however, arthroscopic removal is commonly performed after radiographic diagnosis. Conservative therapy is appropriate for most nonarticular fragments. Clinical signs should always dictate the appropriate course of treatment—in general, type I plantaroproximal P1 tuberosity fragments, dorsoproximal P1 fragments, and type II–II sagittal ridge fragments should be treated with arthroscopic removal.

PROXIMAL SESAMOID BONE FRACTURES AND SESAMOIDITIS
Introduction

Foals are susceptible to most configurations of proximal sesamoid bone fractures described in adults, including apical, midbody, basilar, abaxial, and comminuted fractures. Apical (**Fig. 6**) and basilar (**Fig. 7**) fractures are most common in foals.[16] Biaxial (**Figs. 8** and **9**) and bilateral, uniaxial midbody transverse proximal sesamoid fractures have also been described in young foals (<2 months) running to keep up with their dams in the pasture.[17] These fractures occur secondary to muscle fatigue, which results in hyperextension of the fetlock joint and sesamoid bone fracture secondary to the strong tensile pull of the suspensory apparatus.

Whereas proximal sesamoid bone fractures are most common in foals less than 2 months of age, sesamoiditis is a condition predominantly affecting yearlings to 2-year-old horses. Sesamoiditis refers to inflammation of the proximal, abaxial aspect of the proximal sesamoid bones. Pain and inflammation are thought to originate from the insertion of the suspensory ligament branches on the sesamoid bones, and this condition may involve multiple limbs and/or multiple bones.

Patient Evaluation Overview

Proximal sesamoid bone fractures

The degree of lameness in young foals with proximal sesamoid bone fractures is variable and based on fracture configuration. Foals with small or minimally displaced proximal sesamoid bone fractures may only present with slight lameness or severe lameness that quickly resolves and can be easily overlooked.[18] Foals with larger, uniaxial proximal sesamoid bone fractures typically present with fetlock swelling, joint effusion, and moderate lameness. Palpation of the affected sesamoid bone and flexion of the joint may elicit pain. Diagnosis is based on clinical and radiographic examination; however, radiodensity and contrast may be poor in young foals due to limited ossification, especially of apical, basilar, or abaxial fragments. Ultrasound

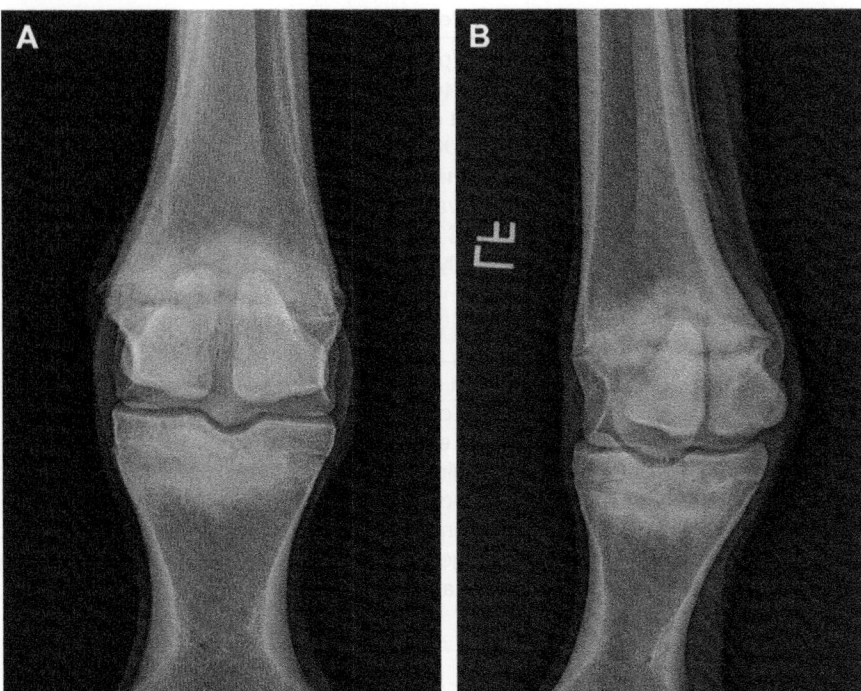

Fig. 6. (*A*) Dorsopalmar and (*B*) dorsomedial palmarolateral oblique radiographs of the left front fetlock of a 5-month-old Thoroughbred filly, revealing a minimally displaced apical sesamoid fracture of the medial proximal sesamoid bone. (*A*) Lateral is to the right. This filly presented with lameness secondary to bilateral apical fractures of the forelimb medial proximal sesamoid bones. Box stall confinement was recommended.

may be a useful adjunctive modality, and some fractures may become more radiographically apparent 7 days to 10 days after injury.

Biaxial fractures, resulting in significant distraction, lameness, and gross instability of the suspensory apparatus, occur when young foals gallop to exhaustion (see **Fig. 9**). Foals are at highest risk of biaxial and midbody transverse fractures when turned out with their dams into a large paddock after a spell of box stall confinement. For this reason, mares and foals should be gradually reintroduced to turnout after a period of stall rest, and mares that run excessively should be kept in smaller paddocks until foals have had an opportunity to strengthen their proximal sesamoid bones. When biaxial midbody fractures occur, lameness is typically severe, resulting in a dropped fetlock due to suspensory apparatus disruption.

Sesamoiditis
In horses with sesamoiditis, the affected proximal sesamoid bones may be enlarged, painful to direct palpation, and mild-to-moderate lameness may be present; however, radiographic evidence of sesamoiditis may be present in the absence of lameness. The diagnosis is confirmed radiographically, and oblique projections are most useful for demonstrating new bone production on the abaxial and palmar/plantar surfaces of the sesamoids. Sesamoiditis is characterized by enlarged vascular channels or an increased number of vascular channels (**Fig. 10**).[19] The suspensory ligament and distal sesamoidean ligaments may also be affected.

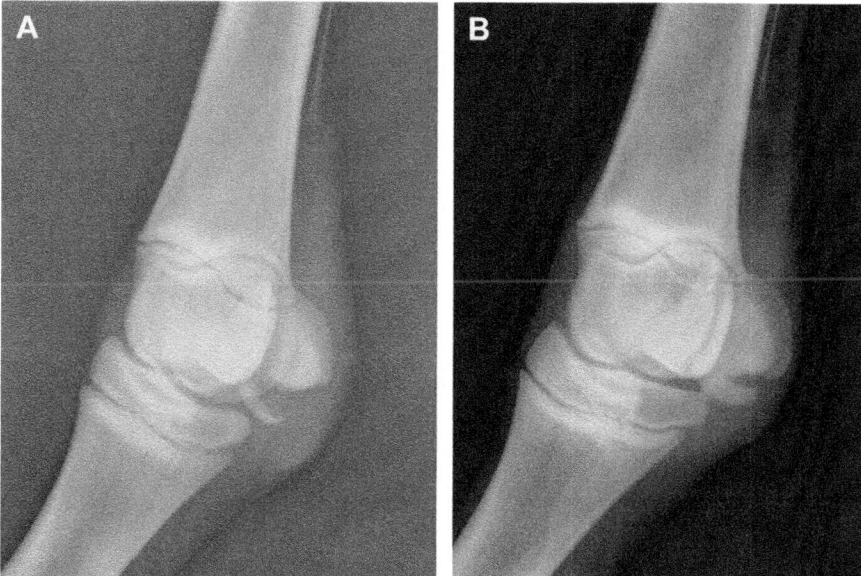

Fig. 7. (*A*) Dorsomedial palmarolateral oblique projection of the right front fetlock of a 3-week-old Thoroughbred foal with a displaced basilar sesamoid bone fracture treated with exercise restriction. (*B*) Follow-up radiographs 2 months later reveal fracture remodeling and evidence of healing. In young foals, these fractures can heal with an acceptable functional result, although the affected sesamoid bone remains elongated radiographically. (*Courtesy of* Dr Alan Nixon, Ithaca, NY; with permission.)

Pharmacologic Treatment Options

When proximal sesamoid bone fractures cause significant lameness, anti-inflammatories/analgesics are indicated in the acute postinjury period to encourage weight bearing and to prevent breakdown of the contralateral limb.[17] Options include phenylbutazone, firocoxib, and meloxicam (**Table 1**). Nonsteroidal anti-inflammatories may also be indicated in the acute phases of sesamoiditis. There may be some rationale for the use of tiludronate or other bisphosphonates in the treatment of sesamoiditis in horses over the age of 2; however, information on efficacy is lacking.[20]

Nonpharmacologic Treatment Options

Proximal sesamoid bone fractures

Conservative therapy, consisting of stall confinement for 1 to 2 months, followed by a graduated turnout regimen, is the treatment of choice for the majority of proximal sesamoid bone fractures in foals.[16,20] Unlike adult horses, proximal sesamoid fractures in foals typically progress to bony union. Even when 1 sesamoid bone is affected by fracture fragment distraction, young foals may heal adequately with conservative treatment alone (see **Fig. 7**). These fractures typically heal with an elongated appearance to the proximal sesamoid bone.

Coaptation via casting or splinting is generally contraindicated due to the risk of development of flexor tendon laxity; however, application of a dorsal splint may be necessary to provide support to the fetlock joint and to prevent fracture distraction in cases of suspensory apparatus disruption (see **Fig. 8**).[16,17] Foals with biaxial proximal sesamoid bone fractures can be managed with splints to salvage for breeding or

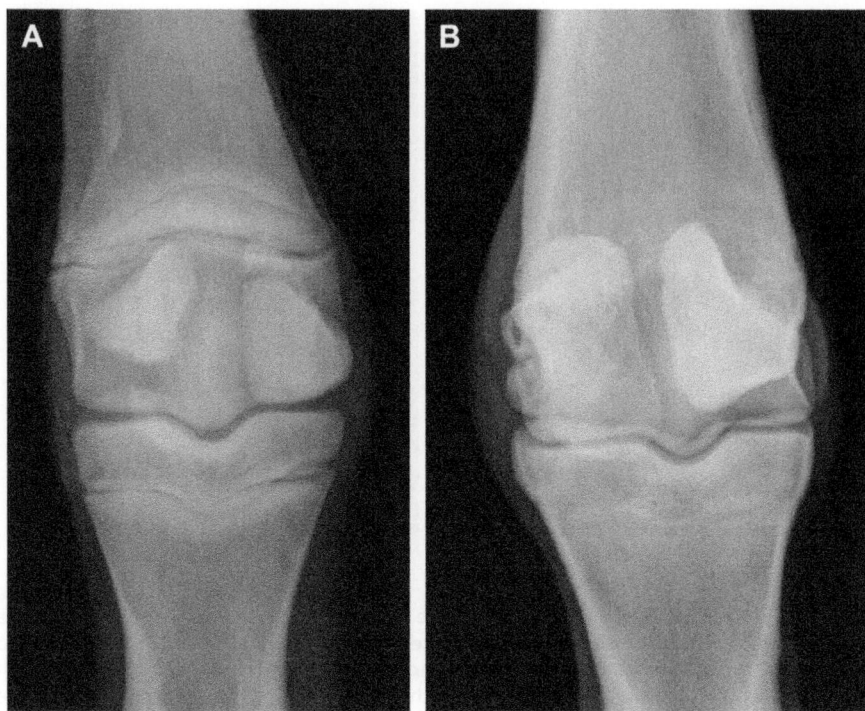

Fig. 8. (*A*) Dorsopalmar projection revealing biaxial proximal sesamoid bone fractures of the left front fetlock in a 4-week-old Thoroughbred foal. Lateral is to the right. An apical fracture of the lateral proximal sesamoid bone and a basilar fracture of the medial proximal sesamoid bone are present. (*B*) Dorsopalmar projection 8 months later revealing healing of the proximal sesamoid bone fractures with slight elongation of the lateral proximal sesamoid and significant elongation and distal remodeling of the medial proximal sesamoid bone. These fractures were treated conservatively. (*Courtesy of* Dr Alan Ruggles, Lexington, KY; with permission.)

pasture soundness.[17] Bandages should be inspected daily and reapplied every 2 days to 3 days to prevent sores and splint complications. As the fetlock joint regains stability, splints can be adjusted to gradually increase loading by lowering the fetlock.[17]

Sesamoiditis
Treatment of sesamoiditis is challenging and involves exercise restriction, followed by a slow and gradual return to activity, often over 6 months to 8 months. Alternating cold and hot compresses may be useful in the acute phases of inflammation, and shock wave therapy has been used to treat pain in acute sesamoiditis.[21]

Surgical Treatment Options
Surgical treatment of proximal sesamoid bone fractures is rarely indicated in young foals. Indications for surgical repair include cases of biaxial fracture with complete disruption of the suspensory apparatus, significant fracture distraction, and a dropped fetlock.[16] Although lag screw fixation is the preferred method of internal fixation for proximal sesamoid bone fractures in adults,[22] suturing with high tensile-strength flexible fiber[20] or stapling[16] may be more appropriate for the soft bone in foals. When biaxial proximal sesamoid bone fractures are accompanied by gross medial-lateral

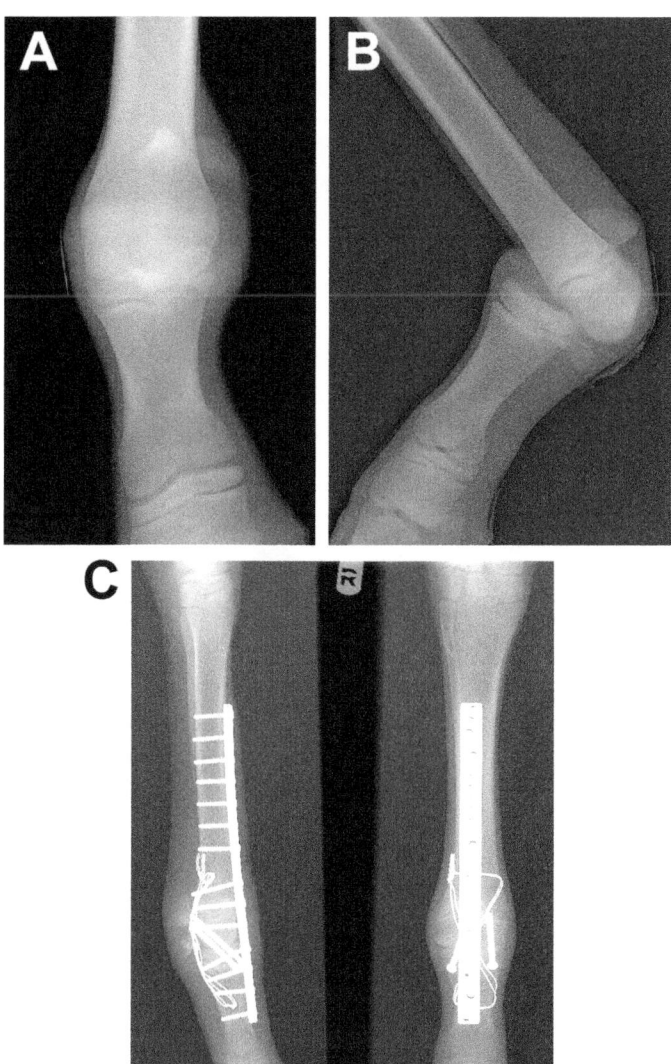

Fig. 9. (*A*) Dorsopalmar projection revealing biaxial midbody proximal sesamoid bone fractures of the right front fetlock in a 4-week-old Thoroughbred foal. Lateral is to the right. (*B*) Lateromedial projection revealing dorsal luxation of the P1 secondary to biaxial proximal sesamoid bone fractures and associated disruption of the suspensory apparatus and collateral ligaments. (*C*) Fetlock arthrodesis was performed using a 14-hole dynamic compression plate and figure-of-eight tension band wire as a salvage procedure. (*Courtesy of* Dr Alan Ruggles, Lexington, KY; with permission.)

instability and luxation of the fetlock joint, fetlock arthrodesis may be performed as a salvage procedure (see **Fig. 9**).

Treatment Resistance/Complications

Proximal sesamoid bone fractures with significant distraction or those that occur in older foals may heal via fibrous instead of bony union. Although foals may not be

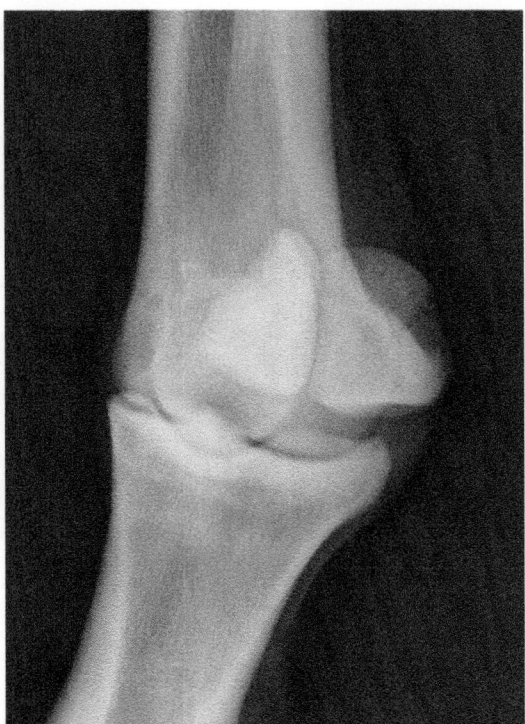

Fig. 10. Dorsomedial palmarolateral oblique projection of the right front fetlock of an 11-month-old Thoroughbred colt with sesamoiditis. Radiographs revealed 3 parallel vascular channels in the apical and proximal midbody of the medial proximal sesamoid bone, in addition to a wide (>2 mm) midbody vascular channel opening to an irregular, wedge-shaped lucent region. This is classified as grade 3 sesamoiditis using the modified Spike-Pierce scale. (*Courtesy of* Dr Christina Cable, Lansing, NY; with permission.)

lame, fractures healing via fibrous union are more likely to have persistent thickening of the fetlock joint and restricted range of motion.[18]

Evaluation of Outcome and Long-term Recommendations

Proximal sesamoid bone fractures
The prognosis for young foals with simple, uniaxial proximal sesamoid bone fractures is good for healing with box-stall confinement alone.[18] The bones may heal with an

Table 1 Nonsteroidal anti-inflammatory medications used in foals	
Medication	**Dosage**
Phenylbutazone	2.2 mg/kg IV/PO twice a day
Firocoxib	0.1 mg/kg PO once a day
Meloxicam	0.6 mg/kg PO twice a day

Data from Hovanessian, Davis JL, McKenzie HC 3rd, et al. Pharmacokinetics and safety of firocoxib after oral administration of repeated consecutive doses to neonatal foals. J Vet Pharmacol Ther 2013;37:243–51; and Raidal SL, Edwards S, Pippia J, et al. Pharmacokinetics and safety of oral administration of meloxicam to foals. J Vet Intern Med 2013;27(2):300–7.

elongated appearance, but the prognosis for athletic function is good. If there is significant fracture distraction or severe distortion of the proximal sesamoid bones, restricted fetlock motion and lameness may ensue.[20] Foals sustaining biaxial proximal sesamoid bone fractures can heal with or without surgical treatment; however, the prognosis for high-level athleticism or racing is guarded. With appropriate treatment, these foals can achieve breeding or pasture soundness.

Sesamoiditis
The prognosis for racing soundness or high-level athletic performance is unfavorable. In 1 study evaluating 2-year-old Thoroughbreds at in-training sales, the odds of starting a race or earning money were lower for horses with sesamoiditis compared with horses without radiographic abnormalities.[23] A radiographic diagnosis of severe (grade 3–4) sesamoiditis using the modified Spike-Pierce scale in yearling Thoroughbreds was associated with a 5-times greater risk of developing clinical suspensory ligament branch injury in the adjacent branch during training.[24]

Classification of sesamoiditis via modified Spike-Pierce scale[19]
- Grade 1: no significant defects
- Grade 2: any number of parallel vascular channels <2 mm (conical opening on abaxial margin permitted)
- Grade 3: 1 or 2 abnormally shaped linear defects >2 mm in width
- Grade 4: 3 or more abnormally shaped linear defects >2 mm in width

Summary/Discussion
Proximal sesamoid bone fractures occur in young foals, with apical and basilar sesamoid fractures most common. Conservative management with stall rest is appropriate for the majority of foal proximal sesamoid bone fractures, and most fractures heal via bony union. Displaced fractures heal with an enlarged sesamoid, but most of these horses can go on to perform athletically. Young foals (<2 months) galloping with their dams to the point of exhaustion may sustain multiple sesamoid fractures and/or biaxial proximal sesamoid fractures. Midbody fractures with complete suspensory apparatus disruption may require surgical repair and coaptation to achieve pasture soundness.

Sesamoiditis is a condition primarily affecting yearling to 2-year-old horses in training, although it can also be diagnosed in foals. The diagnosis is confirmed radiographically by the presence of enlarged vascular channels or an increased number of vascular channels in the proximal sesamoid bones. Horses with severe radiographic evidence of sesamoiditis have an unfavorable prognosis for racing soundness or high-level athletic performance.

DISTAL PHALANX FRACTURES
Introduction
Distal phalanx fractures are classified into 7 distinct fracture types in the horse (**Table 2**).[25] Type VII fractures are unique to foals. Type VII fractures occur commonly and may not be associated with any localizing clinical signs. Type IV extensor process fractures are the second most common distal phalanx fracture type in foals. Although other fracture types can occur in foals, they are rare.

Type VII fractures (osseous bodies or ossicles)
Type VII distal phalangeal fractures are sometimes referred to as osseous bodies, or ossicles.[26] These are nonarticular fractures of the solar margin of the distal phalanx, originating at the incisure separating the proximal and distal palmar/plantar process

Table 2
Classification of distal phalanx fracture types

Fracture Type	Description
I	Nonarticular fractures of the palmar/plantar processes
II	Oblique, articular fractures of the palmar/plantar processes
III	Articular, midsagittal fractures
IV	Extensor process fractures
V	Comminuted fractures
VI	Nonarticular, solar margin fractures
VII[a]	Nonarticular, solar margin fractures dorsal to the palmar/plantar processes

[a] Foal-specific fractures.

angles.[27] From the incisure, these fractures continue dorsally 1 cm to 3 cm before exiting at the solar margin, forming a semilunar wedge of bone adjacent to the palmar/plantar process (**Fig. 11**). Type VII fractures are common on Thoroughbred breeding operations, most commonly recognized between 2 weeks and 5 months of age.[28] The prevalence of these fractures has been reported to range anywhere from 19%[26] to as high as 74%[29] in a recent longitudinal study. The prevalence seems highest in Thoroughbred foals, potentially due to the hoof conformation of this breed.[29] Type VII fractures most likely represent acute, traumatic fractures; however, other proposed etiologies include separate centers of ossification and developmental orthopedic disease. Other factors implicated in these fractures include hard footing and over trimming.

Type IV fractures

Type IV fractures are articular, involve the extensor process and occur predominantly in the front feet (**Fig. 12**). Fractures can be either traumatic or developmental in origin. When present bilaterally, they are thought to be a manifestation of osteochondrosis or a separate center of ossification.[30] The size of the fragment can vary considerably, but

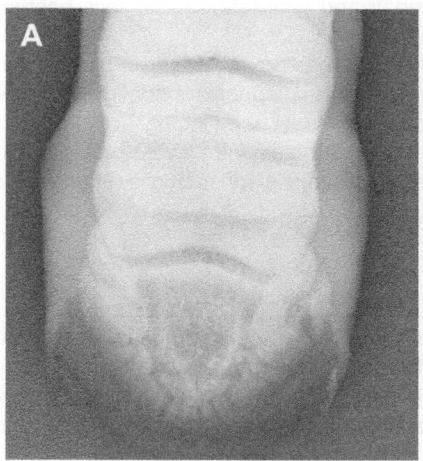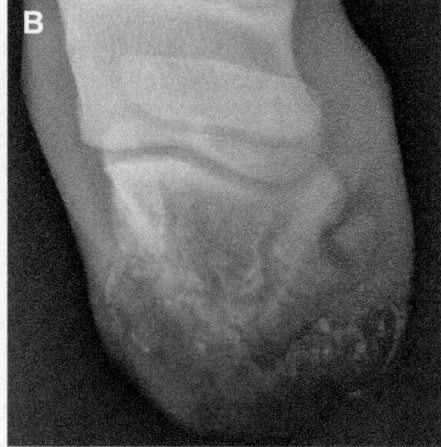

Fig. 11. (*A*) A 45° dorsoproximal palmarodistal radiographic projection, revealing a type VII fracture of the left forelimb in a 4-month-old Appendix Quarter Horse colt. Lateral is to the right. (*B*) A 45° dorsoproximolateral palmarodistomedial oblique projection in the same forelimb, clearly delineating the type VII fracture. (*Courtesy of* Dr Ashlee Watts, College Station, TX; with permission.)

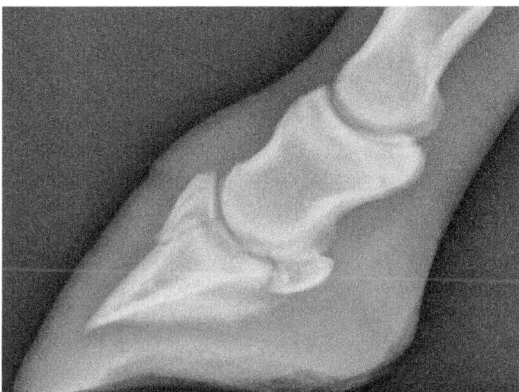

Fig. 12. Acute, minimally displaced type IV fracture of the left front coffin bone of a young Thoroughbred filly. Despite the significant size of this fragment, bony union is typically achieved in young foals with conservative treatment. (*Courtesy of* Dr Alan Nixon, Ithaca, NY; with permission.)

moderate-to-large fragments are commonly observed in foals. Some investigators have proposed that these moderate-sized fractures are a variation of the traumatically induced, nonunion osseous bodies similar to type VII fractures foals.[26]

Other fractures

Type III fractures have also been described in foals. Foals with these fractures are typically acutely, severely lame with distal interphalangeal joint effusion. Whereas these fractures typically result in significant synovitis and performance-limiting distal interphalangeal joint arthritis in adult horses, radiographic healing and return to soundness after stall confinement have been reported in a small number of foals treated with these types of fractures.[28] Type VI solar margin fractures are less common in foals than adults. Type VI fractures may be seen in foals with contracted tendons or flexural deformities of the metacarpophalangeal/metatarsophalangeal and proximal and distal interphalangeal joints, which subject the dorsal hoof wall and distal phalanx to increased concussive forces (**Fig. 13**).

Patient Evaluation Overview

Type VII palmar/plantar process fractures do not necessarily cause lameness and may be detected as incidental findings radiographically. If clinical signs are present, they may include limb abduction to unload the lateral aspect of the foot, increased digital pulses, and reaction to medial-to-lateral hoof wall compression at the quarters/heels.[16] If lameness is present, it is likely more noticeable on sharp turns. Type VII fractures are more common in the forelimb than the hind limb, and the lateral wing is affected more commonly than the medial wing in the forelimb. Biaxial and bilateral fractures are not uncommon. In the hind limb, there is an equal distribution between medial and lateral plantar process fractures. Type VII fractures may be detectable on a lateromedial or 45° dorsoproximal palmarodistal projection; however, a 45° dorsoproximal palmarodistal oblique projection is most sensitive for diagnosis of these fractures (see **Fig. 11**).

Although type IV (extensor process) fractures involve the articular surface of the distal interphalangeal joint, they may only cause mild or transitory lameness in foals. Clinical signs may include slight swelling around the coronary band and

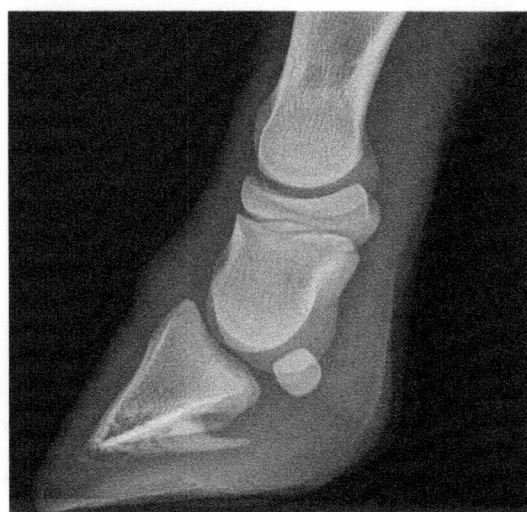

Fig. 13. Lateromedial radiograph of the left front foot of an 11-day-old foal with a type VI fracture of the distodorsal border of the coffin bone. Flexural deformity of the fetlock and pastern joints resulted in increased weight-bearing on the dorsal aspect of the hoof wall, predisposing to this solar margin fracture. (*Courtesy of* Dr Norm Ducharme, Ithaca, NY; with permission.)

increased digital pulses. The diagnosis is confirmed radiographically, typically with a lateromedial projection (see **Fig. 12**). Other articular distal phalangeal fractures typically result in acute-onset lameness. Sensitivity to medial-to-lateral hoof wall compression is one of the most reliable clinical signs for distal phalangeal fractures in foals, and the source of lameness can be confirmed with perineural diagnostic anesthesia.

Pharmacologic Treatment Options

When significant lameness is present, anti-inflammatories/analgesics are indicated. Options include phenylbutazone, firocoxib, and meloxicam (**Table 1**).

Nonpharmacologic Treatment Options

The typical treatment recommendation for distal phalanx fractures in foals is exercise restriction in a stall or small paddock with soft footing. For type VII fractures, stall rest is recommended until the foal is sound. If no lameness or clinical signs are noted, treatment may be unnecessary.

Surgical Treatment Options

Surgical treatment is not indicated for nonarticular distal phalangeal fractures in foals, unless there is abscessation and septic pedal osteitis. Surgery is rarely indicated for articular distal phalangeal fractures in foals. Unlike adults, most distal phalanx fractures in foals proceed to bony union without extensive osteoarthritis or lameness.[28] In rare cases, arthroscopic surgery may be indicated. Arthroscopic removal may be appropriate for type IV fractures that do not show evidence of radiographic healing and for which clinical signs persist. In adults, large, minimally displaced, acute extensor process fractures can be repaired by internal fixation with a 3.5-mm Association for Osteosynthesis/Association for the Study of Internal Fixation (AO/ASIF) cortical screw.[31] Internal fixation of a nondisplaced type IV fracture in a 4-month-old foal, combined with inferior check ligament desmotomy to treat flexural deformity of the distal interphalangeal joint, has been reported with a successful outcome.[32] Trauma to the extensor process resulting in multiple fragments, persistent distal interphalangeal joint effusion and lameness is an indication for surgery in foals (**Fig. 14**). Although lateromedial, dorsopalmar/plantar, and oblique projections are typically sufficient, CT may provide additional information about fragment number and location as well as damage to the articular surface of the distal phalanx.

Treatment Resistance/Complications

Rigid coaptation of the foot with a shoe, cuff, or cast is not indicated in foals due to the propensity for foal feet to quickly develop contracture[16] (**Fig. 15**).

Evaluation of Outcome and Long-term Recommendations

Type VII fractures have a good to excellent prognosis for healing and long-term soundness. Radiographic fracture healing has been documented as early as 4 weeks in

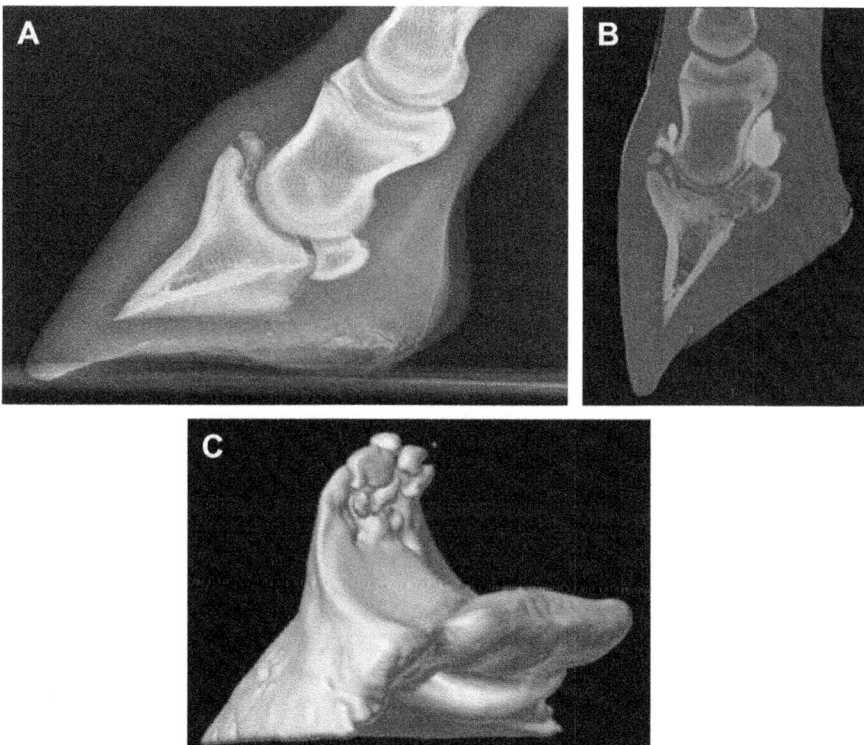

Fig. 14. (*A*) Lateromedial radiograph of the right hind foot of a 6-month-old Warmblood foal, revealing significant bony remodeling in the dorsal aspect of the distal interphalangeal joint associated with the extensor process and articular surface of the distal phalanx. (*B*) Contrast CT was used to delineate the distal interphalangeal joint, revealing fibrous union of several osteochondral fragments to the extensor process. (*C*) A 3-D CT reconstruction reveals numerous osteochondral fragments with an irregular articular surface of the coffin bone and a small bone cyst. The osteochondral fragments were removed arthroscopically. (*Courtesy of* Dr Norm Ducharme, Ithaca, NY; with permission.)

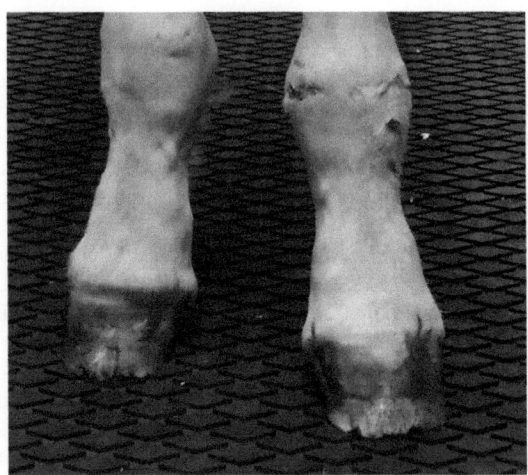

Fig. 15. Bilateral forefoot contracture in a 4-month-old Paint foal secondary to glue-on shoe application. Shoes, cuffs or foot casts are not indicated for distal phalanx fractures in foals due to the propensity for foals to develop contracted feet.

1 foal with acute lameness.[26] In another study, radiographic union and soundness were evident at 8 weeks and 10 weeks after diagnosis.[28]

Summary/Discussion

Type VII fractures are nonarticular fractures of the distal phalanx, which are unique to foals, occurring most commonly in Thoroughbred foals between 2 weeks and 5 months of age. Rarely causing lameness or clinical signs, these fractures are frequently diagnosed as incidental radiographic findings. The prognosis for radiographic healing and return to soundness is excellent. Type IV fractures also occur in foals, are most common in the forelimbs, and may be present bilaterally—possibly a manifestation of osteochondrosis or a separate center of ossification. Type III and other articular coffin bone fractures also occasionally occur in foals. Overall, the prognosis for soundness after distal phalangeal fractures is better for foals than adults. Conservative management is appropriate for most fracture types in foals.

REFERENCES

1. Barclay WP, Foerner JJ, Phillips TN. Lameness attributable to osteochondral fragmentation of the plantar aspect of the proximal phalanx in horses: 19 cases (1981-1985). J Am Vet Med Assoc 1987;191(7):855–7.
2. Sønnichsen HV, Kristoffersen J, Falk-Rønne J. Joint mice in the fetlock joint–osteochondritis dissecans. Nord Vet Med 1982;34(11):399–403.
3. Theiss F, Hilbe M, Fuerst A, et al. Histologic evaluation of intraarticular osteochondral fragments. Pferdeheilkunde 2010;26(4):541–52.
4. Nixon AJ, Pool RR. Histologic appearance of axial OC plantar palmar P1 fragments. J Am Vet Med Assoc 1995;207(8):1076–80.
5. Jacquet S, Robert C, Valette JP, et al. Evolution of radiological findings detected in the limbs of 321 young horses between the ages of 6 and 18months. Vet J 2013;197(1):58–64.
6. Declercq J, Hauspie S, Saunders J, et al. Osteochondral fragments in the metacarpo- and metatarsophalangeal joint and their clinical importance Osteochondrale

fragmenten in het kogelgewricht en hun klinisch belang. Vlaams Diergen Tijds 2011; 80:271–80.

7. Fortier LA, Foerner JJ, Nixon AJ. Arthroscopic removal of axial osteochondral fragments of the plantar/palmar proximal aspect of the proximal phalanx in horses: 119 cases (1988-1992). J Am Vet Med Assoc 1995;206(1):71–4.

8. Grondahl AM. (Norwegian C of VMON. The incidence of bony fragments and osteochondrosis in the metacarpo- and metatarsophalangeal joints of Standardbred trotters: a radiographic study. J Equine Vet Sci 1992;33(1):18–21.

9. Nixon AJ. Phalanges and the metacarpophalangeal and metatarsophalangeal joints. In: Auer JA, Stick JA, editors. Equine surgery. 4th edition. St Louis (MO): Elsevier Saunders; 2012. p. 1300–25.

10. Declercq J, Martens A, Bogaert L, et al. Osteochondral fragmentation in the synovial pad of the fetlock in Warmblood horses. Vet Surg 2008;37(7):613–8.

11. Mc Ilwraith CW, Voorhees M. Management of osteochondritis dissecans of the dorsal aspect of the distal metacarpus and metatarsus. Proc Am Assoc Equine Pract 1990;35:547–50.

12. Raidal SL, Edwards S, Pippia J, et al. Pharmacokinetics and safety of oral administration of meloxicam to foals. J Vet Intern Med 2013;27(2):300–7.

13. Hovanessian N, Davis JL, McKenzie HC III, et al. Pharmacokinetics and safety of firocoxib after oral administration of repeated consecutive doses to neonatal foals. J Vet Pharmacol Ther 2013;37:243–51.

14. McIlwraith CW, Nixon AJ, Wright IM. Diagnostic and surgical arthroscopy of the metacarpophalangeal and metatarsophalangeal joints. In: McIlwraith CW, Nixon AJ, Wright IM, editors. Diagnostic and surgical arthroscopy in the horse. 4th edition. China: Mosby Elsevier; 2015. p. 111–74.

15. Wright IM, Minshall GJ. Identification and treatment of osteochondritis dissecans of the distal sagittal ridge of the third metacarpal bone. Equine Vet J 2014;46(5): 585–8.

16. Hunt RJ. Lameness in foals. In: Baxter GM, editor. Adams and Stashak's lameness in horses. 6th edition. Chichester (West Sussex): Wiley-Blackwell; 2011. p. 1165–73.

17. Honnas CM, Snyder JR, Meagher DM, et al. Traumatic disruption of the suspensory apparatus in foals. Cornell Vet 1990;80(2):123–33.

18. Ellis DR. Fractures of the proximal sesamoid bones in Thoroughbred foals. Equine Vet J 1979;11(1):48–52.

19. Spike-Pierce DL, Bramlage LR. Correlation of racing performance with radiographic changes in the proximal sesamoid bones of 487 Thoroughbred yearlings. Equine Vet J 2003;35(4):350–3.

20. Richardson DW, Dyson SJ. Conditions of the proximal sesamoid bones. In: Ross MW, Dyson SJ, editors. Diagnosis and management of lameness in the horse. 2nd edition. St Louis (MO): Saunders; 2011. p. 402–7.

21. Bertone AL. Sesamoiditis. In: Baxter GM, editor. Adams and Stashak's lameness in horses. 6th edition. Singapore: Wiley-Blackwell; 2011. p. 604–6.

22. Busschers E, Richardson DW, Hogan PM, et al. Surgical repair of mid-body proximal sesamoid bone fractures in 25 horses. Vet Surg 2008;37(8):771–80.

23. Meagher DM, Bromberek JL, Meagher DT, et al. Prevalence of abnormal radiographic findings in 2-year-old Thoroughbreds at in-training sales and associations with racing performance. J Am Vet Med Assoc 2013;242(7):969–76.

24. McLellan J, Plevin S. Do radiographic signs of sesamoiditis in yearling Thoroughbreds predispose the development of suspensory ligament branch injury? Equine Vet J 2014;46(4):446–50.

25. Bertone AL. Fractures of the distal phalanx. In: Nixon AJ, editor. Equine fracture repair. 1st edition. Philadelphia: W.B. Saunders; 1996. p. 146–52.

26. Kaneps AJ, O'Brien TR, Redden RF, et al. Characterisation of osseous bodies of the distal phalanx of foals. Equine Vet J 1993;25(4):285–92.

27. Dyson SJ. The distal phalanx and distal interphalangeal joint. In: Ross MW, Dyson SJ, editors. Diagnosis and management of lameness in the horse. 2nd edition. St Louis (MO): Elsevier Inc; 2011. p. 349–66.

28. Yovich JV, Stashak TS, DeBowes RM, et al. Fractures of the distal phalanx of the forelimb in eight foals. J Am Vet Med Assoc 1986;189(5):550–4.

29. Faramarzi B, Mcmicking H, Halland S, et al. Incidence of palmar process fractures of the distal phalanx and association with front hoof conformation in foals. Equine Vet J 2015;47(6):675–9.

30. Furst AE, Lischer CJ. Foot. In: Auer JA, Stick JA, editors. Equine surgery. 4th edition. St Louis (MO): Elsevier; 2012. p. 1264–99.

31. McIlwraith CW, Nixon AJ, Wright IM. Arthroscopic surgery of the distal and proximal interphalangeal joints. In: McIlwraith CW, Nixon AJ, Wright IM, editors. Diagnostic and surgical arthroscopy in the horse. 4th edition. China: Mosby Elsevier; 2015. p. 316–43.

32. MacLellan KNM, MacDonald DG, Crawford WH. Lag screw fixation of an extensor process fracture in a foal with flexural deformity. Can Vet J 1997;38(4):226–8.

Physeal Fractures in Foals

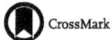 CrossMark

David G. Levine, DVM*, Maia R. Aitken, DVM

KEYWORDS

- Physis • Fracture • Internal fixation • External coaptation • Foal

KEY POINTS

- Physeal fractures are common musculoskeletal injuries in foals.
- Careful evaluation of the patient, including precise radiographic assessment, is paramount in determining the options for treatment.
- Prognosis for physeal fractures varies depending on location, age of patient and timeliness of referral.

INTRODUCTION

The term physis is historically defined as "a common term used to describe the epiphyseal growth plate" of long bones.[1] It is also commonly called the growth plate or, more appropriately, the metaphyseal growth plate because elongation of the bone is done by lengthening the metaphysis and not the epiphysis. The term physis is most appropriate when dealing with physeal fractures because some fractures deal with the cartilaginous plate and some deal with the adjacent bone. Physis covers all of these fracture types.

During rapid growth of the immature animal, the physis provides a weak point in the bone where fractures can occur. Fracture configuration, treatment, and prognosis differ depending on the location and type of fracture sustained. Physeal fractures have been historically classified using the Salter Harris classification system.

Salter Harris Classification System
- Type 1: A fracture through the zone of hypertrophied cells only, without involvement of the adjacent epiphysis or metaphysis.
- Type 2: A fracture through the physis across part of the width of the bone and through the metaphysis, leaving a segment of metaphysis attached to the epiphysis.
- Type 3: A fracture through the physis across part of the width of the bone and through the epiphysis, entering the joint.
- Type 4: A fracture across the epiphysis, growth plate, and a portion of the metaphysis perpendicular to the plane of the physis.
- Type 5: A crushing or compression fracture of the growth plate with little or no displacement.

University of Pennsylvania, Department of Clinical Studies New Bolton Center, 382 W Street Road, Kennett Square, PA 19348, USA
* Corresponding author.
E-mail address: dglevine@vet.upenn.edu

Vet Clin Equine 33 (2017) 417–430
http://dx.doi.org/10.1016/j.cveq.2017.03.008
0749-0739/17/© 2017 Elsevier Inc. All rights reserved.

Although the Salter Harris system is the most common classification system to describe physeal fractures, it does not fit all physeal fractures. Although many of the physes in the horse are under compressive loads (compression physis), there are some physes at attachment sites of soft tissue structures (ie, olecranon) that are under tensile loads (tension physis). The Salter Harris system is not equipped to describe fractures of the tension physis and, therefore, simple anatomic description of these fractures is preferred by the authors.

PATIENT ASSESSMENT

Similar to most conditions, a good history and thorough physical examination is of utmost importance. History of how the fracture occurred, as well as the age of the patient and duration of fracture, can help determine the prognosis in several cases.

Physical examination will give information regarding patient stability and safety, as well as additional information that can aid in determination of prognosis. Whether the fracture is new or old, the condition of overlying soft tissue structures, as well as the overall health of the patient, can guide the course of action.

Careful initial patient assessment, including heart rate, mucous membrane color, hydration status, and capillary refill time, can determine if the patient is stable or hypovolemic. Shock from trauma may occur although blood loss that from fractured long bones is generally not a major concern for foals with physeal fractures because these fractures do not involve the diaphysis. Young foals with fractures may also not be able to nurse effectively and can rapidly become dehydrated and possibly hypoglycemic. If available, initial hematology and serum biochemical analysis, including packed cell volume, total solids, blood glucose, and lactate measurements, can aid in assessing the foal's level of hydration and volume status. Fluid therapy should be administered as determined to stabilize a patient before treatment or shipping.

Radiographs should be obtained before stabilization if appropriate and available. Very unstable limbs or injuries in the field, where radiography is unavailable, should be stabilized to the best ability of the clinician.

Wounds should be cleaned, investigated, and addressed before shipping. In most cases, open fractures have a decreased prognosis compared with closed fractures. Appropriate antimicrobial therapy and tetanus prophylaxis should be considered in open fractures before transport and treatment.

Stabilization of the limb before transport can prevent further injury; however, it cannot be stressed enough that improper stabilization can exacerbate the initial injury, which may lead to decreased prognosis, depending on the degree of fracture propagation or continued soft tissue injury. **Fig. 1** can help guide stabilization techniques, though the authors would recommend the use of a modified Robert-Jones as opposed to the traditional Robert-Jones bandage. Splint material can be made from a variety of household items if specialized equipment is not available. The best splint material is lightweight and strong, providing stability without excessive weight. Polyvinyl chloride (PVC) pipe cut in half lengthwise is commonly used and is a lightweight and rigid material. Wood, especially 2 by 4 inch boards, is too heavy and often can lead to more injury. Splints should be applied over a light bandage that protects the skin and soft tissues. Application of a splint over a large or heavily padded bandage increases the distance from the bone to the splint, thereby decreasing the effectiveness of the splint. A light elastic bandage can also be placed over the splint as an additional protective layer, to avoid the foal injuring adjacent structures or limbs.

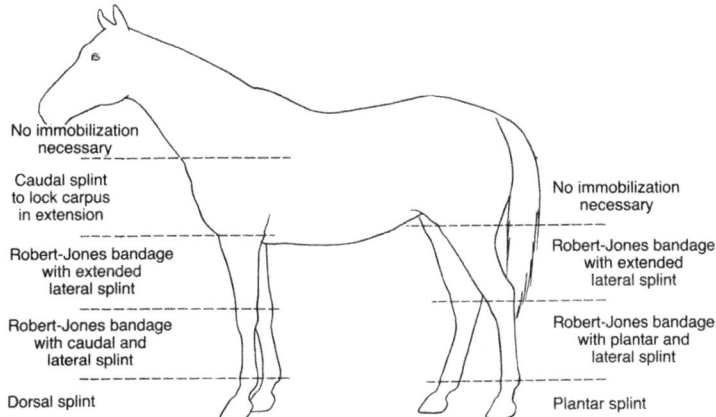

Fig. 1. Guidelines for splint placement based on fracture location. (*From* Mudge MC, Bramlage LR. Field fracture management. Vet Clin Equine 2007;23:123; with permission.)

FRACTURE TREATMENT AND PROGNOSIS BY LOCATION
Digits or Phalanges

Physeal fractures of the digit in foals are rare. To the authors' knowledge, there are no case reports in the literature of fractures involving the middle phalanx, although physeal fractures of the proximal physis of the middle phalanx are possible and may be managed similar to proximal phalangeal fractures. Proximal physeal fractures of the proximal phalanx have been reported but are limited to 7 cases.[2–8] In the 2 larger retrospective case studies on physeal fractures, the proximal phalanx was the affected bone in only 4 in 160 cases, demonstrating the relative rarity of this fracture.[2–4] In the proximal phalanx, Salter Harris type 2 and 3 fractures are the most common, with 1 reference to a type 4 fracture (**Figs. 2** and **3**).

Treatment of proximal phalangeal fractures can be divided into conservative and surgical methods:

- Conservative: Application of external coaptation to the lower limb, in the form of a rigid cast or bandage, is a reasonable technique for minimally displaced fractures or the reported type 3 fractures. Due to the rapid growth and healing potential in foals, this type of external coaptation should only be required for a short amount of time. In the authors' opinion, 4 to 6 weeks of rigid coaptation, with an additional several weeks of limited exercise, should be adequate to allow healing of a minimally displaced proximal phalangeal fracture. Prolonged coaptation should be avoided because this can lead to tendon laxity in the foal.
- Surgical: Internal fixation techniques including screws, screws and wire, and plate fixation can be used to reduce and stabilize the proximal physis. Only 2 cases are reported with surgical repair of a proximal physeal fracture of the proximal phalanx, although undoubtedly more have been repaired in practice.[7,9] Because the proximal physis accounts for less than 2 cm of total growth of the limb, loss of this growth potential is not overly concerning.[10]

Prognosis in the current literature is guarded to poor for athletic outcome in proximal phalangeal physeal fractures.[2–9] This may be due to conservative management in most of these cases, with development of osteoarthritis in the future. This is especially evident in type 3 fractures with joint involvement. Due to the overwhelming number of

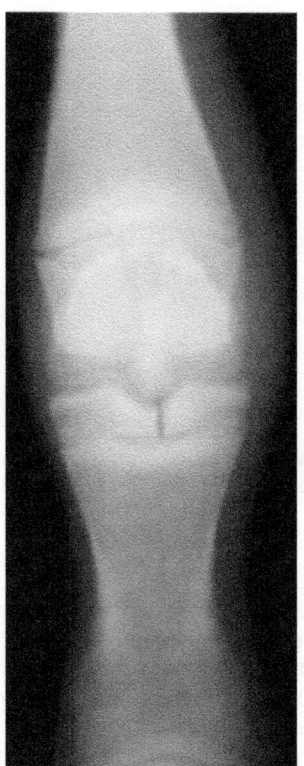

Fig. 2. Dorsoplantar projection showing a Salter Harris type 3 fracture of the proximal phalanx.

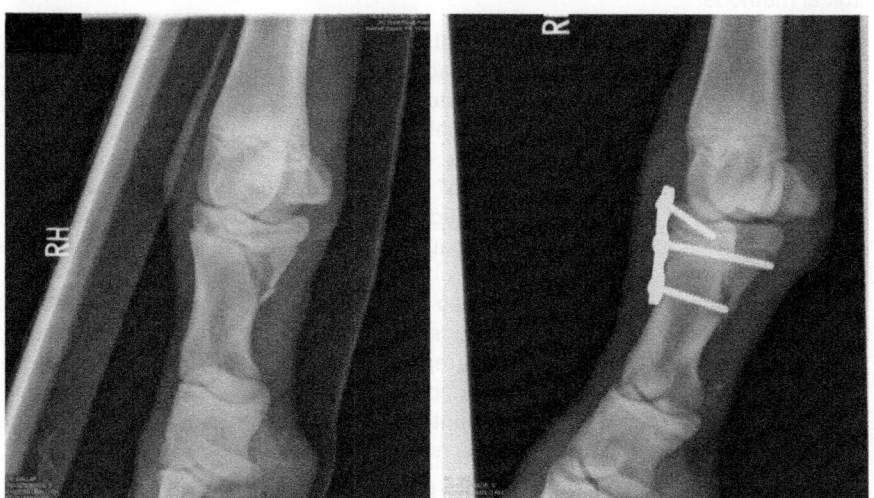

Fig. 3. Preoperative (*left*) and postoperative (*right*) radiographs of a Salter Harris type 2 fracture of the proximal phalanx showing internal fixation using a 3-hole narrow 4.5 mm Limited Contact Dynamic Compression Plate (LC-DCP).

cases that have been managed conservatively in the literature, this may not accurately determine prognosis for current cases. With the advancement of imaging and surgical guidance afforded by intraoperative computed tomography, these fractures may be more accurately surgically reduced using minimally invasive techniques, leading to a more favorable outcome in the future.

Metacarpus or Metatarsus

Salter Harris fractures of the distal metacarpal or metatarsal physis accounted for 10% of all physeal fractures in the largest retrospective on the subject.[2] Type 2 fractures accounted for all but 1 of these fractures, which is in agreement to other case reports as well as the authors' experience.[2–4,11] These fractures often occur traumatically in weanling to suckling foals that are stepped on while recumbent (**Fig. 4**).

Treatment can be divided into conservative and surgical methods:

- Conservative: Application of rigid half limb cast or bandage is a reasonable technique for minimally displaced fractures of young foals (younger than 2 months). This can be maintained for 2 to 3 weeks, followed by lighter coaptation for an additional 2 to 3 weeks.
- Surgical: Older foals or those with displacement of the fracture should be addressed with internal fixation. This can often be accomplished with lag screw fixation across the metaphyseal component after anatomic alignment. Care should be taken in young foals to minimize fixation across the distal physis because elongation of the metacarpus accounts for a substantial amount of total limb length and can lead to shortening of the limb. This surgical correction is usually combined with a rigid external coaptation technique for the first few weeks after repair. Other techniques of screw and wire fixation, as well as plate fixation, are possible but usually not necessary to achieve healing.

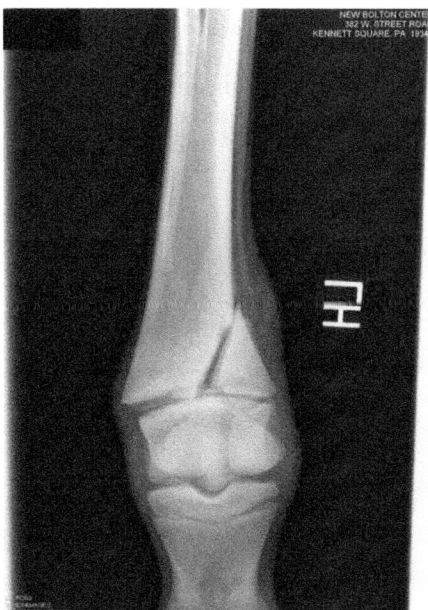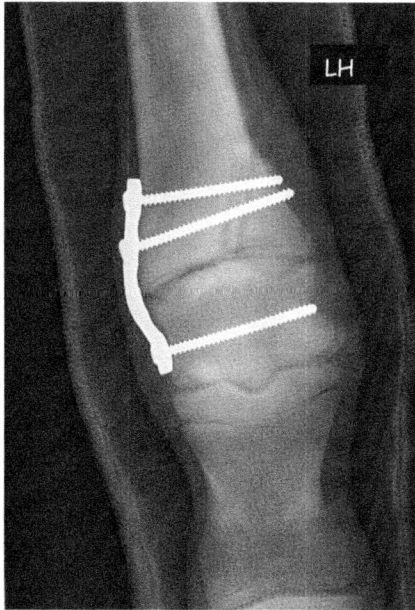

Fig. 4. Preoperative (*left*) and postoperative (*right*) radiographs of a Salter Harris type 2 fracture of the distal metatarsus repaired using a 4-hole narrow 4.5 mm LC-DCP.

Prognosis for metacarpal or metatarsal physeal fractures is good. Initial data showed metacarpal fractures to have a better prognosis than metatarsal fractures; however, because most of the metatarsal fractures were repaired surgically, whereas the metacarpal fractures were repaired conservatively, a direct comparison cannot be made.[2–4] Both conservative and surgical techniques can achieve acceptable outcomes if chosen for the correct fractures. There is a single case report of an older foal with a displaced fracture that was able to achieve a successful union when managed conservatively.[11] Despite healing in this case, poor athletic outcome was the result, demonstrating that, although healing can be achieved with coaptation if finances are limited, anatomic alignment is the key for an athletic outcome.

Radius

Physeal fractures of the radius can be distinguished between proximal and distal physeal fractures. Although current literature,[12,13] and the authors' experience would say that proximal physeal fractures are more common, Embertson and colleagues[2,3] report similar numbers of proximal and distal fractures. Both proximal and distal physeal fractures can occur when a foal becomes entrapped and struggles, or by being kicked in the upper portion of the limb. Metaphyseal and diaphyseal fractures of the radius are more common than physeal fractures of the radius. The method of treatment depends largely on which physis is affected. Though conservative management with external coaptation may be attempted in very young foals with distal radial physeal fractures, most radial physeal fractures require surgical intervention.

Proximal physeal fractures often involve the proximal ulna (**Fig. 5**). Type 1 and type 2 fractures are most common, although type 3 fractures can occur.[2,3,13–15] The most common and recommended method of treatment is surgical repair, specifically plate fixation of the ulna incorporating the proximal radius. This can be combined with an additional plate applied to the lateral aspect of the radius if more stabilization is necessary. Plates bridging the physis in young foals should be removed as soon as deemed possible to avoid bridging the proximal radial physis. Earlier reports did not show a favorable prognosis for radial physeal fractures but more recent reports suggest that the prognosis is good for return to athletic function as long as physeal growth is spared and correct anatomic reduction is achieved.[2,3,13–15] In a recent report on

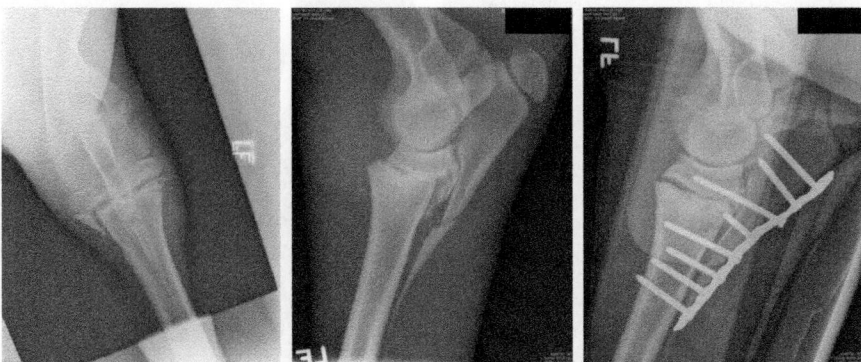

Fig. 5. Preoperative and postoperative radiographs of a typical proximal radial physeal fracture (Salter Harris type 2) that also involves an ulnar fracture. This was repaired using an 8-hole narrow 4.5 mm LCP.

ulna fractures from the authors' clinic, 3 of the fractures involved the proximal radial physis (2 Salter Harris type 2 and 1 Salter Harris type 3). All were sound for intended use following treatment[15] except 1 foal that was sound and in use but subsequently developed unrelated neurologic disease and was euthanized.

Distal physeal fractures are less common and are most often type 1 or type 2 fractures of the distal radius. These can be treated in young foals with external coaptation or with screw and wire fixation (transphyseal screw and wire) similar to that used for angular limb deformity. These screws and wires should be removed as soon as deemed safe (3–4 weeks) to salvage growth at the distal physis. With correct anatomic reduction and without destruction of the distal physis, this type of fracture should have a good prognosis.

Ulna

The proximal physis of the ulna or olecranon is a tension physis. Fractures of this physis are a common type of physeal fracture accounting for 15% of all physeal fractures in a large retrospective study.[2] The classification system for proximal ulnar fractures uses the system in place for olecranon fractures in which type 1a is a Salter Harris type 1 fracture type and a type 1b is a Salter Harris type 2 fracture. Type 1a fractures are much more common than type 1b fractures. Foals with this fracture often assume the position of a dropped elbow and inability to fix the carpus, similar to adults with olecranon fractures (**Fig. 6**).

Conservative management of these physeal fractures should be reserved for foals that have minimal displacement and are able to ambulate on the limb without coaptation. Several weeks of stall confinement may allow healing in foals, although most fractures diagnosed will require some type of internal fixation. Several techniques have been described for surgical repair of proximal ulnar physeal fractures including[14]

- Tension band wire fixation
- Curved plate fixation
- Hook plate fixation.

The challenge in this surgical repair is the small amount of bone to engage at the proximal aspect of the ulna and the tensile forces of the triceps muscle that distract the ulnar apophysis. To achieve as much purchase in the proximal fragment, the plate is bent over the proximal ulna, or wires are used to wrap and engage the proximal fragment.

Prognosis for repair of any ulnar fracture is good, with the proximal physis being no exception. Reports of all types of ulnar fractures indicate between 72% and 85% success, depending on the report and the technique.[12,14–17] These reports are usually not exclusive to physeal fractures of the ulna but prognosis is good if purchase and stability of the proximal fragment can be obtained.

Humerus

Physeal fractures of the humerus accounted for 15% of total fractures in the same retrospective study on the subject.[2] Most (~65%) of these fractures were of the distal humerus (**Fig. 7**). Proximal humeral physeal fractures are uncommon and, although Embertson and colleagues[2] included a single Salter Harris type 2 fracture, the authors have primarily seen Salter Harris type 3 fractures with involvement of the scapulohumeral joint surface. Depending on the location of the fracture, conservative of surgical management may be pursued:

- Conservative management of proximal humeral physeal fractures can be attempted if minimal displacement is noted and there is no involvement of the

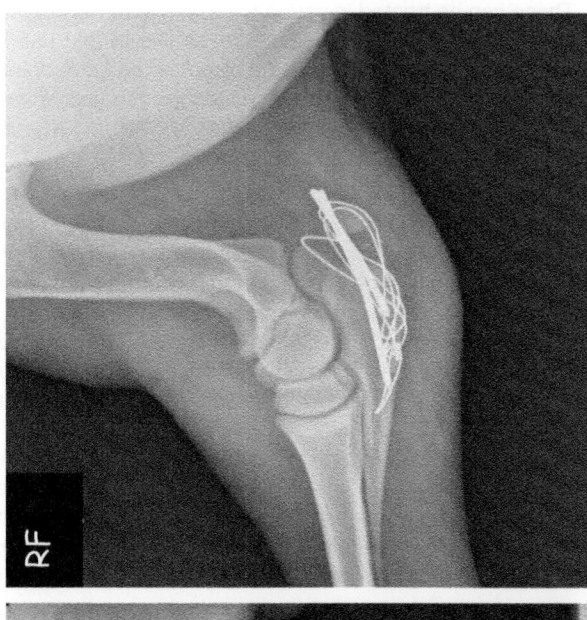

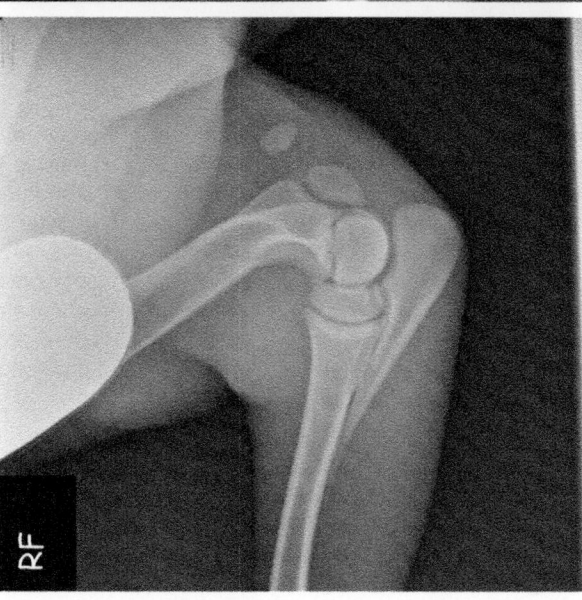

Fig. 6. Preoperative (*left*) and postoperative (*right*) radiographs of a Salter Harris type 1 fracture of the proximal ulna. Note the displacement of the apophysis due to tension from the triceps muscle. Repair was performed using 2 pins and 4 figure-of-8 stainless steel wires.

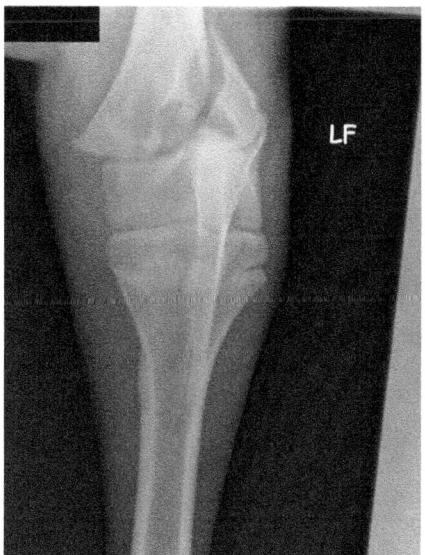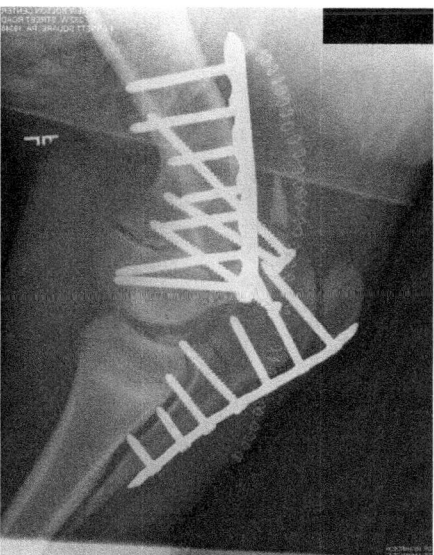

Fig. 7. Preoperative (*left*) and postoperative (*right*) radiographs of a distal humeral physeal fracture (Salter Harris type 2). This fracture was approached via an ulnar osteotomy and repaired with 3 screws placed in lag fashion and a 7-hole broad 4.5 mm locking compression plate (LCP). The osteotomy was repaired using a 7-hole narrow 4.5 mm LCP.

scapulohumeral joint. Coaptation of the humerus is impossible and conservative management would include stall confinement. Conservative management should not be attempted in distal humeral physeal fractures.

- Surgical: Distal fractures should be treated with internal fixation. The shape and forces applied to the distal humeral physis makes fixation challenging. In the study by Embertson and colleagues,[2] none of the 7 foals with distal humeral physeal fractures survived. Many attempts have been made to fix distal physeal humeral fractures, including rush pins, pins and wire, lag screw fixation, and plate fixation. Most of these cases resulted in euthanasia. One case report of a foal with a distal humeral fracture repaired by ulnar osteotomy and locking compression plate (LCP) fixation was successful.[18] The superior strength of the LCP, as well as the approach to the joint via the ulnar osteotomy, may have led to the success in this single case. This surgical approach and plate fixation using the LCP can be attempted in the future for foals with distal humeral fractures. The anatomic shape of the proximal humerus makes fixation of proximal physeal fractures difficult to attempt in larger foals.

Due to the poor reported outcomes in the literature of both proximal and distal physeal fractures of the humerus, prognosis in these cases is guarded to poor. Fixation can be attempted for valuable animals with distal humeral physeal fractures, with the knowledge that many may not survive.

Scapula

Physeal fractures of the scapula are uncommon and represent only 7% of total fractures in the study by Embertson and colleagues.[2] Of interest is that these fractures were more likely to be type 1 fractures than any other physeal fracture reported. There are limited reports on distal scapular physeal fractures in horses. Of these reports, only 1 foal returned to soundness.[2] All foals were treated conservatively and the 1 foal that eventually regained soundness was substantially younger at 4 months old than the average age of 9.5 months.

Because distal scapular physeal fractures involve the supraglenoid tubercle, it is reasonable to extrapolate data from the literature regarding this type of fracture in older horses. Many of these horses can be managed surgically with fragment removal or with partial biceps tenotomy, or with tension band wiring in combination with lag screw compression. Although this has not been reported for distal physeal fractures, it could be attempted in the right cases. Because this has not been reported in the literature, it is still considered a guarded to poor prognosis for returning to soundness after distal scapular physeal fractures in foals, with younger foals and minimally displaced fractures carrying a more favorable prognosis.

Tibia

Physeal fractures of the tibia accounted for 10% of all fractures in the study by Embertson and colleagues,[2] with more fractures occurring in the distal physis than the proximal physis. In the authors' opinions, proximal physeal fractures are now substantially more common, with distal physeal fractures being a rarity in the foal. Current literature supports this theory in that there has been much published on repair of proximal physeal fractures in the foal but minimal publications describing distal fracture repair.[19–22]

Proximal tibial physeal fractures are almost always a Salter Harris type 2 fracture with the metaphyseal spike on the lateral aspect of the limb (**Fig. 8**). These fractures occur most likely with a kick to the lateral aspect of the limb while weight-bearing. The lateral kick provides tension to the medial aspect of the physis,

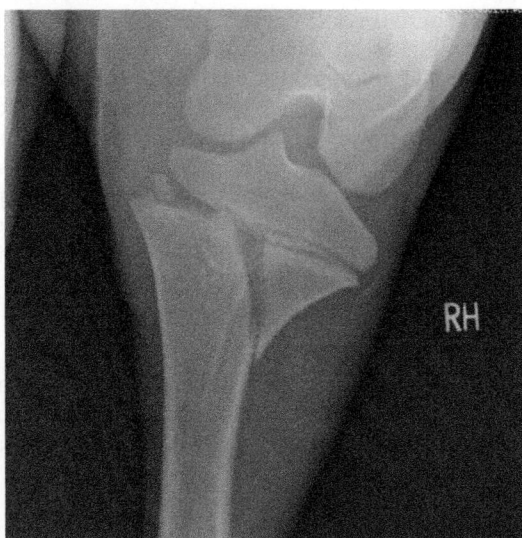

Fig. 8. Typical appearance of a proximal tibial physeal fracture, Salter Harris type 2, with a lateral metaphyseal spike.

creating the fracture that will propagate across the physis from medial to lateral. Because the fracture approaches the lateral aspect of the physis, bending forces on the limb will distract the fracture and create a lever arm, which will propagate the fracture along the lateral metaphysis leaving the lateral aspect of the physis intact.

Treatment of proximal physeal fractures has been accomplished with multiple types of internal fixation, including lag screws, pinning, and wire fixation, as well as lateral and medial plate fixation. The most biomechanically secure fixation is a plate placed on the medial aspect of the tibia because of the tension surface on this side of the limb, despite the limited amount of soft tissue coverage of this area. Furthermore, plate placement may not be possible medially. Soft tissue coverage is always a concern with regard to surgical planning, and the relative lack of soft tissue coverage lends to increased postoperative infection. In young animals with this type of fracture, healing is rapid and the plate can be removed in 6 to 8 weeks to allow continued physeal growth.

Prognosis for return to soundness is good with internal fixation. Implant infection and secondary implant failure are the most common complications, with larger foals, and open fractures carry a worse prognosis.

Distal physeal fractures of the tibia are rare and most commonly are Salter Harris type 2 fractures involving the lateral metaphysis. Limited data are published on this type of fracture. The prognosis from the study by Embertson and colleagues[2] is poor, with only 1 horse becoming sound.

Treatment of this fracture type is guided by the displacement of the fracture, as well as the size and age of the animal. Young horses with minimally displaced fractures can be managed with external coaptation for a period of 3 to 6 weeks with decreasing cast or bandaging, and increasing exercise, during healing. With larger foals or with displacement of the fracture, lag screw fixation in combination with tension band wiring can be used to repair the fracture. The shape of the distal tibia requires creativity when repairing these fractures and limits what can be repaired in more comminuted or displaced fractures. Prognosis should still be regarded as guarded, with displaced fractures of the distal tibial physis.

Femur

Physeal fractures of the femur are common and accounted for 30% of all physeal fractures in the study by Embertson and colleagues.[2] They can be separated into proximal and distal fractures, with approximately even distribution found in the literature.

Proximal physeal or femoral capital physeal fractures can be challenging to diagnose in the foal. Lameness is localized to the upper limb or coxofemoral joint, and good quality radiographs are required to diagnose this fracture. This is often done under general anesthesia or heavy sedation in a young foal, with manipulation of the limb and multiple radiographs occasionally required to see the displacement of the fracture. These fractures can occur as Salter Harris type 1 to 3, with type 1 and 2 being the most common (**Fig. 9**). Fracture configuration does not routinely change the treatment or outcome.

Treatment involves internal fixation in most cases. Conservative management has been attempted in foals and does not result in a favorable outcome. Surgical repair is challenging and requires skill (and some luck) to reduce the fracture adequately and provide enough stability to avoid implant failure. Lag screw fixation is the most common technique, using multiple lag screws to reduce and stabilize the capital femoral head.[23–25] Prognosis is guarded in these cases, with younger and lighter animals having a better prognosis.

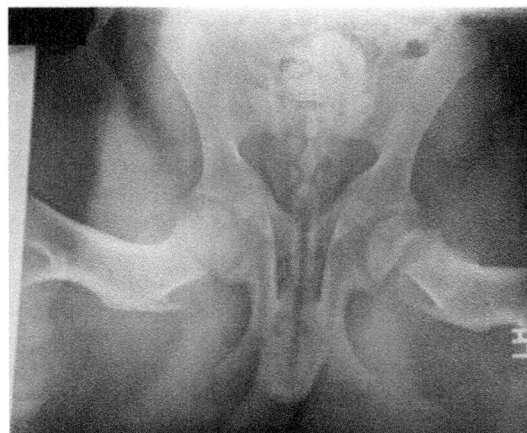

Fig. 9. Ventrodorsal projection obtained under general anesthesia showing a Salter Harris type 1 fracture of the left proximal femoral physis.

Salter Harris type 2 fractures are the most common seen in the distal femoral physis (**Fig. 10**). The metaphyseal spike is most commonly caudal, although a large cranial metaphyseal spike is also seen.[23] These fractures can be confused with stifle lesions in foals and are quite unstable.

Treatment includes internal fixation using a combination of techniques. The dynamic condylar screw plate is among the strongest fixations for this type of fracture, although many techniques and plate configurations have been used, including the locking compression plate and flared condylar repair plates.[23,26,27] Prognosis is guarded for this fracture for several reasons. In general, fractures of the femur are often comminuted fractures with significant soft tissue swelling, making both the surgical approach and the ability to achieve stability difficult. Postoperative implant infection and

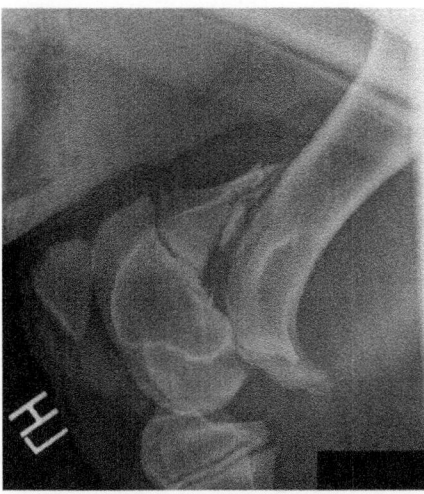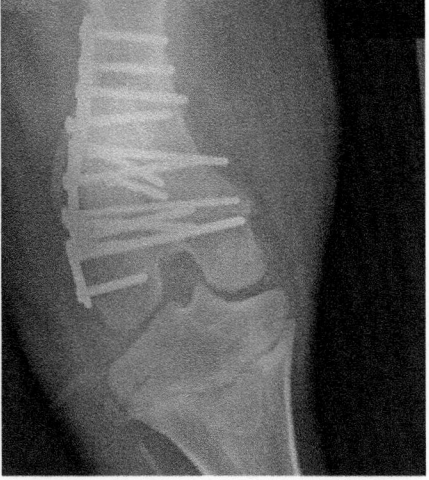

Fig. 10. Preoperative (*left*) and postoperative (*right*) radiographs of a Salter Harris type 2 fracture of the distal femur repaired with 5 screws placed in lag fashion and a 9-hole broad 4.5 mm LCP.

subsequent instability are other complicating factors of femoral fracture repair. In foals, distal physeal fracture repair inevitability involves early closure of the growth plate and a shortened limb. This is acceptable as a salvage procedure but is not likely to result in an athletic animal.

SUMMARY AND DISCUSSION

Long bone fractures in foals that involve the physes have varying degrees of prognosis, depending on the bone involved, the type of fracture, and the damage to the surrounding structures. In general, prompt diagnosis and treatment leads to more favorable outcomes. The difficulties in managing these cases involve the degree of growth left in the affected limb, instability of the fracture, surrounding soft tissue damage, and surgical accessibility to the fracture site. However, though there are exceptions to this rule, given the rapid bone growth that does occur in the foal, if a physeal fracture can be appropriately stabilized, healing should occur.

REFERENCES

1. Dorland WA. Dorland's illustrated medical dictionary. Philadelphia: Saunders; 2007.
2. Embertson RM, Bramlage LR, Gabel AA. Physeal fractures in the horse I. Classification and incidence. Vet Surg 1986;15(3):223–9.
3. Embertson RM, Bramlage LR, Herring DS, et al. Physeal fractures in the horse II. Management and outcome. Vet Surg 1986;15(3):230–6.
4. Auer JA. Frakturen beim wachsend Fohlen und deren Behandlung Teil I: Epiphysenfrakturen. Pferdeheilkunde 1986;2(6):353–70.
5. Auer JA. Physeal fracture of the proximal phalanx in foals. Equine Vet Ed 2015; 27(4):183–7.
6. Orsini JA, Grenager N, Carr J, et al. What's your diagnosis. J Am Vet Med Assoc 2006;228(3):353–4.
7. Van Spijk JN, Furst AE. Minimally invasive plate osteosynthesis of a Salter Harris type 2 fracture of the proximal phalanx in a filly. Equine Vet Ed 2015;27(4):179–82.
8. Markel MD, Richardson DW. Noncomminuted fractures of the proximal phalanx in 69 horses. J Am Vet Med Assoc 1985;186(6):573–9.
9. Ross MW. The hindfoot and pastern. In: Ross MW, Dyson SJ, editors. Lameness in the horse. St Louis (MO): Elsevier; 2011. p. 479–80.
10. Fretz PB, Cymbaluk NF, Pharr JW. Quantitative analysis of long-bone growth in the horse. Am J Vet Res 1984;45:1602–9.
11. Amaniti EM, Diakakis N, Patsikas M, et al. Conservative management of a distal epiphyseal metacarpal fracture in a skyros pony. J Equine Sci 2008;19(3):57–61.
12. Watkins JP. Radius and ulna. In: Auer JA, editor. Equine surgery. St Louis (MO): Elsevier; 2012. p. 1363–78.
13. Sanders-Shamis M, Bramlage LR, Gable AA. Radius fractures in the horse: a retrospective study of 47 cases. Equine Vet J 1986;18(6):432–7.
14. Auer JA, Struchen CH, Weidmann CH. Surgical management of a foal with a humerus radius ulna fracture. Equine Vet J 1996;28(5):416–20.
15. Jacobs CC, Levine DG, Richardson DW. Use of locking compression plates in ulnar fractures; 18 cases. Vet Surg 2017;46(2):242–8.
16. Donecker JM, Bramlage LR, Gabel AA. Retrospective analysis of 29 fractures of the olecranon process of the equine ulna. J Am Vet Med Assoc 1984;15(2):183–9.
17. Swor TM, Watkins JP, Bahr A, et al. Results of plate fixation of type 1b olecranon fractures in 24 horses. Equine Vet J 2003;35(7):670–5.

18. Ahern BJ, Richardson DW. Distal humeral Salter Harris (type II) fracture repair by an ulnar osteotomy approach in a horse. Vet Surg 2010;39:729–32.
19. Wagner PC, DeBowes RM, Grant BD, et al. Cancellous bone screws for repair of proximal growth plate fractures of the tibia in foals. J Am Vet Med Assoc 1984; 184(6):688–91.
20. Watkins JP, Auer JA, Taylor TS. Crosspin fixation of fractures of the proximal tibia in three foals. Vet Surg 1985;14(2):153–9.
21. Godoy RF, Filgueiras RR, Gontijo LA, et al. Treatment of a periarticular tibial fracture in a foal with a hybrid external fixator. Vet Surg 2009;38:650–3.
22. Bramlage LR. Tibia. In: Auer JA, editor. Equine surgery. St Louis (MO): Elsevier; 2012. p. 1409–14.
23. Richardson DW. Femur and pelvis. In: Auer JA, editor. Equine surgery. St Louis (MO): Elsevier; 2012. p. 1442–52.
24. Smyth GB, Taylor EG. Stabilization of a proximal femoral physeal fracture in a filly by use of cancellous bone screws. J Am Vet Med Assoc 1992;201(6):895–8.
25. Hunt DA, Snyder JR, Morgan JP, et al. Femoral capital physeal fractures in 25 foals. Vet Surg 1990;19(1):41–9.
26. Byron CR, Stick JA, Brown JA, et al. Use of a condylar screw plate for repair of a Salter Harris type 3 fracture of the femur in a 2 year old horse. J Am Vet Med Assoc 2002;221(9):1292–5.
27. Orsini JA, Buonanno AM, Richardson DW, et al. Condylar buttress plate fixation of femoral fracture in a colt. J Am Vet Med Assoc 1990;197(9):1184–6.

Diagnosis and Treatment Considerations for Nonphyseal Long Bone Fractures in the Foal

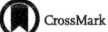 CrossMark

Kati Glass, DVM, Ashlee E. Watts, DVM, PhD*

KEYWORDS

- Fracture • Emergency management • Coaptation

KEY POINTS

- Many long bone fractures that are not considered repairable in the adult horse are repairable in the foal. This is largely because of reduced patient size and more rapid healing in the foal.
- When there is no articular communication, the long-term prognosis for athletic function can be very good.
- Emergency care and transport of the foal with a long bone fracture is different than the adult.

INTRODUCTION

With advancements in veterinary care, procedures, and surgical implants, many fractures that were once considered "not fixable" in the adult horse can now be repaired with good outcomes. However, there are many long bone fractures that are still considered irreparable or unlikely to succeed in the adult horse because implant failure is expected to outpace bony healing. In the foal, smaller size and a faster rate of healing translate to successful outcomes for many of these long bone fractures. The purpose of this article is not to inform on how long bone fracture repair in the foal is performed. Rather, it is to outline differences that exist between the foal and the adult horse in emergency fracture management, surgical options, and long-term outcome. It is important for the veterinary practitioner to recognize these differences when discussing options with horse owners after identifying long bone fractures in the foal. When long bone fractures occur in the foal and surgical fixation is to be pursued, there are

The authors have no commercial or financial disclosures related to this article.
Department of Large Animal Clinical Sciences, College of Veterinary Medicine & Biomedical Sciences, Texas A&M University, 4475 TAMU, College Station, TX 77843-4475, USA
* Corresponding author.
E-mail address: awatts@cvm.tamu.edu

Vet Clin Equine 33 (2017) 431–438
http://dx.doi.org/10.1016/j.cveq.2017.03.013
vetequine.theclinics.com

several considerations in emergency care, splinting, and transport that are different to the adult that should be kept in mind.

SCAPULA

Complete scapular fractures that cause axial instability can occur in the neck or body and occur most commonly secondary to direct trauma from kicks, collisions, or falls in the young horse. Fracture will result in acute, severe lameness, an unwillingness to advance the limb and usually significant swelling over the shoulder. Crepitation and pain on palpation of the shoulder region may be appreciated. Radiographs made in the field are usually successful at diagnosing the fracture due to the foal's small size. Radiographic projections should include medial to lateral and craniolateral to caudolateral oblique views (**Fig. 1**). Differentials include humeral fracture, soft tissue trauma, scapular fracture that does not cause axial instability, suprascapular nerve injury, and depending on the age of the foal, infection of musculoskeletal structures. When fracture is not recognized in the acute stages, swelling will subside, lameness will persist, and marked muscle atrophy of the supraspinatous and infraspinatous muscles will occur either due to injury to the suprascapular nerve or to disuse.

Successful repair of complete neck and body fractures with open reduction and internal fixation in young horses has been reported using both dynamic compression plates and locking compression plates.[1–3] When the fracture is nonarticular, surgical options can provide a good prognosis for future athletic performance (**Fig. 2**). When neck or body fractures are minimally displaced and nonarticular and the foal is willing to bear some weight, complete healing can occur with stall confinement alone but is very likely to result in an unsatisfactory outcome due to prolonged lameness and resultant severe support limb abnormalities.

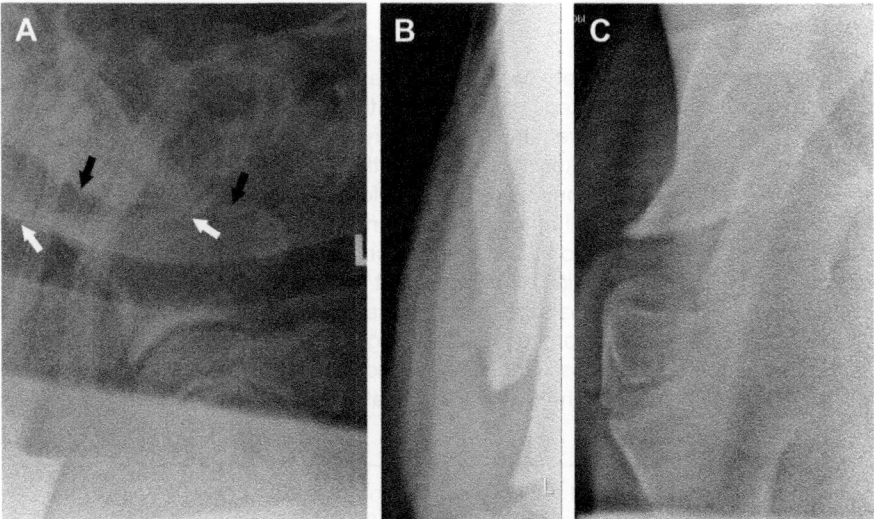

Fig. 1. Standing radiographic projections of a 3-month-old warmblood filly with a simple, short oblique, complete, closed, medially and caudally displaced scapular neck fracture. (*A*) Medial to lateral projection showing the distal (*white arrows*) and proximal (*black arrows*) ends of the fracture. (*B*) Cranial to caudal projection with a small portion of the scapulohumeral joint and the proximal fragment. (*C*) Cranial-medial to caudal-lateral oblique projection demonstrates the fracture well.

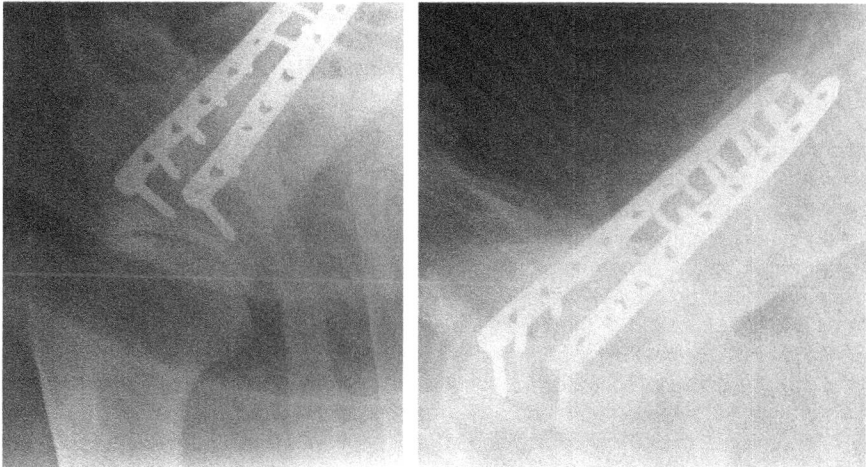

Fig. 2. Lateral to medial radiographs of the scapulohumeral joint of the same horse in **Fig. 1** four years later at a prepurchase examination. The mare was in work, sound, negative to joint flexion, and considered suitable for the intended purpose (dressage). (*Courtesy of* Dr Clifford Honnas, Texas Equine Hospital; with permission.)

In preparation of a foal with a scapular fracture for transport to a surgical facility, external coaptation is not recommended, similar to that in the adult horse.[4] External coaptation is not recommended because there is no way to additionally stabilize these fractures, and there is a low likelihood of the fracture becoming open due to lack of coaptation because of the large surrounding muscle mass and close proximity to the body.

ULNA

Fractures of the olecranon of the ulna are common in the foal and are covered in detail (see David G. Levine and Maia R. Aitken's article, "Physeal Fractures in Foals," in this issue). Ulnar fractures will be briefly discussed in this article because they are sometimes seen in concert with radial fractures and may be difficult to differentiate from radial or humeral fracture. With ulnar fracture, there is usually acute, severe lameness, swelling, and pain on palpation of the elbow region. When subsequent to a kicking injury, superficial wounds are often present. A dropped elbow appearance is common due to either disruption of the triceps apparatus or pain. Medial to lateral and cranial to caudal radiographs of the elbow with the limb pulled craniad are used to confirm the diagnosis and rule out fracture of the humerus or radius.

Conservative care with confinement and splinting as needed to prevent carpal contracture is occasionally performed with success in nondisplaced olecranon fractures in foals. Conservative approaches with long-term splinting to fix the carpus in the treatment of displaced fractures are rarely attempted. Both displaced and nondisplaced fractures of the olecranon of the ulna are relatively easily repaired surgically with good long-term outcomes.

Because foals are likely to become recumbent during transport, foals with displaced olecranon fractures can be safely shipped without external coaptation, unlike the adult horse that should have the carpus fixed in extension for transport. This is especially true when radiographs have not been obtained and humeral fracture has not been ruled out, as splinting a humeral fracture can worsen soft tissue injury. For nondisplaced olecranon fractures, external coaptation to fix the carpus might reduce the risk of progression to a displaced fracture.

RADIUS

In contrast to the adult horse, fractures of the radius are commonly repaired with good outcomes in the foal. This is in part because radial fractures in the foal tend to be simple oblique fractures or simple spiral fractures as opposed to the highly comminuted fractures more commonly seen in the adult radius. The presenting signs will depend on the fracture location. When very proximal, the presenting signs can be very similar to that of an olecranon fracture and will commonly occur in combination with fracture to the ulna and/or luxation of the elbow joint (Monteggia fracture).[5] When fractures are located mid diaphyseal or distal, there is usually marked swelling of the forearm and carpus and visible instability of the limb. Routine orthogonal radiographs are used to determine fracture configuration and prognosis of surgical repair.

Although repair of complete, displaced radial fracture is rarely pursued in adult horses, foals less than 1 year of age have a good prognosis following open reduction and internal fixation techniques.[5] In a recent report, weanlings and foals were found to be 18 times more likely to survive to discharge following surgical repair of radial fractures.[5] Among horses aged less than 1 year of age, 86% managed surgically had a positive outcome.[5] Similarly, successful outcomes have been achieved in young horses after surgical repair of Monteggia fracture (fracture of the radius and ulna with luxation of the humeroradial joint).[6] When appropriate intraoperative or postoperative technique is performed to ensure coordinated radius and ulnar elongation during longitudinal bone growth, the development of elbow subluxation can be avoided.[7,8] When elongation is prevented, the distal physis will usually compensate, resulting in minimal limb length discrepancy between the left and right forelimbs (**Fig. 3**).

Fractures of the radius are at a great risk of becoming open, and thus, bandaging and external coaptation are extremely important. External coaptation would be similar to that in the adult horse.[4,5] The ultimate goal in splinting is to prevent abduction of the limb, which forces the sharp bone ends through the thin soft tissues on the medial aspect of the forearm. This is achieved via a rigid caudal splint to the elbow and a lateral splint to the shoulder.

TIBIA

Fractures of the tibia will be very similar to fractures of the radius in that there will be acute, non-weight-bearing lameness, significant soft tissue swelling, instability of the limb, and a high likelihood of fracture fragments damaging the medial aspect of the limb. Routine orthogonal radiographs are used to determine fracture configuration and prognosis of surgical repair. Like the radius, tibial fractures in the foal are also frequently simple oblique or spiral configurations that are relatively easily surgically repaired when they remain closed. Thus, coaptation of the limb to prevent abduction of the limb will be of the utmost importance. Similar to radial fractures, a lateral splint to the croup to prevent abduction and protect the thin medial soft tissues is of paramount importance. A customized rigid caudal splint contoured to the limb to the level of the stifle (casting tape laid on the caudal aspect of the bandaged limb in accordion style of multiple layers, for example) will provide additional stability.

THIRD METACARPAL/METATARSAL FRACTURES

Complete fractures of the third metacarpal (MC3) and third metatarsal (MT3) bones account for approximately one-third of all long bone fractures in the equine patient.[9]

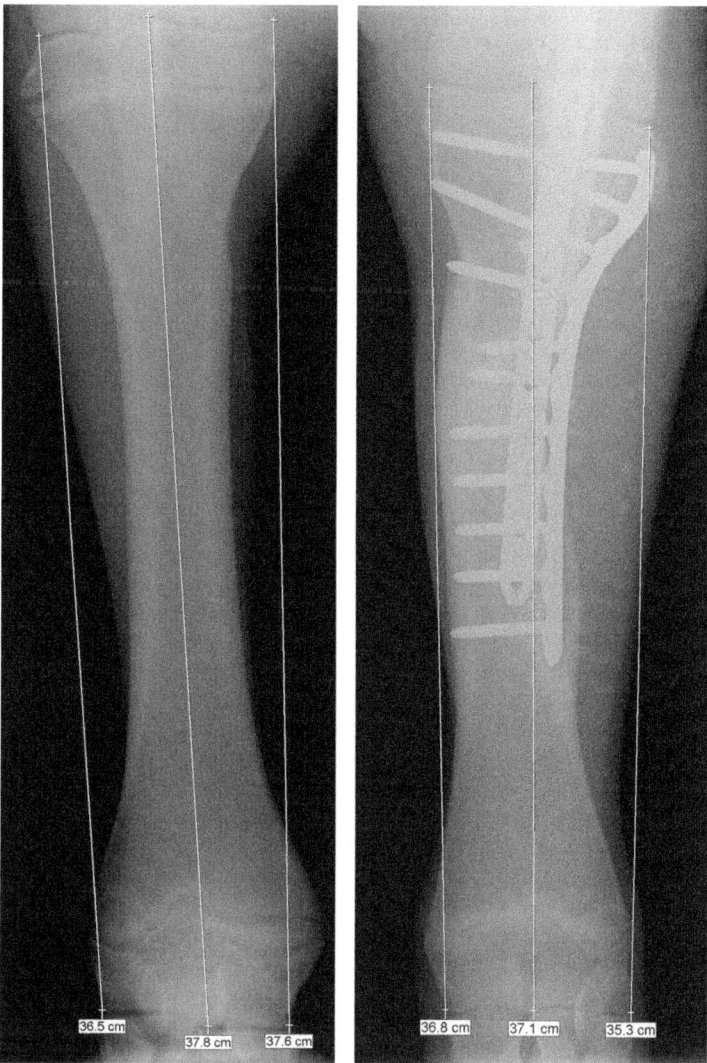

Fig. 3. Cranial to caudal radiographs of the right and left radii of an 18-month-old Arabian filly. Open reduction and internal fixation of fractures of the left proximal diaphyseal radius, distal ulna, and olecranon were performed 16 months before. Despite prevention of proximal radial or ulnar elongation of the limb by the surgical implants, the length of the left radius is similar to that of the right radius. This was due to compensatory growth of the distal radial physis.

In contrast to the more commonly comminuted fracture of the adult horse, fractures of MC3/MT3 in the foal are usually simple and secondary to direct trauma.[10] Diagnosis can be made on physical examination, and routine orthogonal radiographs are used to determine fracture configuration and prognosis of surgical repair.

Foals have a much higher survival rate (91%) after surgical fixation of the metacarpus (tarsus) than mature horses (30%),[11] and when fractures are nonarticular, the long-term outcome for athleticism is good. Significant associations have been revealed between survival and bodyweight, with body weights greater than 320 kg being a major risk factor for an unsuccessful outcome.[11]

Because of a near lack of soft tissue coverage other than skin, these fractures are commonly open or at great risk for becoming open. Therefore, these fractures should be stabilized as soon as possible with external coaptation. External coaptation would be similar to that in the adult horse and should include a lateral splint to the elbow/stifle as well as a caudal splint to the elbow or a plantar splint to the point of the hock.[4,11]

HUMERUS AND FEMUR

Fractures of the humerus and femur are relatively common in the foal as compared with the adult horse. There will be crepitation, moderate to marked soft tissue swelling, inability to use the limb, and pain on manipulation of the limb. For the humerus, there will be a dropped elbow appearance, and the carpus and fetlock will generally be flexed. For the femur, there will sometimes be upward fixation of the patella due to the shortening of the quadriceps musculature. Both are confirmed with radiographs. For the humerus, standing medial to lateral and craniomedial to caudolateral oblique projections are diagnostic. For the femur, heavily sedated or anesthetized medial to lateral projections made in recumbency with the affected side down and on the radiographic receptor and the contralateral limb abducted out of the way of the radiographic beam are diagnostic.

Conservative management of humeral or femoral fractures can occasionally be successful in foals, but it is very likely that severe support limb complications will occur. Complications include varus deformity of the support limb, carpal contracture of the affected limb, and less commonly, support limb laminitis.

Open reduction and internal fixation of humeral and femoral fractures in foals, using stacked pin, dynamic compression or locking compression plate, or intramedullary interlocking nail fixation, has been successful in achieving survival to discharge and future athletic performance.[12–14] Success is related to age and weight of the foal, with foals less than or equal to 3 months of age more likely to survive a femoral fracture repair and foals less than or equal to 220 kg more likely to survive humeral fracture repair.[14,15] Overall, survival to hospital discharge in foals surgically treated for fracture of the humeral and femoral diaphysis is approximately 50%.[14,15]

There is relatively good experimental evidence for use of the intramedullary, interlocking nail fixation of humeral and femoral fractures in foals to prevent collapse of the fracture fragments while minimizing bending and rotational forces.[14] Healing of femoral osteotomies was complete within 6 months among a group of 6 foals following placement of intramedullary, interlocking nail fixation.[16] The clinical use of this specifically designed implant has yielded results equal to or better than previously reported outcomes following open reduction and internal fixation of humeral and femoral fractures.[14]

Emergency coaptation for humerus and femoral fractures is not recommended. This is because it is not possible to adequately stabilize the affected area, and attempts at stabilization only serve to increase the weight of the distal limb and encourage the foal to engage in weight bearing. Increased use of the limb results in the possibility for increased soft tissue and neurovascular damage (specifically the femoral vasculature adjacent to femoral fractures and radial nerve damage adjacent to humeral fractures) that may significantly worsen the prognosis.[14]

GENERAL EMERGENCY CARE AND TRANSPORT

Emergency stabilization and coaptation of the foal fracture patient are similar in most fractures to that of the adult and have been outlined above for each fracture location.

Medical management and transport of the foal with axial instability of a long bone have a few key points that contrast to the care of an adult horse with similar fracture. Because of their smaller size, reduced capability to recruit energy reserves, and the potential for immunologic compromise (immunoglobulin G [IgG] <400 mg/dL), systemic supportive care is paramount.[4] The IgG status of the foal should be investigated in neonates with unknown after-parturient IgG results. Antimicrobial administration should be initiated promptly. It is recommended to be in contact with your referral facility and surgeon before selecting antimicrobial medications, allowing for selection of an antimicrobial regimen to be continued in the hospital without the need for switching unnecessarily. Intravenous fluid therapy is necessary when the fracture results in a reluctance or inability to nurse.

Emergency transportation of the foal should be well planned. Every effort should be made to minimize emotional stress to the foal, which is unlikely to be accustomed to shipping. The foal should be transported with the mare if not weaned and a companion horse if weaned. Efforts to transport the foal with the mare or a companion horse are particularly important if transport duration will be prolonged. Unlike the adult horse, healthy foals up to 1 year of age will elect to lie down during transport, and foals with long bone fractures should have the option to lie down if possible. Open box stalls with the mare and foal together should be avoided when it is feasible to separate them without undue stress to the mare or foal. Ideally, the mare should be confined within the trailer (ie, the front slant, or stall within the trailer) and able to see and/or touch the foal while the foal travels recumbent on an adjacent deeply bedded area of shavings or straw. An attendant traveling with the foal can help minimize movement and struggling of the foal during transport, but the safety and legality of this should be considered before making this recommendation. Particular caution should be paid to mare handling if it is suspected that a kick from the mare resulted in the foal's fracture.

REFERENCES

1. Bukowiecki CF, van Ee RT, Schneiter HL. Internal fixation of comminuted transverse scapular fracture in a foal. J Am Vet Med Assoc 1989;195(6):781–3.
2. Shamis LD, Sanders-Shamis M, Bramlage LR. Internal fixation of a transverse scapular neck fracture in a filly. J Am Vet Med Assoc 1989;195(10):1391–2.
3. Kamm J, Quinn G, Zwanenberg D. Fixation of a complete scapular neck fracture in a foal using two 3.5 mm locking compression plates. Equine Vet Educ 2015; 29(4):180–3.
4. Mudge MC, Bramlage LR. Field fracture management. Vet Clin North Am Equine Pract 2007;23(1):117–33.
5. Stewart S, Richardson D, Boston R, et al. Risk factors associated with survival to hospital discharge of 54 horses with fractures of the radius. Vet Surg 2015;44(8): 1036–41.
6. Jalim S, McKinnon A, Russell T. Repair of a type IV Monteggia fracture in a foal. Aust Vet J 2009;87(11):463–6.
7. Clem MF, DeBowes RM, Douglass JP, et al. The effects of fixation of the ulna to the radius in young foals. Vet Surg 1988;17(6):338–45.
8. Stover SM, Rick MC. Ulnar subluxation following repair of a fractured radius in a foal. Vet Surg 1985;14(1):27–31.
9. McClure SR, Watkins JP, Glickman NW, et al. Complete fractures of the third metacarpal or metatarsal bone in horses: 25 cases (1980-1996). J Am Vet Med Assoc 1998;213(6):847–50.

10. Schneider R, Jackman B. Fractures of the third metacarpus and metatarsus. In: Nixon AJ, editor. Equine fracture repair. Philadelphia: WB Saunders; 1996. p. 179–94.

11. Bischofberger A, Fürst A, Auer J, et al. Surgical management of complete diaphyseal third metacarpal and metatarsal bone fractures: clinical outcome in 10 mature horses and 11 foals. Equine Vet J 2009;41(5):465–73.

12. Carter B, Schneider R, Hardy J, et al. Assessment and treatment of equine humeral fractures: retrospective study of 54 cases (1972–1990). Equine Vet J 1993;25(3):203–7.

13. Rakestraw PC, Nixon AJ, Kaderly RE, et al. Cranial approach to the humerus for repair of fractures in horses and cattle. Vet Surg 1991;20(1):1–8.

14. Watkins J. Etiology, diagnosis, and treatment of long bone fractures in foals. Clin Tech Equine Pract 2006;5(4):296–308.

15. Hance S, Bramlage L, Schneider R, et al. Retrospective study of 38 cases of femur fractures in horses less than one year of age. Equine Vet J 1992;24(5): 357–63.

16. McClure S, Watkins J, Ashman R. In vivo evaluation of intramedullary interlocking nail fixation of transverse femoral osteotomies in foals. Vet Surg 1998;27(1): 29–36.

Moving?

Make sure your subscription moves with you!

To notify us of your new address, find your **Clinics Account Number** (located on your mailing label above your name), and contact customer service at:

Email: journalscustomerservice-usa@elsevier.com

800-654-2452 (subscribers in the U.S. & Canada)
314-447-8871 (subscribers outside of the U.S. & Canada)

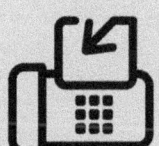

Fax number: 314-447-8029

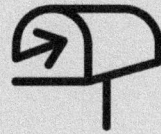

Elsevier Health Sciences Division
Subscription Customer Service
3251 Riverport Lane
Maryland Heights, MO 63043

*To ensure uninterrupted delivery of your subscription, please notify us at least 4 weeks in advance of move.

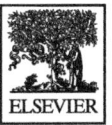

Printed and bound by CPI Group (UK) Ltd, Croydon, CR0 4YY

18/10/2024

01775988-0001